7th EDITION

Larone's Medically Important Fungi

A GUIDE TO IDENTIFICATION

7th EDITION

Larone's Medically Important Fungi

A GUIDE TO IDENTIFICATION

Founding Author
Davise H. Larone, MT(ASCP), PhD, D(ABMM), F(AAM)
Weill Cornell Medicine
New York, New York

Lars F. Westblade, PhD, D(ABMM)
Weill Cornell Medicine
New York, New York

Eileen M. Burd, PhD, D(ABMM)
Emory University Hospital
Emory University School of Medicine
Atlanta, Georgia

Shawn R. Lockhart, PhD, D(ABMM), F(AAM)
Centers for Disease Control and Prevention
Atlanta, Georgia

Gary W. Procop, MD, MS
American Board of Pathology
Tampa, Florida
Cleveland Clinic Lerner College of Medicine
Cleveland, Ohio

With
Thomas J. Walsh, MD, PhD (hon), F(IDSA), F(AAM), F(ECMM), F(AAAS)
Center for Innovative Therapeutics and Diagnostics
Richmond, VA

ASM
PRESS

WILEY

Copublication by the American Society for Microbiology and John Wiley & Sons, Inc.

Limit of Liability/Disclaimer of Warranty
While the publisher and author have used their best efforts in preparing this book, they make no representations or warranties with respect to the accuracy of completeness of the contents of this book and specifically disclaim any implied warranties or merchantability of fitness for a particular purpose. No warranty may be created or extended by sales representatives or written sales materials. The publisher is not providing legal, medical, or other professional services. Any reference herein to any specific commercial products, procedures, or services by trade name, trademark, manufacturer, or otherwise does not constitute or imply endorsement, recommendation, or favored status by the American Society for Microbiology (ASM). The views and opinions of the author(s) expressed in this publication do not necessarily state or reflect those of ASM, and they shall not be used to advertise or endorse any product.

Editorial Correspondence:
ASM Press, 1752 N Street, NW, Washington, DC 20036-2904, USA

Registered Offices:
John Wiley & Sons, Inc., 111 River Street, Hoboken, NJ 07030, USA

For details of our global editorial offices, customer services, and more information about Wiley products, visit us at www.wiley.com.

Wiley also publishes its books in a variety of electronic formats and by print-on-demand. Some content that appears in standard print versions of this book may not be available in other formats.

Library of Congress Cataloging-in-Publication Data

Names: Westblade, Lars F. (Lars Frederick), 1976- author. | Westblade, Lars
    F. (Lars Frederick), 1976- author. | Burd, Eileen M., 1956- author. |
    Lockhart, Shawn R., 1966- author. | Procop, Gary W., author. | Larone,
    Davise Honig, 1939- author. | Walsh, Thomas J., M.D. author. | Larone,
    Davise Honig, 1939- Larone's medically important fungi.
Title: Larone's medically important fungi : a guide to identification /
    Lars F. Westblade, Eileen M. Burd, Shawn R. Lockhart, Gary W. Procop
    with Davise H. Larone and Thomas J. Walsh.
Other titles: Medically important fungi
Description: 7th edition. | Hoboken, NJ : Wiley-ASM Press, [2023] |
    Preceded by Larone's medically important fungi / Thomas J. Walsh,
    Randall T. Hayden, Davise H. Larone ; illustrated by Davise H. Larone.
    6th edition. [2018].
Identifiers: LCCN 2023011203 (print) | LCCN 2023011204 (ebook) | ISBN
    9781683674405 (cloth) | ISBN 9781683674412 (adobe pdf) | ISBN
    9781683674429 (epub)
Subjects: MESH: Fungi—pathogenicity | Fungi—cytology | Mycology |
    Laboratory Manual
Classification: LCC QR245 (print) | LCC QR245 (ebook) | NLM QW 25 | DDC
    616.9/6901—dc23/eng/20230615
LC record available at https://lccn.loc.gov/2023011203
LC ebook record available at https://lccn.loc.gov/2023011204

Cover: *Curvularia* sp. on Sabouraud dextrose agar at 30°C for 5 days. Black woolly colony. Microscopic structures consist of septate hyphae and simple or branched conidiophores that are bent or knobby at points of conidium formation. Conidia are large, usually contain four cells, and eventually appear curved due to swelling of a central cell. Illustration by Davise H. Larone.

Cover design: Wiley

Set in 11/13 pt Sabon LT Std by Straive, Chennai, India

SKY10087996_101624

Dedicated with love
To Angela, Henry, and Elaine. (LFW)

Dedicated with love
To Rebekah and Larisa. All my heart. (EMB)

Dedicated with love
To my wife Kathleen and to my parents Bob and Dotti for enabling me to become a scientist. (SRL)

In loving memory of Delonda B. Procop (née MacDonald), Mom –
When Dad passed too soon, you bore the mantle of mother and father. Thank you for the moral compass, the blue-ribbon baking, making our house a home, and so much more. (GWP)

Dedicated with love
With all my heart to Marie, Emma, and Laura Walsh, and with loving memory of John, Frances, and Margaret Walsh. (TJW)

Dedicated with love
To Ronit, Jessie, and Beth, and with loving memory to John D. Lawrence. (DHL)

Contents

PART II

Identification of Fungi in Culture   73

PART III
Basics of Molecular Methods for Fungal Identification   379

Staining Methods   431

Media   441

List of Tables

Preface to the Seventh Edition

Every edition of *Larone's Medically Important Fungi: A Guide to Identification* has been written with the needs of the reader foremost in mind so that the identification of fungi encountered in the clinical laboratory is logical, understandable, and enjoyable for all medical mycologists and those interested in this fascinating field. The goal has never been to compete with larger texts, but to present information in a format so arranged that a medical mycologist can reach a possible identification knowing only the colony and microscopic morphology of an isolated organism. This format, which has proven so successful, is maintained in this edition. Further, with each new edition a major accompanying goal is to expand the reader's knowledge and provide contemporary information regarding emerging fungal pathogens and their associated properties.

This edition introduces four new authors: Lars F. Westblade, Eileen M. Burd, Shawn R. Lockhart, and Gary W. Procop. Each brings a unique perspective and area of expertise, and all have worked in close collaboration to honor the work of Davise H. Larone, the founding author, while striving to update this important diagnostic resource.

Both Part I, "Direct Microscopic Examination of Clinical Specimens", and Part II, "Identification of Fungi in Culture", are expanded to include several new organisms. In addition, many organism descriptions have been updated, and some organisms have been regrouped to better reflect their biology. The various reference sections in previous editions are now consolidated into a single reference section, and references for many organisms are updated. Part III, the "Basics of Molecular Methods for Fungal Identification" section, and Part IV, the "Laboratory Technique" section have also been carefully reviewed and revised to ensure information is current and universally applicable to the practicing medical mycologist.

Due to the flurry of molecular taxonomic studies applied to medically important fungi, taxonomy and nomenclature adjustments continue to be hotly debated topics in medical mycology. These changes can cause confusion especially when viewed by patient-facing colleagues. We have endeavored to provide clarity by highlighting the name suggested for clinical reporting in the banner heading associated with each organism description. We have also included additional taxonomic and nomenclature information in a newly introduced feature, "Taxonomy Notes," that is associated with organism descriptions as needed. The information presented in "Taxonomy Notes" provides continuity with earlier names and presents revised names. We are mindful that for those organisms whose names have been revised, yet not adopted for clinical reporting in this edition, eventual accumulation of data that may lead to improved diagnosis and treatment of our patients may warrant acceptance of the revised names.

As this edition goes to press we are already considering the next! As such, we seek feedback from readers and all comments, suggestions, or requests aimed at fulfilling the needs of the readership will be most appreciated.

February, 2023

Preface to the First Edition

More than ever, clinical laboratory personnel with limited experience in mycology must culture and identify fungi isolated from clinical specimens. Even after attending a course in the subject, technologists often need guidance in identifying the great variety of organisms encountered in the lab. With the advent of proficiency testing by local and national organizations, technologists have a need and opportunity to practice and increase their skills in the medical mycology laboratory.

Most classic texts, though rich in information, are arranged according to the clinical description of the infection; the textual discussion of any particular fungus can be located only from the index or table of contents. Since the technologist doesn't know the name of an unidentified fungus and usually has little or no knowledge of the clinical picture, these texts are at best difficult to use effectively. The unfortunate result is the all-too-common practice of flipping through an entire mycology textbook in search of a picture that resembles the organism under examination. Such a practice may make the more accomplished mycologist's hair stand on end, but it is a fact to be acknowledged.

This guide is not meant to compete with these large texts, but to complement them. The material here is so arranged that the technician can systematically reach a possible identification knowing only the macro- and microscopic morphology of an isolated organism. Reference can then be made to one of the classic texts for confirmation and detailed information.

Many possible variants of organisms are found under several categories of morphology and pigment. The outstanding characteristics are listed on the page(s) apportioned to each organism, and references are suggested for further information and confirmation (see How To Use the Guide).

Medically Important Fungi avoids the jargon so commonly and confusingly used in most mycology books. Drawings are used wherever possible to illustrate organisms described in the text. To ensure clarity, a glossary of terms is included, as well as a section on laboratory techniques for observing proper morphology. Another section includes use of the various media, stains, and tests mentioned in the book.

The actinomycetes, although now known to be bacteria rather than fungi, are included because they are frequently handled in the mycology section of the clinical laboratory.

It is believed that this guide will enable students and medical technologists to culture and identify fungi with greater ease and competency and in so doing to develop an appreciation of the truly beautiful microscopic forms encountered.

I wish to acknowledge with gratitude the encouragement and advice received from my co-workers at Lenox Hill Hospital, and Dr. Norman Goodman, Mr. Gerald Krefetz, Mr. Bill Rosenzweig, Ms. Eve Rothenberg, Dr. Guenther Stotzky, Mr. Martin Weisburd, Dr. Irene Weitzman, and Dr. Marion E. Wilson.

Davise H. Larone
New York
December, 1975

Acknowledgments

We extend our gratitude to numerous colleagues and friends for their support and generosity in helping to bring this edition to completion: Jake Cochran, Centers for Disease Control and Prevention (CDC), Atlanta, GA; David Ellis, University of Adelaide, Adelaide, Australia; Brendan Headd, CDC; Jos Houbraken, Westerdijk Fungal Biodiversity Institute, Utrecht, Netherlands; Sarah Kidd, National Mycology Reference Centre, SA Pathology, Adelaide, Australia; John McQuiston, CDC; Bobbi Pritt, Mayo Clinic, Rochester, MN; Ilan Schwartz, Duke University, Durham, NC; Amir Seyedmousavi, National Institutes of Health (NIH), Bethesda, MD; Nathan Wiederhold, UT Health San Antonio, TX; and Adrian Zelazny, NIH.

As acknowledged in previous editions, almost all the organisms shown microscopically and/or as cultured colonies were prepared in the Mycology Laboratory of NewYork-Presbyterian/Weill Cornell Medical Center (NYP/WCMC), New York, NY. We will forever be indebted to the staff of the NYP/WCMC Mycology Laboratory for their enormously significant contributions over the years. Dr. Stephen Jenkins, Weill Cornell Medicine (WCM), New York, NY has always provided encouragement, and shared many puns along the way (and we didn't pay a hyphae for them!). Additionally, Karen Acker, WCM; Melissa Cushing, WCM; Kathy Fauntleroy, NYP/WCMC; Rebecca Marrero Rolón, WCM; Jacob Rand, WCM; Selma Salter, NYP/WCMC; and Michael Satlin, WCM have all offered valuable advice and been incredibly supportive.

We are also grateful to the many colleagues who assisted with the preparation of previous editions, not least Dr. Sanchita Das, NIH for her role in initially writing and subsequently updating the section entitled "Basics of Molecular Methods for Fungal Identification" (Part III) in the 5th and 6th editions, respectively; Randall Hayden, St. Jude Children's Research Hospital, Memphis, TN for his extensive work on the 6th edition; and Pat Kuharic of the Photography Department of WCM for preparing photographs and photomicrographs.

Throughout the course of working on this new edition we were fortunate to meet and befriend three wonderfully talented artists: Ken Fasano, Ann Hoffenberg, and Robin Jess. With passion and diligence they have faithfully created illustrations for this new edition and, as one will see, their work is nothing short of astounding.

We deeply appreciate members of ASM Press. Christine Charlip, Director, provided unwavering support for the 7th edition. She has an unshakable belief that *Larone's Medically Important Fungi: A Guide to Identification* is an essential component of ASM Press's clinical microbiology repertoire and worked tirelessly to ensure this new edition came about smoothly. We are also extremely thankful for Megan Angelini, Managing Development Editor. Indeed, where would this new edition be without Megan? The answer is simple, nowhere. Through her dedication, industriousness, intellect, and kindness she has shepherded this edition to completion. At every point along this incredible journey her insight has proven invaluable. Without doubt, Megan's name deserves to be on the cover of this edition. Thank you, Megan!

Last, but by no means least, we acknowledge every medical microbiologist who pursues identification of fungal pathogens from increasingly complex populations of patients. We hope that the descriptions on these pages help you navigate the unique challenges of fungal identification and inspire a sense of wonder for the world of medical mycology. Thank you for your devotion and commitment to this field and the patients you serve.

About the Authors

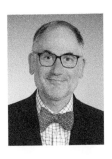

Lars F. Westblade, PhD, D(ABMM) is the Director of the Clinical Microbiology Service at NewYork-Presbyterian/Weill Cornell Medical Center and Associate Professor at Weill Cornell Medicine with a primary appointment in the Department of Pathology and Laboratory Medicine and a secondary appointment in the Division of Infectious Diseases, Department of Medicine. He earned his doctoral degree from the University of Birmingham in the United Kingdom, and completed a fellowship in medical and public health laboratory microbiology at Washington University School of Medicine in St. Louis.

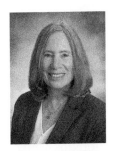

Eileen M. Burd, PhD, D(ABMM) is the Director of the Clinical Microbiology Laboratory at Emory University Hospital and Professor at Emory University School of Medicine with a primary appointment in the Department of Pathology and Laboratory Medicine and a secondary appointment in the Department of Medicine, Division of Infectious Diseases. She earned her doctoral degree from the Medical College of Wisconsin in Milwaukee and was the Division Head of Microbiology at Henry Ford Hospital in Detroit, Michigan prior to joining the faculty at Emory University in 2007.

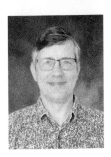

Shawn R. Lockhart, PhD, D(ABBM), F(AAM) is the Senior Clinical Laboratory Advisor in the Mycotic Diseases Branch at the Centers for Disease Control and Prevention. He earned his doctoral degree from the University of Kentucky and completed his clinical microbiology fellowship at the University of Iowa Hospitals and Clinics. He directs the CDC training course in mold identification.

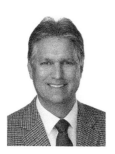

Gary W. Procop, MD, MS is the CEO of the American Board of Pathology and Professor of Pathology at the Cleveland Clinic Lerner School of Medicine. He remains a Consulting Staff for the Institute of Pathology and Laboratory Medicine, where he served as Medical Director for the Mycology Laboratory for more than two decades. He earned his doctoral degree from the Marshall University School of Medicine. His residency in anatomic and clinical pathology was completed at Duke University and his medical microbiology fellowship at the Mayo Clinic.

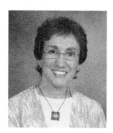

Davise H. Larone, MT(ASCP), PhD, D(ABMM), F(AAM) is the founding author of *Larone's Medically Important Fungi: A Guide to Identification* and Professor Emerita at Weill Cornell Medicine in the Department of Pathology and Laboratory Medicine and the Department of Clinical Microbiology and Immunology. From 1997 to 2008, she served as Director of the Clinical Microbiology Laboratories of The NewYork–Presbyterian/Weill Cornell Medical Center. Prior to that, she was for many years at Lenox Hill Hospital, New York, rising from technologist to Chief of Microbiology. During that period, in 1985, she received her PhD in Biology/Microbiology from New York University. Her interest in clinical mycology dates from the 1970s. Her undergraduate degree was in Medical Technology from the University of Louisville, but her love for drawing led her to study art on the side. The combination of her organizational skills and her art background resulted in the first edition of this book in 1976. The subsequent editions in 1987, 1995, 2002, 2011, and 2018 all feature Dr. Larone's elegant drawings. Dr. Larone has served on numerous standards, advisory, editorial, educational, and examination boards/committees. Over the years, she has presented more than 100 workshops and lectures in 52 cities in the United States and in 14 cities in nine other countries. She has received numerous awards for teaching and for contributions to clinical mycology.

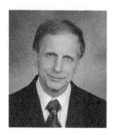

Thomas J. Walsh, MD, PhD (hon), F(IDSA), F(AAM), F(ECMM), F(AAAS) is the Founding Director for the Center for Innovative Therapeutics and Diagnostics, and serves as the Henry Schueler Foundation Scholar, Investigator of Emerging Infectious Diseases of the Save Our Sick Kids Foundation; Adjunct Professor of Microbiology & Immunology, University of Maryland School of Medicine; Adjunct Professor of Pathology, The Johns Hopkins University School of Medicine; and Visiting Professor, Infectious Diseases and Medical Mycology, Aristotle University School of Medicine. He earned his doctoral degree from the Johns Hopkins University School of Medicine, and completed 10 years of postdoctoral training at Johns Hopkins University School of Medicine, University of Maryland School of Medicine, and National Cancer Institute leading to Boards in Medicine, Oncology, and Infectious Diseases.

Basics

Larone's Medically Important Fungi: A Guide to Identification, 7th Edition.
Lars F. Westblade, Eileen M. Burd, Shawn R. Lockhart, and Gary W. Procop.
© 2023 American Society for Microbiology. DOI: 10.1128/9781683674436.

BASICS

How To Use the Guide

Before beginning to use the guide, the reader should understand several points.

Fungi often appear different in living hosts than they do in cultures. Part I (pp. 15–72) is designed as a guide for preliminary identification of fungi seen on direct microscopic examination of clinical specimens.

In Part II (pp. 73–378), the descriptions of the macroscopic and microscopic morphologies of the cultured fungi pertain to those on Sabouraud dextrose agar (SDA) unless otherwise specified. SDA may not be as regularly used for primary isolation of fungi directly from specimens as it was in the past, due to evidence that it is not as supportive as once believed. Fortunately, the descriptions can also be applied to growth on alternative media.

Many moulds begin as white mycelial growths, and coloration occurs at the time of conidiation or sporulation. Hence, organisms are listed under their most likely color(s) at maturity, when the typical microscopic reproductive formations are more readily observed.

In Parts I and II, when feasible, organisms are arranged in an order based on morphologic similarities (rather than alphabetical order) to facilitate convenient comparison.

This book is a *guide to identification*. Standard texts and our suggested references should be used for additional information concerning clinical disease, history, ecology, immunology, and therapy.

As molecular assays are increasingly being employed for identification of fungi, the basics of these methods and their utility in the clinical mycology laboratory are discussed in Part III (pp. 379–401).

Instructions for general laboratory procedures, i.e., collection of specimens, direct microscopic preparations, primary isolation, slide cultures, special tests, maintenance of stock cultures, and the like, are given in Part IV (pp. 405–430). Staining methods are described on pp. 431–440; the preparation and use of media are on pp. 441–467.

Any terms used that may not be familiar to the reader can most likely be found in the Glossary on pp. 477–488.

Once the organism has been properly collected, cultured, isolated, and observed microscopically, use of the guide is quite simple.

1. Note the morphology of the unknown fungus.
   a. Is it a filamentous bacterium, yeast/yeastlike thermally dimorphic, or a thermally monomorphic mould?
   b. Record color of surface and reverse (underside) of colony.
2. Using the initial "Guide to the Identification of Fungi in Culture" on pp. 75–104, refer to a page that shows drawings of the microscopic morphologies of organisms having the appropriate macroscopic appearance. Here one may see either the exact organism under examination or several possibilities.
3. Proceed to the page given in parentheses under the likely organism(s) to find more detailed information, including pathogenicity, rate of growth, colony morphology, an enlarged drawing of the microscopic appearance, a photomicrograph, and references for additional information. Where applicable, there will be reference to tables and image appendix figures and discussions of tests or characteristics that may help to differentiate extremely similar organisms.
4. Ordinarily, based on macroscopic and microscopic morphology the identification will be quite certain and the level (i.e., to genus or, where possible, species) more than sufficient for clinical management. However, for those fungi routinely only identified to genus level, if species-level identification is requested, further consultation with the clinical microbiology laboratory/medical director and/or the clinical team taking care of the patient may be required to understand if identification to species level is clinically warranted. If any doubt remains, or if the morphologic identification is uncertain, the organism should be sent to a reference laboratory for confirmation of identification as discussed in the following section.

Use of Reference Laboratories and Regulations for Transport

Laboratories generally do not have difficulty identifying most commonly encountered fungi using standard identification methods. However, rare or atypical fungi can be difficult to identify, even for a very experienced microbiologist or medical technologist. Few laboratories can perform the highly specialized or rarely used tests that are often needed for identification of unusual yeasts or moulds.

When the identification of a clinically significant isolated fungus is uncertain, a reputable commercial reference laboratory of proven competency can be used to complete the identification. A reference laboratory can also be utilized if identification to species level is needed and requires methods that are not available in the source laboratory. Some reference laboratories also offer antifungal susceptibility testing if it is requested and not available in-house.

Cultures sent to reference laboratories should be pure, young, and actively growing on agar slants. Petri plates should not be transported. The reference laboratory can provide specific requirements on the labeling and transport of isolates. Personnel involved in packing and shipping infectious substances must receive training in the proper procedures, and the training must be maintained and documented.

The regulations for transport of infectious substances and biological substances are developed and issued by several major authorities: the International Civil Aviation Organization (ICAO) (a United Nations [UN] agency), the International Air Transport Association (IATA), the United States Department of Transportation (DOT), and the United States Postal Service (USPS). Regulations from these agencies are in substantial agreement with one another but instructions change frequently and it is necessary to repeat training periodically. Employers must determine what training is needed and approve the training program or course according to the IATA Dangerous Goods Regulations (available for purchase at https://www.iata.org/en/publications/store/infectious-substances-shipping-regulations/) and the Code of Federal Regulations (49 CFR 171-180 available at https://www.ecfr.gov/current/title-49/subtitle-B/chapter-I/subchapter-C/part-171).

Infectious substances are classified as either Category A or Category B. Because of the differences in the hazards posed by Category A and Category B infectious substances, there are separate packaging, labeling, and documentation requirements. The definition of each category and the instructions for packing and shipping isolates from humans follow below.

A **Category A Infectious Substance** is an infectious substance in a form capable of causing permanent disability or life-threatening or fatal disease in otherwise healthy humans or animals when exposure to it occurs. At the time of this writing, the only fungus expressly listed in Category A is *Coccidioides immitis* (includes *Coccidioides posadasii*), in cultured form. Other fungi may, with careful consideration of risk, qualify as Category A. If there is doubt as to whether or not an isolate meets the criteria for Category A, it must be handled as a Category A infectious substance.

Category A infectious substances must be triple-packaged and cannot be sent by domestic mail. The packaging consists of a leakproof primary receptacle, leakproof secondary packaging, and outer packaging of adequate strength to protect the contents under the intended shipping conditions. The instructions for packing Category A organisms are as follows.

1. The tube containing the slanted culture must be made of glass, metal, or plastic and should be labeled with the organism identification (in general terms if the identification is unknown). It must be securely closed and rendered leakproof by positive means (such as heat seal or metal crimp); if a screw cap is used, it must be secured with adhesive tape, paraffin sealing tape, or manufactured locking closure. The culture tube is considered the "primary receptacle."

2. Position enough packing and absorbent material at the top, bottom, and sides of the culture tube to prevent breakage and to absorb the entire volume of the culture in case of leakage. If more than one tube is being transported, each one must be wrapped individually to ensure that contact between them, and consequent breakage, is prevented.

3. Insert the wrapped culture tube(s) into durable, watertight "secondary packaging." Either the primary receptacle or the secondary container must be made of fiberboard or other equivalent material that is certified for ability to withstand an increased amount of pressure (95 kPa) as well as temperatures in the range of −40°C to +55°C (−40°F to 130°F) if it is to be shipped by air. Although several culture tubes may be placed in a single secondary container, the total contents cannot exceed 50 ml (or 50 g) on passenger aircraft. For Category A infectious substance shipments being carried on a cargo-only aircraft, the total contents per package cannot exceed 4 liters or 4 kg.

4. Attach an itemized list of the contents of the primary receptacle(s) to the outside of the secondary packaging. The list should include the UN number, proper shipping name of the infectious substance (i.e., infectious substance affecting humans) with the technical name (i.e., identification of the infectious substance) in parentheses. For example, "UN2814, Infectious substance affecting humans (*Coccidioides immitis/posadasii* culture)." When the identification of the infectious substance is unknown but suspected of meeting the criteria

for inclusion in Category A, the words "suspected Category A infectious substance" must be shown in parentheses following the proper shipping name on the itemized list of contents as well as on the Shipper's Declaration as described below.

5. Place the secondary package(s) in an outer shipping container with a smallest external dimension that measures at least 3.9 × 3.9 inches (100 × 100 mm) and is constructed of sturdy material that meets the strict UN specifications for shipping Category A substances.

The outer shipping container must show the diamond hazard label with the biohazard symbol (i.e., three crescents superimposed on a black circle), an inscription indicating "In case of damage or leakage immediately notify Public Health Authority," and the number 6 in the bottom corner. The following must also be present: a label showing the proper shipping name, "Infectious Substance Affecting Humans," and the UN2814 marking; the UN package certification mark affixed by the packaging manufacturer that provides information on how, when, and where the packaging was manufactured and approved; sender's name and address; and recipient's name and address. Orientation arrows are required if the package contains >50 ml of infectious substance. These labels are not required for Category B packages.

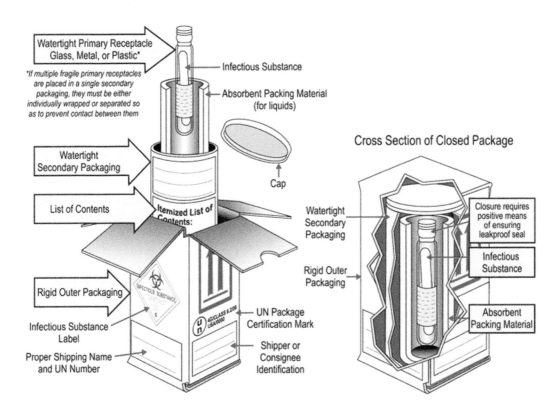

Category A packaging

BASICS

A completed Shipper's Declaration must accompany shipment of a Category A substance. The necessary form has vertical red "candy stripes" along the left and right edges. Most carriers require that the form be typed (not handwritten). FedEx Corporation (https://www.fedex.com/content/dam/fedex/us-united-states/services/ShippersDecColumnsColorPrinter.pdf) and IATA (https://www.iata.org/en/programs/cargo/dgr/shippers-declaration/), as well as other vendors, provide online software to generate the form. A color printer is required. Enter all information including the proper shipping name for the infectious substances being shipped. The technical name in parenthesis is required in association with the proper shipping name. If the identification of the infectious substance is not known but is suspected to be Category A, the complete entry would be "Infectious Substance, affecting humans (Suspected Category A, Infectious Substance)". A 24 hours a day, 7 days a week emergency response telephone number must be supplied; it must be monitored by a person (not an answering machine or message service) who has access to information concerning the hazards, and actions required, in case of human exposure to the contents of the shipment. This role can be filled by an agency or commercial company that provides this service.

A **Category B Infectious Substance** is an infectious substance that does not meet Category A criteria. The proper shipping name for this type of infectious substance is "Biological Substance, Category B."

Triple packaging is required for packing Category B infectious substances. Instructions are very similar to those for Category A, but differ in the following ways.

- The primary receptacle does not require sealing by a positive means.
- The maximum allowable volume per primary receptacle is 1 liter (4 kg).
- The secondary packaging must be leakproof and siftproof, but may be a sealed plastic bag or other intermediate packaging.
- Either the primary or secondary container must be pressure resistant for transport by air.
- There are no UN manufacturing specifications for the outer packaging, but it must be rigid and strong enough for its intended use and able to pass a 3.9-foot drop test.
- The outer shipping container must show a label showing the proper shipping name (i.e., Biological Substance, Category B), and the UN3373 marking. The name and telephone number of a responsible person who is available throughout the shipping process may be placed on the outer packaging or on a document such as an air waybill.
- The Shipper's Declaration for Dangerous Goods is not required.
- An emergency response telephone number is not required.

Materials for Category A and Category B packaging that have the required secondary and outer components and meet the pressure and temperature requirements are commercially available and can be obtained from many suppliers.

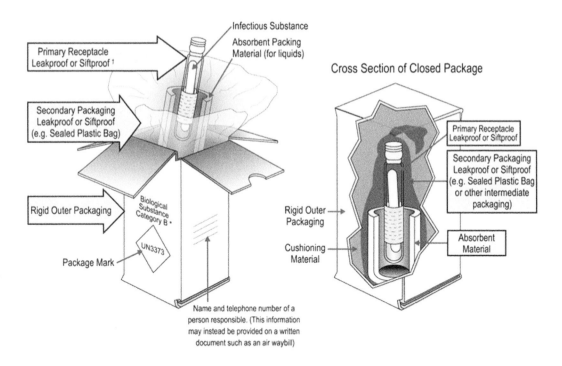

Primary Receptacle
Leakproof or Siftproof [1]

Infectious Substance

Absorbent Packing
Material (for liquids)

Secondary Packaging
Leakproof or Siftproof
(e.g. Sealed Plastic Bag)

Rigid Outer Packaging

Biological
Substance
Category B •

UN3373

Package Mark

Name and telephone number of a
person responsible. (This information
may instead be provided on a written
document such as an air waybill)

Cross Section of Closed Package

Primary Receptacle
Leakproof or Siftproof

Secondary Packaging
Leakproof or Siftproof
(e.g. Sealed Plastic Bag
or other intermediate
packaging)

Rigid Outer
Packaging

Cushioning
Material

Absorbent
Material

Category B packaging

Safety Precautions

Since many fungi produce conidia or spores that easily become airborne, precautions are essential to prevent contamination of the laboratory environment and infection of personnel.

- If at all possible, laboratories culturing filamentous fungi should ideally be in a separate room with negative air pressure; the minimum alternative is a designated separate space in the open microbiology laboratory.
- A suitable biological safety cabinet (BSC); e.g., Class II BSC, must be used when dealing with moulds. Yeast cultures can be handled on the bench in the same manner that bacterial cultures are routinely handled.
- Care must be taken not to spatter infectious material by careless sterilization of wire needles or loops. Use of a benchtop microbiology incinerator is one way to avoid this hazard. Sterile disposable implements provide the best solution by also eliminating the need to sterilize.
- All used implements and any supernatants should be placed in a vessel containing disinfectant.
- Sharps (e.g., scalpels) should be disposed of in a sharps disposal container.
- If plates are used, shrink seals should be employed. Screw-cap tubes of slanted media should be used if *Blastomyces* spp., *Cladiophialophora bantiana*, *Coccidioides* spp., or *Histoplasma capsulatum* are suspected and for subsequent manipulations upon identification, or if a culture of any fungus is to be mailed or otherwise transported to another laboratory.
- Plates and slants should be observed for growth before opening.
- A lactophenol cotton blue preparation should be made of all moulds before setting up a slide culture; do not make slide cultures of isolates that may be *Blastomyces* spp., *C. bantiana*, *Coccidioides* spp., or *H. capsulatum*. These organisms can usually be identified on well-prepared lactophenol cotton blue preparations.
- All contaminated materials must be autoclaved before being discarded.

- Laboratory coats must be worn at all times in the work area.
- Gloves should be worn when manipulating a mould culture that is possibly a dermatophyte; when the task is completed, hands and wrists must be washed well (removing watches and bracelets).
- Personnel must wash their hands thoroughly with a disinfectant soap after handling any mycology cultures.
- The work area must be cleaned with disinfectant at least daily.
- Mouth pipetting must not be done.
- There can be no smoking, drinking, eating, gum chewing, application of cosmetics, insertion of contact lenses, or use of personal mobile devices (e.g., cellular phones and tablet computers) in the laboratory.
- A culture must never be sniffed to determine whether it has an odor; the typical *Streptomyces* spp. can be smelled from afar.

For further information, see
Meechan and Potts (ed.), 2020
Miller et al., 2012
Wooley and Byers (ed.), 2017

BASICS

Taxonomy and Nomenclature

In 2011, a landmark development in the field of fungal taxonomy occurred: the concept of "one fungus/one name." Throughout the past century, pleomorphic fungi had been defined with two different names based upon the phenotypic identification of the sexual state (teleomorph) or the asexual form (anamorph). With the advent of numerous advances in molecular taxonomy, the teleomorphic and anamorphic stages of several medically important fungi were confirmed to be the same organism.

Recognizing the unique dilemma posed by the identification of pleomorphic fungi having two names, the Nomenclature Section meeting of the International Botanical Congress in Melbourne, Australia, in July 2011 recommended the discontinuation of the dual nomenclature system for fungi with anamorphic and teleomorphic forms. Known as the "Amsterdam Declaration on Fungal Nomenclature," this recommendation resulted in a historic revision of the International Code of Botanical Nomenclature. Becoming effective on January 1, 2013, the principle of "one fungus/one name" assigned priority to the oldest genus/species name independently of whether the organism was originally described as the anamorph or teleomorph.

Furthermore, the widespread introduction of DNA sequencing technologies has driven definition of taxonomic relationships that were not recognized using phenotypic identification. These developments have enabled clinical microbiologists to better understand the relatedness of fungal pathogens and more accurately communicate their identification, particularly at the genus/species level. In parallel with these advances, the International Society for Human and Animal Mycology (ISHAM) Working Group on Fungal Taxonomy issued a report advocating for nomenclatural stability among the medically important fungi, while enthusiastically supporting continued research in fungal taxonomy. Underscoring that a given genus/species name conveys critical information on epidemiology, clinical manifestations, treatment, and prognosis for management of a patient, clear communication of a microbiological diagnosis is essential.

There have been revisions in fungal nomenclature since the last edition of *Larone's Medically Important Fungi* that may impact laboratory identification of medically important fungi. As the fundamental purpose of this book is to provide a practical resource for clinical laboratory diagnosis, we have attempted to address fungal nomenclature in three ways: (i) in the detailed descriptions of Part II we include our recommendation for reporting fungi as the organism banner heading name (which is typically the most recent name), while also noting recent earlier names; (ii) where applicable, we retain the more clinically recognized organism name, notably for members of the genera *Aspergillus* and *Candida*, but also include other recognized names given their increased use; and (iii) where practical we list members of species complexes (i.e., morphologically indistinguishable but genetically distinct species) designated due to the increased use of molecular diagnostics in medical mycology. To that end, we encourage reporting organisms to species complex level (e.g., *Aspergillus fumigatus* species complex) unless data related to the clinical significance of a particular member of the species complex is available or emerges, or if required for epidemiological or infection control purposes. All this information is distilled in the individual organism detailed descriptions of Part II with newly introduced "Taxonomy Notes", as needed. Recognizing that names of fungi may change, we also provide links to the following resources:

http://www.mycobank.org/
https://mycology.adelaide.edu.au/
http://www.fungaltaxonomy.org/
http://www.clinicalfungi.org/
http://www.ncbi.nlm.nih.gov/Taxonomy/Browser/wwwtax.cgi

The advances made in the fields of fungal taxonomy and nomenclature will help to further augment our understanding of the relatedness and identification of medically important fungi. As with all medical science, confirmation of the observations and validation of the epidemiological, clinical, pathogenic, and therapeutic implications are important criteria for acceptance into the lexicon of medical mycology.

For further information, see
Borman and Johnson, 2021
Brandt and Lockhart, 2012
de Hoog et al., 2013
de Hoog et al., 2015
Hawksworth, 2011
Warnock, 2017
Warnock, 2019

PART I
Direct Microscopic Examination of Clinical Specimens

Larone's Medically Important Fungi: A Guide to Identification, 7th Edition.
Lars F. Westblade, Eileen M. Burd, Shawn R. Lockhart, and Gary W. Procop.
© 2023 American Society for Microbiology. DOI: 10.1128/9781683674436.pi

Introduction

Specimens submitted to the mycology laboratory should predominantly consist of skin, tissue, or normally sterile body fluids. Swabs may be used to confirm the clinical diagnosis of mucosal infections, such as vulvovaginitis or oropharyngeal candidiasis, but should <u>not</u> be used in the attempt to diagnose deep-seated fungal infections. This is because when invasive fungal elements, such as hyphae, are present in tissue, the fungi intercalate between tissue structures or are encased within an inflammatory reaction (e.g., a cryptococcoma). The fungi in these instances are not easily disrupted and collection by swabbing may result in a failure to recover the etiologic agent in culture (i.e., a false-negative culture result). Ideally, specimens should be obtained prior to the initiation of antifungal therapy to optimize recovery.

The direct examination of clinical specimens, be it by histopathology, cytology, or KOH/calcofluor white is complementary to culture and important for several reasons.

- It may provide the physician with a rapid diagnosis and information regarding the possible need for treatment.

  This is particularly important, as severely ill individuals may be thought to have a bacterial or viral infection. The identification of fungal elements within tissue and associated with an inflammatory response confirms a fungal etiology and directs the appropriate therapy.

- It is helpful in determining the significance of an organism that may later be definitively identified on culture. If the cultured organism is one that is only sometimes pathogenic and it is seen on direct microscopic examination in appreciable numbers, it is more likely to be involved in a disease process and not merely present as a contaminant.

- Observation of unique fungal elements may indicate the need for special media, additional specimens from other sites, and/or molecular or serologic studies.

- All too often, tissue sections are submitted to the anatomic pathology laboratory in fixative, rendering the specimens unsuitable for culture. In these situations, the direct microscopic examination of the tissue plays the principal role in diagnosis.

Multidisciplinary quality initiatives, which include microbiologists, surgeons, and anatomic pathologists, should be considered within an institution to help assure that excised tissues are submitted for both histopathology and culture, as both are important for optimal patient care.

- Some organisms do not grow *in vitro*, or do not grow well, rendering direct microscopic examination an important method of detection and identification.

It is not uncommon for microbiologists to be asked to examine tissue sections from the anatomic pathology laboratory when a fungal infection is suspected or apparent. To attain an acceptable level of comfort and expertise in this responsibility, it is imperative to understand the tissue reactions to mycoses. To familiarize the microbiologist with the histologic responses to fungal infection, the following pages present definitions of pertinent terms, descriptions of the various tissue reactions, and a discussion and table of the histochemical stains that may be employed.

The Guide to Interpretation of Direct Microscopic Examination is intended for use as a quick guide in reading direct smears as well as tissue sections. It is intended to allow rapid comparative viewing of the possible interpretations of the structures in the specimen and to direct the reader to the appropriate pages for more detailed descriptions of the direct microscopic appearance of each of the mycoses.

The detailed description of each mycosis includes (i) the etiologic agent(s), (ii) the common anatomic site(s) of infection, (iii) the tissue reactions most commonly produced, (iv) the microscopic morphology of the organism, and (v) a line drawing and photomicrograph of the organism on direct microscopic examination. There are some infections wherein the direct microscopic examination yields a relatively certain identification of the organism (e.g., cryptococcosis). In other instances, the fungal elements present may simply afford some further categorization of the fungus present (e.g., a hyalohyphomycosis versus a mucormycosis). Although definitive identification may not be possible in such instances, this additional differentiation may be clinically important. For example, all Mucorales are innately resistant to voriconazole, so appropriate categorization, even to this level, guides therapy. Definitive identification usually relies on culture-based methods, although molecular tools are becoming more commonly used in this area.

As the direct microscopic examination usually does not provide definitive identification of the fungal organism observed, it is of utmost importance to render a report that guides the practitioner as much as possible, with respect to the type of fungus present. This increases the opportunity for appropriate treatment. Standardized templates to attain that goal have been designed for anatomic pathology reports and can be modified for use in the clinical mycology laboratory (Sangoi et al., 2009). Such reports should include comments on the type of fungal elements present, such as yeasts, hyphae, or pseudohyphae with a detailed description of their characteristics. For yeasts, comments should include an approximation of size, variation in size, presence and type of budding, and encapsulation. For hyphae, the description should differentiate mucoraceous (i.e., broad, pauciseptate hyphae), hyaline septate hyphae, and dematiaceous hyphae. Organisms should be noted to be intracellular or extracellular. Reproductive structures, if present, should also be described.

Characteristics of various stains are summarized in Table 1.1 (p. 30). Methods for direct microscopic examination of specimens in the mycology laboratory are outlined in Part IV, pp. 414–416. Staining methods are described in Part IV, pp. 431–440.

For further information and excellent photomicrographs of fungi in tissue, see

Chandler and Watts, 1987
Connor et al., 1997
Guarner and Brandt, 2011
Procop and Pritt, 2014
Salfelder, 1990
Schnadig and Woods, 2009
Schuetz and Walsh, 2015

PART I Direct Microscopic Examination of Clinical Specimens

Histological Terminology

Abscess An abscess is a localized collection of predominantly neutrophils. An abscess, if not drained, will become surrounded by a zone of granulation tissue (i.e., organized), and eventually walled off by fibrous connective tissue that limits further spread of the infection. (Image Appendix Figure 1.)

Calcification Calcification is the result of the host reaction to the pathogen and ultimately results in the deposition of calcium in tissue. This often occurs in lymph nodes and other tissues that contain old granulomas (e.g., an old, calcified histoplasmoma). Calcium often appears as an amorphous purple deposit in H&E-stained sections. Spherical calcifications have been mistaken for yeast, and elongate calcifications (e.g., Gamma-Gandy bodies) have been mistaken for filamentous fungi. Histochemical stains are available (e.g., Von Kossa) that stain some calcium deposits; calcium does not stain with GMS, which is a useful characteristic in this setting. (Image Appendix Figures 14 and 15.)

Caseous necrosis Caseous necrosis is differentiated from coagulative and liquefactive necrosis. Caseous necrosis histologically consists of an eosinophilic amorphous material that stains pink (i.e., eosinophilic) in H&E-stained sections. The remnants of the cells that once occupied that histologic space are not discernable, which differentiates this type of necrosis from coagulative necrosis. (Image Appendix Figures 12 and 13.) This type of necrosis was named based on its white to yellowish "cottage cheese" appearance on gross examination.

Collagen Collagen consists of a family of structural fibrous proteins that provides support in human tissues. New collagen deposition first appears as pink fibers in early wound healing in H&E-stained sections. These fibers coalesce into dense organized bands as wound healing culminates in scar formation. (Image Appendix Figures 7 and 8.)

Connective tissue Connective tissue consists of three components: cells, a glycoprotein matrix, and fibers. Fibroblasts are a predominant cell type in connective tissues and produce both the fibers and the matrix. (Image Appendix Figure 7.) Transient acute and chronic inflammatory cells are also commonly present in loose connective tissue. Collagen and elastic fibers are important structural elements of connective tissues. Connective tissue creates the supportive structure in tissues. Two of the most common forms of connective tissue are loose connective tissue (e.g., subcutaneous tissue), which is supportive of nerves and blood vessels transiting the tissue, and dense connective tissue, such as tendons and ligaments.

Cyst   A cyst is a cavity that is lined by epithelial cells. It usually contains liquid or gelatinous material.

Dermis   The dermis is the broad connective tissue layer of the skin located under the epidermis. (Image Appendix Figure 19.)

Eosinophil   Eosinophils are a type of acute inflammatory white blood cell (WBC), which are readily identified by their bilobed nucleus and pink (i.e., eosinophilic) cytoplasmic granules. The granules of eosinophils are rich in histamine, and therefore important in allergic reactions. Although eosinophilic inflammatory responses are common with helminthic parasitic infections, they also occur in allergic fungal sinusitis and in a minor subset of patients with coccidioidomycosis. (Image Appendix Figure 4.)

Eosinophilic   Eosinophilic is an adjective that describes structures that stain pink with the H&E stain.

Epidermis   The epidermis is the outer layer of the skin, which consists of stratified squamous epithelium with an outermost keratin layer. (Image Appendix Figure 19.)

Epithelioid histiocyte   An epithelioid histiocyte is a cell of monocyte or macrophage origin that has characteristics resembling those of an epithelial cell. It is a relatively large, polygonal cell with a pale nucleus, and pale eosinophilic granular cytoplasm in H&E-stained sections. The ratio of the size of the nucleus to total cell size is ~1:4. They are a part of T-cell mediated granuloma formation, which is generated by some fungal infections (e.g., histoplasmosis) (Image Appendix Figure 5.)

Fibroblast   A fibroblast is an elongated, flattened, spindle-shaped cell with cytoplasmic projections at each end. It is the cell within connective tissue that produces collagen fibers and extracellular matrix. (Image Appendix Figure 7.)

Fibrosis   Fibrosis is a proliferation of fibrous tissue that occurs with the maturation and organization of collagen. These appear as eosinophilic (i.e., pink), smooth, dense collagen bundles, in which fibroblasts may be seen embedded. (Image Appendix Figures 8 and 15.)

Giant cell   A giant cell is a multinucleated cell created by fusion of activated macrophages. Giant cells are commonly seen as a component of granulomas produced in response to certain fungal infections (e.g., coccidioidomycosis), but may also be seen in non-infectious conditions (e.g., foreign body giant cells are seen in the inflammatory response to foreign material in the body). (Image Appendix Figures 9, 10, and 13.)

GMS   The Gomori methenamine silver (GMS) stain results from a silver precipitation reaction that stains fungi and bacteria, and sometimes human tissue elements, black against a green background. It is likely the most commonly used stain for the identification of fungi in human tissues. (Image Appendix Figures 24–26.)

Granulation tissue Granulation tissue is early reparative tissue, composed of capillaries, fibroblasts, newly deposited collagen, and predominantly mononuclear leukocytes. As healing continues, granulation tissue often becomes organized to form fibrous tissue (fibrosis). *Note:* This term should not be confused with "granuloma." (Image Appendix Figure 6.)

Granuloma Granulomas are distinct, T-cell mediated inflammatory patterns consisting of activated macrophages/monocytes (epithelioid histiocyte), occasional giant cells, lymphocytes, and a variable infiltration of neutrophils. These may or may not have an area of central necrosis. Granulomas are produced in response to certain infections, including some fungal infections. Granulomas will become organized, forming a circumscribed pattern of inflammation in which the infectious agent is contained (i.e., histochemical stains will often disclose the etiologic agent in the central, eosinophilic, caseous necrosis). Older granulomas will have an outer fibrous rim, minimal-to-no residual epithelioid histiocytes, and a cuff of residual lymphocytes. The walls of old granulomas usually have foci of calcification, which is evident in radiologic studies. (Image Appendix Figures 10–15.)

H&E The hematoxylin and eosin (H&E) stain is the primary stain in histopathology. H&E-stained tissue sections are examined microscopically to determine if a disease is present and to characterize the nature of that disease (e.g., neoplasia versus infection).

Histiocyte A histiocyte is a large, mononuclear phagocyte that is considered a tissue-based macrophage. (Image Appendix Figure 4.)

Hyperkeratosis Hyperkeratosis occurs when there is an increase in the thickness of the keratin layer of the skin. This may be seen in response to dermatophyte infections.

Hyperplasia Hyperplasia is an abnormal increase in the number of normal cells in the tissue.

Infarct An infarct is an area of tissue that has undergone necrosis as a result of obstruction of the blood supply. (Image Appendix Figure 18.)

Lymphocyte A lymphocyte is a mononuclear leukocyte that has relatively scant cytoplasm, yielding a higher ratio of the size of the nucleus to total cell size (~1:1.2). Some lymphocytes are involved in cell-mediated immunity, whereas other are involved in humoral (i.e., antibody mediated) immunity. Generally, these are involved in a more chronic inflammatory process. (Image Appendix Figures 2 and 4.)

Macrophage A macrophage is essentially a monocyte that resides in tissue; these are also commonly referred to as histocytes. They are large, mononuclear, phagocytic cells involved in immunity.

Monocyte A monocyte is the same WBC type as a macrophage, but it is found in the blood. These cells are large, round-to-oval with a large, curved or horseshoe-shaped nucleus and a moderate amount of cytoplasm. The ratio of the size of the nucleus to total cell size is ~1:3.

Necrosis   Necrosis consists of a spectrum of morphologic changes that follow cell death and tissue destruction. It results from the progressive degenerative action of enzymes and/or virulence factors from microorganisms. Classically, these are separated into coagulative, liquefactive, and caseous necrosis, with the latter being the type seen with certain fungal infections (see Caseous Necrosis, above). (Image Appendix Figures 12, 13, 15, 16, and 17.)

Neutrophil   The neutrophil is a WBC with a multilobulated nucleus that appears as two to four small, round to ovoid nuclei connected by thin filaments of nuclear material. This cell type is also known as a polymorphonuclear leukocyte, commonly called a "poly" or "PMN". It is a granulocytic WBC that is neither eosinophilic nor basophilic. This cell is characteristic of acute inflammation. (Image Appendix Figures 1 and 2.)

Parakeratosis   Parakeratosis describes the persistence of nuclei in the cells of the stratum corneum or keratin layer of the skin, which is normally devoid of nucleated cells. This is a nonspecific finding that is present in a variety of dermatologic disorders.

Parenchyma   Parenchyma is the essential functional tissue of an organ, as distinguished from its supporting connective tissue and nutritive framework (i.e., stroma).

PAS   The Periodic acid-Schiff (PAS) stain highlights the cell walls of fungi, but also stains other molecules in tissue such as glycogen. (Image Appendix Figure 28.)

Plasma cell   A plasma cell is a special type of B-lymphocyte that has differentiated to produce antibodies against a particular pathogen. This cell is recognized by an eccentric nucleus that has a speckled chromatin pattern that has been likened to a clock face. The Golgi complex, next to the nucleus, produces a clear, pale-stained area. The ratio of the size of the nucleus to total cell size is ~1:2. (Image Appendix Figure 4.)

Pseudoepitheliomatous hyperplasia   Pseudoepitheliomatous hyperplasia is an extensive increase in the thickness of the epidermis, which is a response to pathogens such as *Blastomyces*, *Sporothrix*, and the agents of chromoblastomycosis. Although this proliferation is benign, it superficially resembles squamous cell carcinoma for which it has been mistaken.

Splendore-Hoeppli phenomenon   The Splendore-Hoeppli phenomenon consists of an aggregation of eosinophilic proteinaceous material around certain microorganisms in tissue, usually in the setting of a chronic infection. (Image Appendix Figure 20.)

Stratum corneum   The stratum corneum is the outermost layer of the epidermis that consists of flat, denucleated cells that are composed of keratin. (Image Appendix Figure 19.)

Suppurative inflammation   Suppurative inflammation is an acute inflammatory reaction characterized by a large number of neutrophils. Necrotic cells, nuclear (apoptotic) debris, and a large amount of edema fluid are also usually present. (Image Appendix Figures 1 and 2.)

Tissue Reactions to Fungal Infection

After damage of any kind, including infection, the body responds in a fairly predictable manner depending on the immunologic status of the host. Individuals with an intact immune system will have a robust, highly predictable response. Those with a profound immunodeficiency will respond quite differently and this will depend on the specific type of immunologic deficit (e.g., T-cell mediated loss versus neutropenia). To complicate matters even further, individuals receiving immunomodulating therapies (e.g., biologics) will often demonstrate a truncated or partial immune response.

The inflammatory process can be separated into three steps: (i) acute or ongoing (i.e., chronic) infection, (ii) resolving disease, and (iii) remote/residual disease. Acute infection occurs with the contraction of the infection and is heralded by the initial inflammatory response. Fungi such as *Aspergillus* and *Candida* usually generate a neutrophilic response, whereas *Histoplasma* and *Coccidioides* generate a granulomatous response. Neutrophilic debris and/or necrosis are seen as cells and tissue die. If the immune system cannot rid the body of the pathogen, then the disease may become chronic. Granulation tissue follows the resolution of a neutrophilic response, whereas granulomas begin to become fibrotic. Complete resolution of a neutrophilic response may show preservation of the tissue architecture or scarring, depending on the degree of tissue damage that occurred.

While no tissue reactions during this process of inflammation and repair are absolutely diagnostic of a specific organism, particular organisms usually generate a particular inflammatory response. This can be useful if the pathogens are morphologically similar-to-identical, but the inflammatory response is different. One of the best examples of this is *Candida glabrata* and *Histoplasma capsulatum*. *Candida* species generate a neutrophilic response, whereas *Histoplasma* generates granulomas in the immunocompetent and a histiocytic response in the immunocompromised.

The angioinvasive nature of moulds deserves mentioning. This is observed with *Aspergillus*, *Fusarium*, and members of the Mucorales, amongst others. When moulds invade blood vessels, thrombosis (i.e., blood clot formation) and infarction of distal tissues follow. The infarcted tissue is dead and can no longer complete its physiologic function. Additionally, the blood vessel is clotted, which precludes the delivery of antifungal agents to the site of infection. It is for this reason that surgical intervention is often needed in addition to specific antifungal therapy. Angioinvasive moulds are often best visualized at the advancing border of the infarcted or devitalized tissue.

The following are the major tissue reactions observed with fungal infections. Patients who are partially immunosuppressed will have a truncated or modified inflammatory response. Those who are profoundly immunocompromised may simply demonstrate tissue damage, or may have alternate immune cells (e.g., macrophages) involved in the response.

Acute Suppurative Inflammation and Microabscesses

Suppurative inflammation is an acute reaction that is characterized by a predominance of neutrophils. Aggregates of neutrophils form pus, and large aggregates of pus form abscesses. The normal human tissue in which this type of inflammation occurs is often destroyed through a combination of the hydrolytic enzymes of the inflammatory cells and the virulence factors of the pathogen present. The suppurative area, with time, may be walled off by granulation tissue, then fibrous tissue, resulting in an abscess cavity. (Image Appendix Figure 1.)

Chronic Inflammation

A chronic inflammatory infiltrate consisting of lymphocytes, plasma cells, and histiocytes becomes predominant as the acute inflammation resolves. This reaction is nonspecific, and is seen with a variety of fungal infections, as well as with inflammatory reactions caused by other agents. (Image Appendix Figures 3 and 4.)

Granulomatous Inflammation (Granulomas)

The term "granulomatous" refers to a type of inflammation that is characterized by aggregates of large mononuclear cells (i.e., macrophages or histiocytes) some of which will fuse to form multinucleated giant cells. In fungal diseases, as well as in tuberculosis, the nuclei are arranged along the inner periphery of the giant cell; this is termed a Langhans giant cell (Image Appendix Figure 9); in foreign body or tumor giant cells, the nuclei are irregularly placed throughout the cytoplasm. There are a variety of types of granulomas. Although it is not possible to definitively determine the type of infectious agent present from the type of granuloma produced, the specific type of granuloma does raise the likelihood of particular etiologic agents. The most commonly encountered granulomas may be characterized as nonnecrotizing or necrotizing granulomas, based on the absence or presence of central caseous necrosis, respectively. These are sometime referred to as noncaseating and caseating granulomas, respectively, because of the gross appearance of the granulomas on cut section. Nonnecrotizing granulomas may become necrotizing with time and additional maturation

Nonnecrotizing granulomas are commonly associated with nontuberculous mycobacterial infections but may also be seen with some fungal diseases (e.g., early histoplasmosis). A nonnecrotizing granuloma consists of a relatively well circumscribed accumulation of epithelioid macrophages without central necrosis but with associated lymphocytes. (Image Appendix Figures 10 and 11.)

An active necrotizing granuloma is composed of an area of central caseous necrosis surrounded by epithelioid histiocytes with or without giant cells. Histochemical stains for microorganisms may disclose them in the necrosis, the giant cells, or the epithelioid histiocytes. Associated lymphocytes are invariably present. (Image Appendix Figures 12 and 13.)

An old, inactive, fibrotic granuloma retains the area of central necrosis that is surrounded by a fibrous wall that is often calcified. A few epithelioid histiocytes with or without giant cells may remain, depending on the stage of resolution of the granuloma. Histochemical stains for microorganisms may disclose these in the area of central necrosis; these are often nonviable, as judged by the low recovery rate in culture.

Suppurative granulomas are similar to necrotizing granulomas in structure, except the center of the granuloma is composed of neutrophils (i.e., pus), as opposed to necrosis. This type of granuloma has been seen with infections by members of the *Exophiala jeanselmei* species complex, certain mycobacteria (e.g., *Mycobacterium abscessus*) and often is the inflammatory response that is present in patients with cat scratch disease (i.e., *Bartonella henselae* infection).

Pyogranulomatous inflammation is distinct from a suppurative granuloma in that there is usually an admixture of neutrophils and nonnecrotizing granulomas (i.e., aggregates of epithelioid histiocytes). Some lymphocytes are invariably present in the background of any granulomatous reaction. Pyogranulomatous reactions are seen in patients with blastomycosis, chromoblastomycosis, and sporotrichosis.

Necrosis

There is a spectrum of morphologic changes that follow cell death due to progressive degenerative enzymatic action, the sum of these changes is known as necrosis. Histologically, the cytoplasm of the cell shows increased eosinophilia (pink with H&E stain) and may appear vacuolated, whereas the nucleus shrinks (pyknosis), becomes hyperchromatic (i.e., demonstrates increased blueness or basophilia), and fragmentation of the chromatin (karyolysis) and the nucleus itself (karyorrhexis). (Image Appendix Figure 16.)

Caseous necrosis is a form of necrosis that occurs within necrotizing granulomas. This is so named since upon gross examination it demonstrates a cottage cheeselike consistency. Microscopically, this type of necrosis appears homogeneous, amorphous, and finely granular; the remnants of the cells that previously existed in the space are not apparent. This latter feature is in contrast to coagulative necrosis that occurs following an infarct. (Image Appendix Figures 12 and 13.)

Angioinvasion, Infarction, and Necrosis

Mucorales, *Aspergillus* spp., and several other fungi, such as *Scedosporium* spp. and *Fusarium* spp., are angioinvasive moulds. The invasion of a blood vessel occludes the lumen causing thrombosis, which precludes blood flow and causes infarction and coagulative necrosis of the tissue deprived of blood supply. Histologically, angioinvasion appears as hyphae in the blood vessel wall and in the thrombotic material that blocks the lumen of the vessel. The associated infarcted tissue will be almost entirely eosinophilic (i.e., the nuclei of the dead cells do not stain blue). Neutrophils and monocytic cells, as well as a large amount of degenerated cellular debris (i.e., pyknotic debris) are usually present, with the inflammatory cells predominating at the periphery of the infarct. (Image Appendix Figures 17 and 18.)

Splendore-Hoeppli Phenomenon

The Splendore-Hoeppli reaction is a localized immunologic host response to antigens of a variety of infectious agents, including some fungi and bacteria. Splendore-Hoeppli reactions consist of radiating homogeneous, refractile, eosinophilic material that coats the microorganisms. (Image Appendix Figure 20.) Splendore-Hoeppli material, although not invariably present, is most commonly seen coating *Sporothrix*, Entomophthorales, and both bacterial and fungal causes of mycetoma. It is also commonly seen with the nonfilamentous bacteria that cause botryomycosis.

Fungus Ball

A fungus ball results when filamentous fungi colonize a previously formed cavity that has access to oxygen. Any filamentous fungus can cause a fungus ball, but *Aspergillus* species, particularly *A. niger*, are common causes. There is minimal-to-no invasion of the tissues unless the host is immunocompromised. Hyphae and sometimes conidial heads, complete with phialides and conidia, develop. Fungal masses are seen lying freely within the cavity and not attached to the cavity wall. Surrounding tissue reaction may demonstrate findings associated with chronic sinusitis or chronic allergic sinusitis. Crystalline material is commonly present, which represents metabolic byproducts of the fungus present. Oxalate crystals, which have a sheaf-of-wheat appearance, are indicative of the presence of *A. niger*.

Stains

Although some fungi may be seen in tissue with the routinely used H&E stain, some are not, or the details of the fungi are not readily apparent. There are special histochemical stains that enhance the detection and characterization of fungi in histologic sections. The most commonly used stains are summarized in Table 1.1 (p. 30). The Gomori methenamine silver (GMS) stain is the most commonly used and generally the preferred method for the detection of fungi in histologic sections. (Image Appendix Figures 24–26.) This stain may also be applied to smeared material and cytologic preparations. The GMS stain is a nonspecific silver precipitation stain that can stain material other than fungi, which denotes the importance of detailed morphologic assessment to differentiate fungi from debris, foreign material, or even normally present histologic elements (e.g., collagen). If the possibility of a morphologic mimic is considered, then an alternative stain, such as periodic acid-Schiff (PAS), can be useful.

The fluorescent calcofluor white (CFW) stain (p. 434), with or without potassium hydroxide (KOH), is recommended for staining wet preparations of specimens or on smeared and dried material. (Image Appendix Figure 27.) The KOH/CFW combination is far superior to the traditional KOH alone. Although CFW may be used on deparaffinized tissue sections, this application is uncommon.

Some stains are used as supplements to aid in more specific characterization of an organism after detection with a preliminary fungal stain. For example, GMS readily detects yeast in tissue, but the mucicarmine or alcian blue stains can subsequently be performed on the tissue to determine the presence of a polysaccharide capsule, typical of *Cryptococcus* spp. Similarly, GMS will detect the yeast cells of *Blastomyces* (Image Appendix Figure 31) but it will not reliably demonstrate the double contoured cell wall, which is readily apparent with a PAS or H&E stain.

The Fontana-Masson (FM) stain is used for detecting melanin, or its precursors, in cell walls. (Image Appendix Figure 29.) It can be helpful in the rare instances of capsule-reduced (i.e., erroneously termed capsule-deficient) strains of *Cryptococcus neoformans* or *Cryptococcus gattii*, as the melanin in the cell wall will stain dark brown. FM is known to intensely stain dematiaceous fungi in tissue sections; however, other fungi may have a variable but smaller amount of stain uptake. Notably, *Candida*, *Scedosporium*, and most *Fusarium* are consistently negative.

Oddly, *Alternaria*, a dematiaceous mould, has been shown to sometimes fail to stain. Therefore, the interpretation of the FM stain should be considered with all other information available.

See Part IV, pp. 431–440, for further information on the stains most commonly used in the clinical mycology laboratory.

TABLE 1.1 Histochemical stains for fungi and/or filamentous bacteria in tissue

Stain (abbreviation)	Characteristics
Alcian blue	The polysaccharide capsules of *Cryptococcus neoformans* and *Cryptococcus gattii* stain turquoise blue. This stain is less frequently used than mucicarmine for this purpose. The combination PAS/Alcian blue stain, which is commonly used to differentiate mucin in the gastrointestinal tract, is particularly interesting for viewing *Cryptococcus*, as the PAS stains the cell wall red, whereas the Alcian blue stains the capsule blue.
Brown and Brenn (B&B)	This is a tissue Gram stain for bacteria and variably stains fungi. It is useful to highlight the bacterial filaments of the actinomycetes, e.g., *Nocardia*, *Actinomadura*, etc. These stain Gram positive, and, particularly *Nocardia* and *Actinomyces israelii*, demonstrate beading (i.e., foci of more intense staining) along the elongate bacterial filaments.
Calcofluor white (CFW)	The molecule binds to chitin in fungal cell walls. Although it may be used on formalin-fixed, paraffin-embedded tissues, this is rarely done. It is more commonly used for direct examination in mycology, in combination with potassium hydroxide. A fluorescence microscope is required.
Fontana-Masson (FM)	This stains melanin and melanin-like pigments. It stains dematiaceous fungi brown to black. It is most commonly used to confirm fungi as dematiaceous. It is particularly useful in this regard when the dematiaceous pigment is not obvious and the fungus simply appears "dusky." It has also been used to stain actively replicating *Cryptococcus*, which is known to contain small quantities of melanin or melanin precursors in their cell walls. Some have cautioned that some strains of *Aspergillus fumigatus*, *Aspergillus flavus*, *Trichosporon* spp., and some Mucorales may stain variably, but less intensely (Kimura and McGinnis, 1998).
Giemsa	Most organisms (fungi and also bacteria) stain blue-purple with the Giemsa stain. It enables visualization of fungi in bone marrow aspirates, body fluid preparations, and peripheral blood smears.
Gomori methenamine silver (GMS)	Most all fungi, including *Pneumocystis jirovecii*, stain black with GMS against a green background. (Image Appendix Figures 22, 24–26, 31, 35, and 36.) Mucorales will occasionally stain very poorly with the GMS stain. GMS is a nonspecific precipitation stain, so it also stains *Nocardia* and other bacteria. A preparation with too much precipitation (i.e., a heavy stain) stains human cells and tissue elements (e.g., neutrophils and collagen), which makes interpretation difficult. A heavy stain also obscures structural details of fungi.
Hematoxylin and eosin (H&E)	H&E stains some fungi blue (i.e., basophilic); this is a common staining pattern for *Candida* spp. and *Aspergillus*. (Image Appendix Figure 18.) Mucorales commonly stain pink, whereas *Cryptococcus* does not stain at all. Some fungi are readily apparent in H&E-stained sections, whereas others are inapparent and require special histochemical stains (e.g., GMS) for detection. The H&E stain is the primary stain used by histopathologists, and affords a characterization of the host inflammatory response, which can be useful for differentiating morphologically similar fungi (e.g., *Histoplasma capsulatum* and *Candida glabrata*). The phaeoid nature of dematiaceous fungi is often readily apparent in H&E-stained sections. (Image Appendix Figure 30.)

Stain (abbreviation)	Characteristics
Modified acid-fast	The modified acid-fast stain, or Fite stain, uses a weaker acid decolorizer than the Ziehl-Neelsen stain. Filaments of *Nocardia* stain pink and often have a beaded appearance (i.e., foci of more intense staining). (Image Appendix Figure 23.) The filaments are elongate branching bacteria, so are ~1 µm in diameter, which is useful for differentiating these from fungi. These organisms would fail to stain with the full acid-fast stain (i.e., the Ziehl-Neelsen or equivalent), because of a lower concentration of mycolic acids in their cell wall compared with mycobacteria.
Mucicarmine	Mucicarmine is another histochemical stain for mucin, which stains the capsule of *Cryptococcus* pinkish red. (Image Appendix Figure 34.) There are rare reports of some staining of *Blastomyces* and *Rhinosporidium* (Image Appendix Figure 37), but it is unclear if staining was a result of the staining of human mucin.
Periodic acid-Schiff (PAS)	The PAS stain is another commonly used stain for fungi. It stains the fungal cell walls pink-to-red. (Image Appendix Figure 28.) It also stains glycogen rich tissues, such as the liver. When used in these locations, it is often best to include a diastase digestion prior to staining.

Guide to Interpretation of Direct Microscopic Examination

Abbreviations: GMS, Gomori methenamine silver stain; H&E, hematoxylin and eosin stain; PAS, periodic acid-Schiff stain.

Observation	Brief description	Interpretation
	• "Sulfur granules" (30–3,000 µm or more in diameter) • Delicate (<1-µm diameter), branched bacterial filaments • Gram positive and non-acid-fast • Stains with GMS and Giemsa stains but not PAS or Fite (modified acid-fast stain)	ACTINOMYCOSIS (p. 40)
	• Granule (white, yellow, or red) • Narrow (0.5–1 µm in diameter), intertwined bacterial filaments • Gram positive and non-acid-fast • Stains with GMS	ACTINOMYCOTIC MYCETOMA (p. 41)
	• Granules (white, yellow, brown, or black) • Hyphae (2–6 µm in diameter) • Swollen cells are common, especially at the periphery of the granule • Stains with GMS	EUMYCOTIC MYCETOMA (e.g., *Madurella mycetomatis, Trematosphaeria grisea, Cladophialophora bantiana, Scedosporium* spp., *Sarocladium strictum, Phaeoacremonium krajdenii, Actinomadura madurae, Fusarium falciforme*, and *Aspergillus nidulans*) (p. 41)
	• Delicate, narrow (0.5–1.0 µm in diameter) branching, bacterial filaments • Tendency to branch at right angles • Frequently appear beaded or granular • Gram positive • Stains with GMS • Partially acid-fast positive	NOCARDIOSIS (p. 43)

Observation	Brief description	Interpretation
	• Hyaline broad hyphae (3–25 μm in diameter; average, 12 μm) • Pauciseptate (coenocytic) with nonparallel hyphal walls • Branching is nondichotomous, irregular, sometimes at right angles	MUCORMYCOSIS (p. 44)
	• Septate hyaline hyphae (3–12 μm in diameter) • Dichotomous branching at acute angles • Tendency to grow in radial pattern • Hyphae cell walls nearly parallel to one another	ASPERGILLOSIS (p. 45)
	• Septate hyaline hyphae (2–8 μm in diameter) • Hyphae irregular and haphazardly arranged • Branching at 45 and 90° angles • Small phialides and conidia (i.e., adventitious conidia) may form in closed lesions	HYALOHYPHOMYCOSES (e.g., *Paecilomyces* spp., *Purpureocillium lilacinum*, and *Fusarium* spp.) (p. 47)
	• Hyaline, branched, septate hyphae • Hyphae often break up into chains of arthroconidia, particularly within hair shafts • Other conidia do not form in tissue	DERMATOPHYTOSIS (tinea, ringworm) (p. 49)
	• Short, septate hyaline hyphal elements (2.5–4.0 μm in diameter) that may be slightly curved, form short chains • Oval to round, thick-walled, yeast cells (3–8 μm in diameter), often in clusters • Produce buds through small, phialidic collarettes • "Spaghetti and meatball" appearance (clusters of yeasts with short hyphal elements)	TINEA VERSICOLOR (e.g., *Malassezia* spp.) (p. 50)
	• Darkly pigmented, septate hyphae (1.5–3.0 μm in diameter) • Sometimes elongated budding cells (1.5–5.0 μm in diameter) • Occasionally chlamydoconidia	TINEA NIGRA (*Hortaea werneckii*) (p. 51)

Observation	Brief description	Interpretation
	• Brown-pigmented, septate hyphae (2–6 µm in diameter) • Dark, budding, pseudohyphal and yeastlike forms may also occur	PHAEOHYPHOMYCOSIS (e.g., *Curvularia* spp., *Exophiala* spp., *Cladophialophora bantiana*, and others) (p. 52)
	• Sclerotic bodies (5–12 µm in diameter): Brown pigmented Thick walled Have horizontal and vertical septations	CHROMOBLASTOMYCOSIS (e.g., *Fonsecaea* spp., *Phialophora verrucosa, Cladophialophora carrionii*) (p. 53)
	• Yeast cells that vary from round to oval to elongate (2–6 µm in diameter); bud on narrow base • Some characteristically elongated "cigar bodies" (2 × 3 to 3 × 10 µm) may be seen	SPOROTRICHOSIS (p. 54)
	• Yeast cells: Small (2–4 µm in diameter), usually ovoid Budding on a narrow base at the smaller end Characteristically within macrophages or monocytes in active disease Commonly remain clustered when extra-cellular in caseous necrosis	HISTOPLASMOSIS (*Histoplasma capsulatum*) (p. 55)
	• Yeast cells: Small (2–4 µm in diameter), usually ovoid Budding on a narrow base at the smaller end Characteristically within macrophages or monocytes in active disease	EMERGOMYCOSIS (*Emergomyces* spp.) (p. 57)

Observation	Brief description	Interpretation
	• Yeast cells: Round or oval (~3 μm in diameter) Characteristically within macrophages or monocytes May elongate somewhat when extra-cellular Have a central septum; do not bud	TALAROMYCOSIS (formerly peni-cilliosis) (*Talaromyces marneffei* [formerly *Penicillium marneffei*]) (p. 58)
	• Yeast cells: Round to oval (3–30 μm in diameter; usually 8–15 μm) Thick, double-contoured cell wall Budding on a broad base	BLASTOMYCOSIS (p. 59)
	• Yeast cells: Round to oval, large (3–30 μm in diameter) Multiple budding Buds are attached to the parent cell by narrow connections	PARACOCCIDIOIDOMYCOSIS (p. 60)
	• Yeast forms round to oval (6 × 12 μm), under polarized light exhibit "Maltese cross" birefringence • Appear singly or in chains joined with tubelike connections; chains have been likened to rosary or rosario beads	LOBOMYCOSIS (*Lacazia loboi*) (p. 61)
	• Round to oval, budding yeast cells (3–6 μm in diameter) • Branching, septate hyphae and pseudohyphae • Chains of budding cells	CANDIDIASIS (CANDIDOSIS) (p. 62)

Observation	Brief description	Interpretation
	• Round to oval, budding yeast cells (3–6 μm in diameter) • Branching, septate hyphae and pseudohyphae • Arthroconidia	TRICHOSPORONOSIS (p. 64)

	• Yeast cells:
	  Mostly round; some oval (2–20 μm in diameter)
	  Encapsulated
	  Thin walled
	  Budding on a narrow base
		CRYPTOCOCCOSIS (p. 65)

	• Round, ovoid, or collapsed crescent cyst forms (3–5 μm in diameter) on silver stain • Nonbudding • Appear in small clusters on a thick, foamy background • Centrally located comma- or parenthesis-shaped intracystic bodies are pathogno-monic; not evident in every cyst	PNEUMOCYSTOSIS (p. 67)
	• Round or oval sporangia (range, 2–25 μm in diameter) • Round or polyhedral endospores within sporangia or free, resembling non-budding yeast • No budding	PROTOTHECOSIS (p. 68)
	• Spherules (10–100 μm or more in diameter) • Mature spherule relatively thin walled (1–2 μm thick) • Round endospores (2–5 μm in diameter) in mature spherules • Free endospores and immature spherules resemble nonbudding yeast • No budding	COCCIDIOIDOMYCOSIS (p. 69)
	• Large, round sporangia (100–350 μm in diameter when mature) • Sporangia thick walled (~5 μm) • Endospores vary in size (1–10 μm in diameter) • Endospores are arranged in zonal pattern in mature sporangia • Inner surface of sporangial wall and walls of endospores stain with mucicarmine • No budding	RHINOSPORIDIOSIS (p. 70)

Observation	Brief description	Interpretation
	• Large, round adiaconidia (200–400 μm in diameter) • Adiaconidia very thick walled (20–70 μm) • Interior of adiaconidium usually appears empty • No budding	ADIASPIROMYCOSIS (*Emmonsia crescens*) (p. 72)

Detailed Descriptions

Actinomycosis

ETIOLOGIC AGENTS: *Actinomyces israelii* (in humans), *Actinomyces bovis* (in animals), and other *Actinomyces* spp.; occasionally *Arachnia*, *Rothia*, and *Eubacterium* spp.

SITES OF INFECTION: Neck and face area, lung, thoracic cavity, liver, abdomen, pelvis, uterus, multiple systemic sites.

TISSUE REACTION: Typically suppuration with microabscesses containing granules composed of the bacterial filaments. The innermost portion of the wall of the abscess may contain foamy macrophages. Palisading epithelioid macrophages and giant cells often surround the abscess and may be encapsulated by fibrosing granulation tissue. Splendore-Hoeppli material often cover the granules. Draining sinus tracts connecting the abscesses to the body surface are common.

MORPHOLOGY OF ORGANISM: Granules from an abscess or draining sinus tract are 30–3,000 μm or more in diameter and are commonly called "sulfur granules" (due to their yellow color, which resembles elemental sulfur; these, however, do not contain sulfur). When crushed, the granules appear microscopically as opaque masses with peripheral, gelatinous, club-shaped bodies. The granules are composed of numerous delicate (~1 μm in diameter) bacterial filaments that branch (often at right angles) and may exhibit beading (but not as commonly as do *Nocardia* spp.). In some instances, only small groups of branching filaments form instead of the characteristic granules. (Image Appendix Figure 21.) The organisms are Gram positive and non-acid-fast with both the full and modified acid-fast staining methods. These stain well with GMS and Giemsa stains, but the individual filaments may not be apparent with H&E and PAS. Other bacteria may also be present in these infections.

Branching filaments of *Nocardia* spp. are morphologically similar, but most (although not all) *Nocardia* stain partially acid-fast. Culture or molecular studies are required for definitive identification of the etiologic agent.

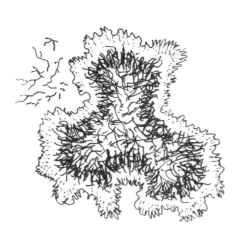

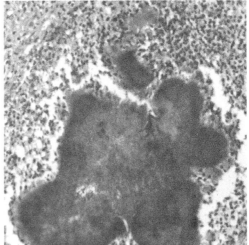

Courtesy of Joan Barenfanger.

Mycetoma (Actinomycotic or Eumycotic)

ETIOLOGIC AGENTS:

Actinomycotic: *Nocardia* spp., *Actinomadura* spp., and *Streptomyces* spp.

Eumycotic: *Scedosporium* spp., *Rhinocladiella* spp., *Madurella* and *Trematosphaeria* spp., *Exophiala jeanselmei* species complex, *Acremonium* and *Sarocladium* spp., *Fusarium* spp., *Curvularia* spp., and occasionally other moulds.

SITES OF INFECTION: Subcutaneous tissue and skin; long-standing infections may involve muscle, fascia, and bone. The infection is most commonly on lower leg or foot, rarely disseminated.

TISSUE REACTION: Similar reactions are seen with all mycetomas, i.e., both actinomycotic and eumycotic. Multiple draining sinus tracts with neutrophilic abscesses containing granules (composed of the etiologic agent) and necrotic debris are characteristic. The abscesses and sinus tracts are surrounded by chronic inflammation consisting of palisading epithelioid macrophages, multinucleated giant cells, lymphocytes, and plasma cells. Between the abscesses is granulation tissue that is usually vascular and contains many inflammatory cells. Splendore-Hoeppli material very often surrounds the granules. Fibrosis may occur in long-standing infections.

MORPHOLOGY OF ORGANISM: The etiologic agent typically organizes into aggregates or tumefactive masses in infected tissue to form granules ranging in size from 25 μm to 5 mm.

- Actinomycotic Mycetoma: Granules (white, yellow, or red) are composed of narrow (1 μm or less in diameter), intertwined filaments that are radially oriented and most numerous at the edge of the granule. *Nocardia* spp. are usually at least partially acid-fast, while *Actinomadura* and *Streptomyces* spp. are not acid-fast. All are Gram positive and stain well with GMS and Giemsa, but individual filaments may not be apparent with H&E or PAS.
- Eumycotic Mycetoma: Granules (white, yellow, brown, or black) contain septate, variously shaped, usually distorted hyphae (2–6 μm in diameter) that are often accompanied by numerous swollen cells; the fungal forms are most commonly visible at the periphery of the granule. (Image Appendix Figure 22.)

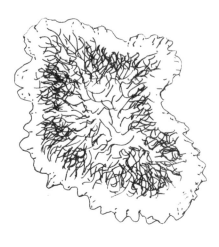

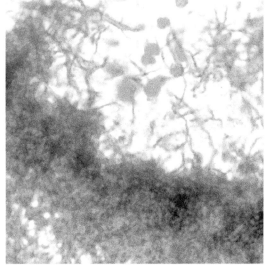

Edge of actinomycotic granule.

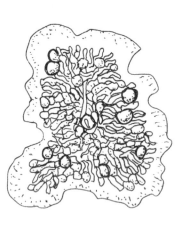

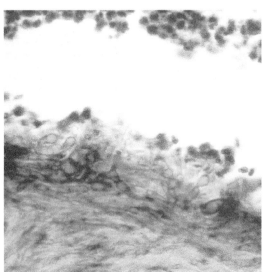

Edge of eumycotic granule.

Nocardiosis

ETIOLOGIC AGENTS: *Nocardia farcinica*, *Nocardia cyriacigeorgica*, *Nocardia nova*, *Nocardia abscessus*, *Nocardia otitidiscaviarum*, *Nocardia brasiliensis*, and occasionally other *Nocardia* spp.

SITES OF INFECTION: Lung, central nervous system, skin and subcutaneous tissue, multiple systemic sites.

TISSUE REACTION: Generally, the reaction is suppurative, sometimes necrotizing. When *N. brasiliensis* is in the subcutis, a mycetomatous-type infection ensues with granule formation, as noted above. Opportunistic infections in immunocompromised patients have poorly defined, variably encapsulated abscesses depending on the degree of neutropenia; granules are not formed in this type of infection. Occasionally, a granulomatous tissue is seen in chronic infections. The Splendore-Hoeppli phenomenon is seen in *Nocardia* mycetomas, but not in nocardiosis of the lungs and central nervous system, which occurs in immunocompromised patients.

MORPHOLOGY OF ORGANISM: Delicate, narrow (0.5–1.0 μm in diameter) bacterial filaments that tend to branch at right angles are seen; rarely, coccobacillary elements may form. Organisms characteristically appear beaded, particularly in Gram stained and modified (i.e., partial) acid-fast stained preparations (e.g., modified Kinyoun stain [p. 432] or another acid-fast stain using a weak acid solution for decolorization). (Image Appendix Figure 23.) The organisms are reliably Gram positive and stain well with GMS; they do not reliably stain with H&E or PAS.

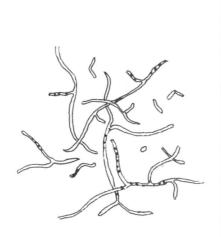
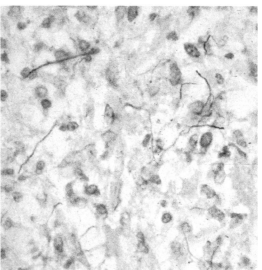

Courtesy of Ron C. Neafie.

Mucormycosis (Zygomycosis)

ETIOLOGIC AGENTS: *Rhizopus* spp., *Mucor* spp., *Rhizomucor* spp., *Lichtheimia corymbifera*, *Apophysomyces elegans*, *Cunninghamella bertholletiae*, and *Saksenaea vasiformis*.

SITES OF INFECTION: Lung, nasal sinus, brain, eye, skin, gastrointestinal tract, and multiple systemic sites.

TISSUE REACTION: Suppurative necrosis and occasionally granulomatous reactions occur. Members of the order Mucorales (p. 195) are angioinvasive (i.e., have a predilection for invasion of blood vessels), causing thrombosis and tissue infarction. These agents must be differentiated from *Aspergillus* spp. and other hyphomycetes that also commonly invade blood vessels. Perineural invasion has also been noted.

MORPHOLOGY OF ORGANISM: The key features are (i) broad hyphae (5–25 µm in diameter; average, 12 µm) with nonparallel walls; (ii) pauciseptate hyphae—the thin walls and lack of regular septation decreases the internal support of these broad hyphae and allows them to become characteristically twisted, collapsed, and folded in a ribbonlike fashion; (iii) branching that is irregularly spaced, nondichotomous, and at various angles (often at right angles) to the parent hypha. (Image Appendix Figure 24.)

The GMS staining of these fungi is variable, with some staining very poorly. Moreover, some strains may be uniformly negative with the GMS stain, and more evident on H&E- or PAS-stained sections.

Note: The microbiology laboratory should be notified as soon as possible if a mucormycete is suspected or seen in tissue, as special measures may be taken to improve its recovery on culture (i.e., teasing the tissue apart for inoculation rather than tissue grinding).

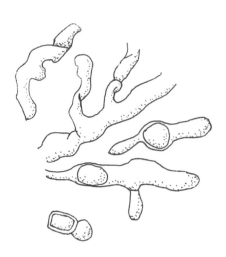
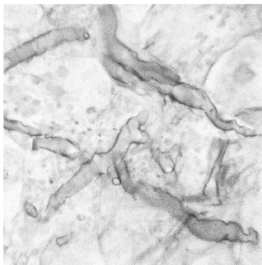

Courtesy of Morris Gordon.

Aspergillosis

ETIOLOGIC AGENTS: *Aspergillus fumigatus*, *Aspergillus flavus*, *Aspergillus niger*, *Aspergillus terreus*, and other *Aspergillus* spp.

SITES OF INFECTION: Lung, paranasal sinuses, ear, eye, skin, brain, heart, and multiple systemic sites.

TISSUE REACTION: Invasive aspergillosis is characterized by an acute inflammatory response (i.e., neutrophils) and necrosis. In severely neutropenic patients, the acute inflammatory response is greatly reduced. A granulomatous response occurs in chronic infections. *Aspergillus* spp. are angioinvasive (i.e., have a predilection for invading blood vessels; see p. 27), causing blockage of blood flow (thrombosis), tissue death and necrosis (infarction), and presence of red blood cells outside of the blood vessels (hemorrhage). Some other hyaline fungi, such as *Fusarium* spp. and *Scedosporium* spp., may cause similar tissue reactions.

Allergic or hypersensitivity aspergillosis may occur in several forms, but most will result in tissue reactions that involve hypersecretion of mucus with neutrophils and eosinophils. Charcot-Leyden crystals are commonly seen in the presence of degranulated eosinophils; these crystals are intensely pink in H&E-stained section, long, narrow, wider at the center, and tapered to a point at each end. Mucus plugs are sometimes expectorated and have concentric layers of eosinophils, epithelial cells, necrotic cellular debris, and Charcot-Leyden crystals.

When fungus balls (aspergillomas; see p. 28) form, the wall of the cavity should be examined for invasion, which is usually absent. Calcium oxalate crystals, if seen within the fungus ball, are indicative of *A. niger*. Other fungi, including other *Aspergillus* spp., may be associated with non-calcium oxalate crystals.

MORPHOLOGY OF ORGANISM: The key features include (i) septate hyphae, mostly 3–6 μm in diameter; (ii) dichotomous branching (i.e., each branch is approximately equal in width to the originating parent hypha) at 45° angles; and (iii) tendency to grow from hematogenous lesions in tissues in a radial fashion, like the spokes of a wheel, with the hyphae appearing nearly parallel to one another. (Image Appendix Figures 25, 26, and 27.) The parallel arrangement is absent if the tissue is not intact or if the specimen is of a more liquid nature.

Aspergillus terreus is unique among clinically relevant aspergilli in having the ability to produce conidia (aleurioconidia) along the hyphae *in vivo* during invasive infection. In chronic lesions, the hyphae of any *Aspergillus* spp. may appear short, distorted, and may be as wide as 12 μm. Conidial heads (vesicle, phialides, and conidia) may occasionally form in areas exposed to air, such as in pulmonary cavities, nasal-sinuses, ear, or skin infections. *Aspergillus niger* is often involved in this type of infection and should be suspected if calcium oxalate crystals are present, as *A. niger* is known to produce large amounts of oxalic acid in this setting.

The hyphae of many other fungi appear similar to the aspergilli in tissue or other clinical specimens; however, there are subtle differences. Nonetheless, definitive microbiological diagnosis is usually made by recovery of the organism in culture followed by phenotypic or genotypic methods. Mucorales have hyphae that are pauciseptate, are commonly broader (up to 25 μm in diameter), show random branching, often appear collapsed and twisted, are irregular and nonparallel, and usually stain lighter with GMS than do the aspergilli. *Candida* spp., in addition to true septate hyphae, form pseudohyphae (typically showing distinct constrictions at the septa) and budding yeast cells. It should be noted, however, that when the hyphae of *Aspergillus* are cut on cross section, they may be mistaken for nonbudding yeast cells. Hyphae of other opportunistic hyaline moulds may be indistinguishable from *Aspergillus* in tissue (see "Miscellaneous Hyalohyphomycoses," p. 47).

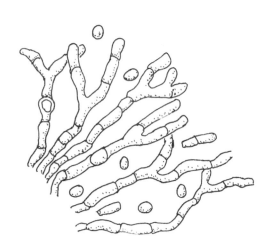
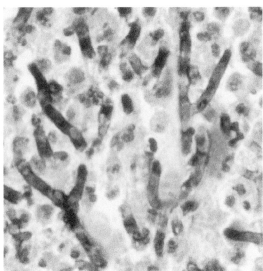

Miscellaneous Hyalohyphomycoses (Other than Aspergillosis)

ETIOLOGIC AGENTS: Any mould that forms colorless, septate hyphae in host tissue, e.g., *Fusarium*, *Paecilomyces*, *Acremonium* and *Sarocladium*, *Scedosporium* and many others.

SITES OF INFECTION: Almost any body site. Several of these moulds produce adventitious conidia in tissue and are much more likely to be recovered in blood culture than is *Aspergillus*.

TISSUE REACTION: The most common tissue responses are acute inflammation and necrosis with occasional granulomatous inflammation. Invasion of blood vessels with subsequent thrombosis and infarction also occurs.

MORPHOLOGY OF ORGANISM: The hyphae are usually irregular and haphazardly arranged, with considerable variation in diameter (2–8 μm). These typically exhibit both 45 and 90° branching. Although these traits suggest an etiologic agent other than *Aspergillus* (p. 327), one cannot reliably differentiate any of these agents from *Aspergillus* in tissue unless there is production of conidia *in situ*; e.g., one may occasionally observe the terminal annelloconidia produced by *Scedosporium* spp. The hyphae of the hyphomycetes differ from the Mucorales in that they are narrower, are regularly septate, and are less prone to ribbon-like folding. These miscellaneous hyphomycetes differ from both the aspergilli and the mucormycetes in that some have the capacity to produce conidia and phialides within a nonaerated deep tissue lesion (*Aspergillus terreus* is the exception to this rule, as it can produce aleuroconidia along the sides of the hyphae). Phialides usually appear as tapering structures (some are slightly flask shaped or bottle necked) along the sides or at the ends of the hyphae; a broad, darkly staining band can be seen on the sides of the neck of the phialide after production of multiple conidia. The conidia commonly have a rounded apex and a flat basal scar when detached; those of *Scedosporium* may be brown. Occasionally, hyphae that are somewhat constricted at the septa, along with the presence of phialoconidia, can resemble the pseudohyphae and budding yeasts seen in candidiasis. Culture or molecular diagnosis is almost always required for definitive identification of the etiologic agent.

For further information, see
Liu et al., 1998

Hyphal elements; courtesy of Wiley Schell.

Conidia formation *in vivo*; courtesy of Wiley Schell.

Dermatophytosis (Tinea, Ringworm)

ETIOLOGIC AGENTS: *Microsporum* spp., *Trichophyton* spp., and *Epidermophyton floccosum*, among other recently described genera.

SITES OF INFECTION: Skin, hair, nails.

TISSUE REACTION: Skin specimens usually show hyperkeratosis and various degrees of acanthosis, parakeratosis, and increased space between the cells (spongiosis). The neutrophilic infiltrate of the epidermis varies in intensity from rare single infiltrating cells to intraepithelial microabscesses. If the skin appendages are involved (e.g., hair follicles), then a suppurative to granulomatous reaction may occur, e.g., Majocchi's granuloma. The etiologic agent is most commonly found in the stratum corneum (i.e., the outermost layer of the epidermis, consisting of keratinized, nonnucleated cells).

MORPHOLOGY OF ORGANISM: All of the dermatophytes appear in the tissue as colorless, branched, septate hyphae that characteristically break up into chains of arthroconidia. Other conidia do not form in tissue. When hair is involved, the pattern of infection depends on the species of dermatophyte; i.e., arthroconidia may form on the outside of the hair shaft (ectothrix type of invasion) or inside the hair shaft (endothrix type). There is also a favic pattern of invasion in which hyphae, arthroconidia, and empty spaces form within the hair shaft.

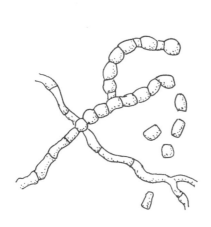 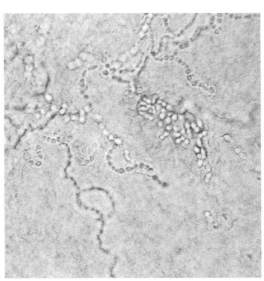

Courtesy of Tomas Roges.

Tinea versicolor

ETIOLOGIC AGENTS: *Malassezia* spp. including *M. furfur*, but not *M. pachydermatis.*

SITES OF INFECTION: The stratum corneum (the outermost layer of the skin); the organisms can therefore be readily seen in skin scrapings.

The etiologic agent can also cause fungemia and occasionally systemic infection (most frequently involving the lung) in patients receiving prolonged infusion of lipid formulation through contaminated central venous catheters (see p. 158).

TISSUE REACTION: Mild to moderate hyperkeratosis and acanthosis are usually seen. The stratum corneum is characteristically splayed giving a "basket weave" morphology. The causative organism is usually seen in the stratum corneum There may be a minimal mononuclear response in the dermis.

It should be noted that *Malassezia* are normal microbiota of the skin. When commensal *Malassezia* are seen in tissue sections, they are associated with the superficial epidermis or skin appendages. These have a "bowling pin" morphology (see below), which is distinctly different from that seen in the setting of tinea versicolor (i.e., the "spaghetti and meatballs" appearance).

MORPHOLOGY OF ORGANISM: Short, slightly curved, septate hyphal elements (2.5–4.0 µm in diameter) typically form in short chains. These are accompanied by clusters of oval to round, thick-walled yeast cells (2.5–8 µm in diameter). This combination produces the so-called "spaghetti and meatballs" appearance. The organisms are routinely observed in skin scrapings with a KOH preparation and/or with calcofluor white; in biopsy specimens, they can be seen with H&E but are best demonstrated by special stains for fungus, preferably PAS to better see the defining lines of the organism. (Image Appendix Figure 28.) The etiologic agents, which are lipid dependent, will grow only on media that have been overlaid or supplemented with olive oil or another long-chain fatty acid.

When *Malassezia* spp. are present as skin commensals or when they are present as a cause of fungemia, which is usually associated with a lipid-containing total parenteral nutrition, they are characteristically round at one end and have a flat collarette at the opposite end through which "buds" are produced. These produce a "bowling pin" appearance; no hyphal elements are produced.

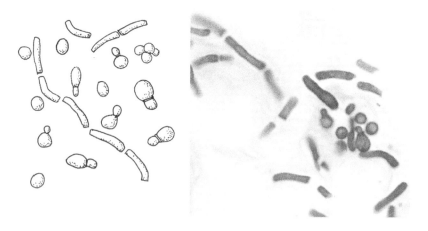

Tinea nigra

ETIOLOGIC AGENT: *Hortaea werneckii.*

SITES OF INFECTION: Palms of hands, soles of feet; rarely on other skin surfaces. Only the stratum corneum (outermost layer of the skin) is involved.

TISSUE REACTION: Mild to moderate hyperplasia and/or hyperkeratosis is seen in the epidermis. A minimal mononuclear cell infiltrate may occur in the dermis. The fungi are easily detected in the stratum corneum.

MORPHOLOGY OF ORGANISM: Darkly pigmented, branched, septate, narrow hyphae (1.5–3.0 μm wide) usually accompanied by elongated budding cells (1.5–5.0 μm in diameter). The organism stains well with the special fungus stains, but the natural pigmentation can be best seen with H&E.

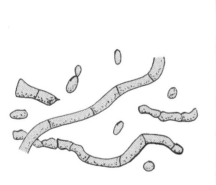
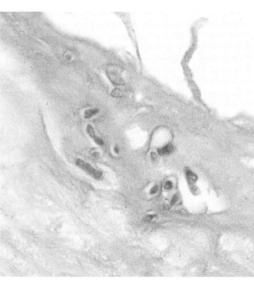

Phaeohyphomycosis

ETIOLOGIC AGENTS: *Exophiala jeanselmei* species complex, *Phialophora verrucosa*, *Phaeoacremonium parasiticum*, *Pleurostoma richardsiae*, *Exophiala dermatitidis*, *Curvularia* spp., *Alternaria* spp., *Cladophialophora bantiana* (in the brain), and a large variety of other dematiaceous fungi.

SITES OF INFECTION: Most commonly in skin and subcutaneous tissue; also occurs in the eye (keratitis), brain (fungal brain abscess), and occasionally in a variety of other body sites. Severe disseminated infection is also reported.

TISSUE REACTION: The more common etiologic agents elicit encapsulated cystic granulomas in the dermis and subcutaneous tissue in immunocompetent hosts (i.e., a phaeohyphomycotic cyst). The center of the granuloma may contain a suppurative exudate surrounded by a wide zone of granulation tissue. Multiple abscesses may occur in early infection. This is usually secondary to inoculation trauma. However, the tissue reaction in immunocompromised patients is truncated and may be devoid of granuloma formation and present with tissue reactions that overlap with those of other invasive mould infections. The less common etiologic agents may produce a dispersed granulomatous inflammation. In cerebral infections, the characteristic inflammatory response is suppurative and granulomatous with abscess formation.

MORPHOLOGY OF ORGANISM: Variably brown- or olivaceous-pigmented hyphae (2–6 μm wide) occur singly or in small aggregates. They often have closely spaced, constricted septations producing a moniliform ("string of beads") appearance. Large, bizarre, thick-walled vesicular swellings (≥25 μm in diameter) resembling chlamydoconidia may be seen along, or at the ends of, the hyphae. Yeastlike cells producing buds singly or in chains are also commonly present, depending on the species. The pigment is usually visible in H&E-stained sections, but is masked by the GMS stain and possibly by the PAS stain. Although the Fontana-Masson stain can be used to further demonstrate melanin in the cell wall, it is usually not necessarily for the detection of pigment with dematiaceous moulds. (Image Appendix Figure 29.) Curiously, instances wherein the Fontana-Masson stain has failed to stain *Alternaria* spp. have been observed.

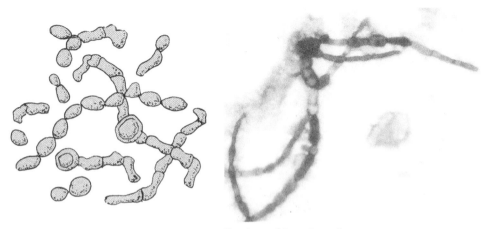

Courtesy of Joan Barenfanger.

Chromoblastomycosis

ETIOLOGIC AGENTS: *Fonsecaea* spp., *Phialophora verrucosa*, *Cladophialophora carrionii*, *Exophiala jeanselmei* species complex, and *Rhinocladiella* spp.

SITES OF INFECTION: Skin and subcutaneous tissue.

TISSUE REACTION: The skin usually demonstrates pseudoepitheliomatous hyperplasia with hyperkeratosis and parakeratosis. Pseudoepitheliomatous hyperplasia has been mistaken for squamous cell carcinoma. A pyogranulomatous inflammatory response (i.e., an admixture of neutrophils and nonnecrotizing granulomas) is typically seen.

MORPHOLOGY OF ORGANISM: Brown-pigmented, round to polyhedral, thick-walled sclerotic bodies (5–12 μm in diameter) having horizontal and/or vertical septations are diagnostic. These structures are also referred to as Medlar bodies or "copper pennies." (Image Appendix Figure 30.) The fungi typically migrate to the surface of the skin and are seen as black dots in the keratin scales; sclerotic bodies are seen microscopically.

The structure and pigment of the organism are usually well demonstrated with H&E stain.

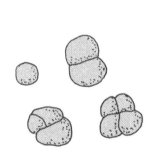
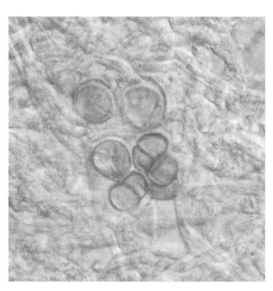

Sporotrichosis

ETIOLOGIC AGENTS: *Sporothrix schenckii* species complex.

SITES OF INFECTION: Skin, subcutaneous tissue, and contiguous lymphatics; rare dissemination to bones, joints, lungs, central nervous system, and other internal organs.

TISSUE REACTION: *Sporothrix schenckii* usually provokes a mixed suppurative and granulomatous inflammatory reaction (i.e., a pyogranulomatous response) that is often accompanied by fibrosis and microabscess formation; this mixed inflammatory reaction is seen in the dermis and subcutaneous tissue as well as in disseminated disease. Splendore-Hoeppli material may encompass the yeast cells. Lesions of cutaneous infections usually exhibit hyperkeratosis, parakeratosis, and pseudoepitheliomatous hyperplasia.

MORPHOLOGY OF ORGANISM: Yeast cells of various sizes and shapes are present. These may be round to oval (usually 2–6 µm in diameter) and often have elongated "pipe stem" buds. Budding is from a narrow base. Characteristic elongated "cigar bodies" may be present and are most commonly seen near the skin surface and in disseminated lesions. In cutaneous lesions, the organisms are usually very sparse, and may be inapparent even with the preferred special stains for this fungus (GMS or PAS).

Sporothrix schenckii, *Candida glabrata*, *Histoplasma capsulatum*, and the more recently described *Emergomyces* spp. appear as small, round or oval cells with narrow-based budding. The neutrophilic infiltrate seen in the mixed suppurative and granulomatous reaction of sporotrichosis is not characteristic of histoplasmosis, but may be present with emergomycosis. *Candida glabrata*, which also appears as small, oval yeast cells, produces a suppurative tissue reaction but does not usually generate granulomas; this fact might assist in differentiating it from *Sporothrix*. Granulomas without a predominant neutrophilic infiltrate are formed in response to both *Histoplasma* and *Emergomyces* infections.

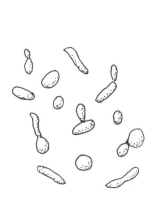
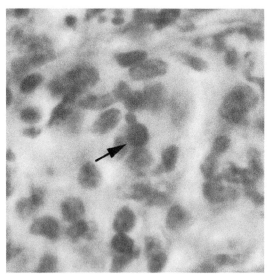

Courtesy of Evelyn Koestenblatt.

Histoplasmosis

ETIOLOGIC AGENT: *Histoplasma capsulatum.*

SITES OF INFECTION: Lung, blood, lymph nodes, bone marrow, liver, spleen, and multiple systemic sites.

TISSUE REACTION: *Histoplasma capsulatum* produces granulomas. Early nonnecrotizing granulomas give way to necrotizing granulomas with centrally located necrosis. Parenchymal necrosis, along with epithelioid and giant-cell granulomas, may result in cavitation. As the infection is contained by the inflammatory response, fibrous tissue replaces the granulomas resulting in fibrocaseous nodules that almost uniformly contain calcifications. (Image Appendix Figures 14 and 15.) Although *Candida glabrata* is similar in size and shape to *H. capsulatum*, the infections differ histologically in that *Candida* almost always produces a suppurative tissue reaction; *Sporothrix schenckii*, which is also a small yeast, differs in commonly producing a mixed suppurative and granulomatous reaction. *Emergomyces* generates a similar inflammatory response.

The inflammatory response in patients with defects in T-cell immunity (e.g., advanced HIV) is distinctly different, as granulomas cannot be formed or are only poorly formed. The macrophage is the primary inflammatory cell to respond in this scenario and are often seen packed with small yeasts.

MORPHOLOGY OF ORGANISM: Small yeast cells (2–4 μm in length) are usually ovoid with budding on a narrow base at the smaller end. The yeasts reproduce within monocytes or macrophages and, when the phagocytic cell dies the yeasts remain in clusters. In Giemsa- or Wright-stained preparations, a pale blue ring (the fungus cell wall) surrounds the darker blue cytoplasm that retracts from the wall, often giving the false impression of a capsule; the chromatin stains dark violet and appears as a crescent-shaped mass within the cell. A halo or pseudocapsule also appears with H&E due to the aforementioned retraction artifact, but the organism stains well and evenly with GMS, but poorly to not at all with PAS.

Differentiation of *Histoplasma* from other small yeasts and a few parasites can be difficult, and differentiation from *Emergomyces* in tissue is not possible, but a few factors may be helpful for other organisms.

- The yeast cells of *Talaromyces marneffei* do not bud; they have a prominent transverse septum and reproduce by fission.
- The yeast cells of *Candida glabrata* stain better with H&E and are basophilic (i.e., stain blueish), and do not demonstrate a pseudocapsule. Also, *Candida* spp. generate a pyogenic tissue reaction, not granulomas.
- *Sporothrix schenckii* causes a pyogranulomatous reaction rather than the purely necrotizing or nonnecrotizing granulomas, as seen in histoplasmosis. In sporotrichosis, the yeast cells are often fewer, and they may be more elongated and variably shaped than those of *Histoplasma*.

- *Cryptococcus* yeast cells are rounder and greatly variable in size. The capsular material of *Cryptococcus* stains with mucicarmine. Although the melanin/melanin-like pigments within the cell walls of cryptococci are not visible with routing H&E staining, they may be accentuated with the Fontana-Masson stain in actively replicating cells. Dead cryptococci within old cryptococcomas usually fail to stain with both mucicarmine and Fontana-Masson.

- The endospores of *Coccidioides* are about the same size as the yeast cells of *Histoplasma*, but the endospores are rounder, do not bud, and are typically accompanied by intact spherules or immature spherules.

- Some protozoans can mimic *Histoplasma* but are different in that they stain entirely with H&E, do not form a pseudocapsule, do not reliably stain with special histologic fungal stains, and do not bud. Additionally, amastigotes of *Leishmania* spp. and *Trypanosoma cruzi* have paranuclear bar-shaped kinetoplasts that can be seen with H&E under oil immersion.

The yeast cells of *Histoplasma duboisii* are 8–15 μm in diameter in tissue, i.e., much larger than those of *H. capsulatum* (2-4 μm), but they are small and identical to *H. capsulatum* when grown on culture. *H. duboisii* is endemic in central and western Africa, most commonly reported in Nigeria.

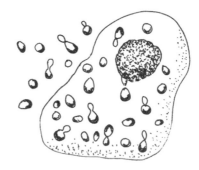

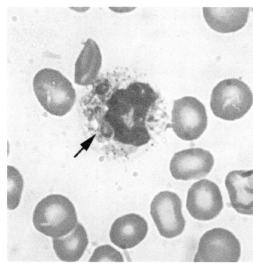

Bone marrow; intracellular.

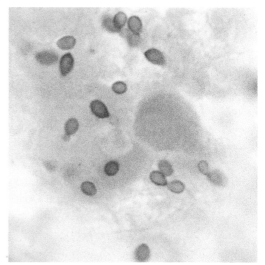

Lung; extracellular; courtesy of Joan Barenfanger.

Emergomycosis

ETIOLOGIC AGENT: *Emergomyces* spp. There are at least five recognized species of *Emergomyces*: *E. canadensis* (North America), *E. pasteurianus* (Africa, Asia, Europe, and India), *E. europaeus* (Europe), *E. africanus* (South Africa), and *E. orientalis* (China and India).

SITES OF INFECTION: The disease caused by *Emergomyces* is similar to histoplasmosis with a primary pulmonary infection that may be contained in the immunocompetent host or may become disseminated in the immunocompromised individual. Reported sites of dissemination include the skin, gastrointestinal tract, liver, bone marrow, and lymph nodes.

TISSUE REACTION: Individuals with an intact immune response form granulomas with or without a substantial neutrophilic infiltrate (i.e., pyogranulomatous inflammation). The inflammatory response varies with the degree and type of compromise to the immune system. The tissue reactions in immunocompromised individuals range from poorly formed granulomas to a predominantly histiocytic response.

MORPHOLOGY OF ORGANISM: The morphologic features of *Emergomyces* in tissue are indistinguishable from those of *Histoplasma capsulatum*. Small (2-4 μm) yeasts with narrow based budding are seen singly or in clusters. These are readily visualized with the GMS stain. A morphology that is indistinguishable from *Histoplasma capsulatum* underscores the importance of culture and/or molecular studies to achieve the appropriate diagnosis.

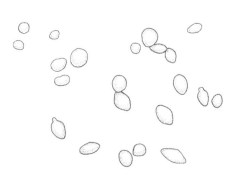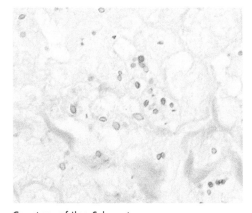

Courtesy of Ilan Schwartz.

For further information, see
Kenyon et al., 2013
Schwartz et al., 2019a

Talaromycosis (Penicilliosis)

ETIOLOGIC AGENT: *Talaromyces marneffei.*

SITES OF INFECTION: Blood, bone marrow, skin, lung, liver, spleen, lymph nodes, multiple systemic sites.

TISSUE REACTION: Talaromycosis is an opportunistic infection of immunocompromised patients that lack T-cell immunity. It has a similar anatomic distribution and inflammatory response as that seen in patients with disseminated histoplasmosis. Yeast cells are found in histiocytes and other phagocytic cells, and a granulomatous response is absent or significantly diminished, depending on the degree of immunosuppression.

MORPHOLOGY OF ORGANISM: Oval to elongate, yeast cells are 2.5–5 μm in length and multiply within histiocytes in tissue or within monocytes in blood or bone marrow. Budding does not occur; a prominent central septum forms, and reproduction is by fission (arthroconidium-like). Outside of histiocytes, yeast cells are up to 8 μm in length, may have several septa, and are sometimes curved. The organisms stain well with GMS or PAS; they give a false impression of having a capsule when stained with H&E, so they can very closely mimic *Histoplasma capsulatum*, especially when intracellular (but the yeast cells of *Histoplasma* reproduce by budding).

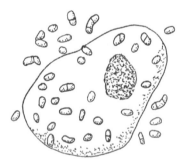

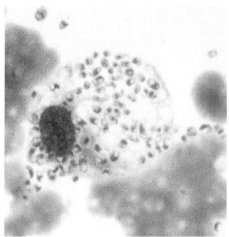

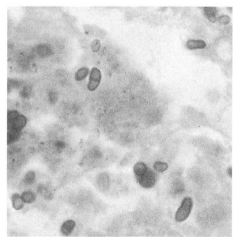

Bone marrow; intracellular; courtesy of William Merz.   Bone marrow; extracellular; courtesy of Ron C. Neafie.

Blastomycosis

ETIOLOGIC AGENT: *Blastomyces dermatitidis* and *Blastomyces gilchristii*

SITES OF INFECTION: Lung, skin, bones, multiple systemic sites.

TISSUE REACTION: *Blastomyces* evokes a pyogranulomatous (i.e., mixed suppurative and granulomatous) response. In young lesions, neutrophils predominate, whereas in older lesions, the suppurative reaction decreases and granulomas, which may contain microabscesses, predominate. Long-standing infections commonly show fibrosis and sometimes cavitation. In skin, pseudoepitheliomatous hyperplasia occurs.

MORPHOLOGY OF ORGANISM: The yeast cells are large (3–30 μm in diameter; most commonly 8–15 μm; there have been several reported cases with yeast cells as large as 40 μm) and round to oval, with sharply defined refractile cell walls that are commonly referred to as "double contoured." The thick wall is seen with H&E and PAS, and it is sometimes lightly colored with mucicarmine stain. The fungus stains with the GMS stain, but the morphology is better appreciated in the H&E stain. Each yeast cell produces only one bud, which is distinctively attached to the parent cell on a very broad base (average, 4–5 μm); the bud characteristically grows to the same size as the parent cell before detaching. (Image Appendix Figures 31 and 32.)

Immature and "sterile" (i.e., empty) spherules of *Coccidioides* may be easily mistaken for yeast cells of *Blastomyces*, especially if two spherules abut one another and give the impression of broad-based budding. Both organisms have thick, refractile walls, but close examination should reveal typical single spherules with endospores with *Coccidioides*.

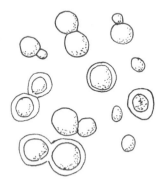 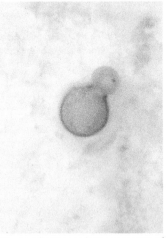 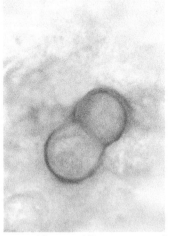

Young blastoconidium; courtesy of Joan Barenfanger.

Mature blastoconidium; courtesy of Joan Barenfanger.

Paracoccidioidomycosis

ETIOLOGIC AGENT: *Paracoccidioides brasiliensis.*

SITES OF INFECTION: Lung, skin, mucous membranes, multiple systemic sites.

TISSUE REACTION: A mixed suppurative and granulomatous inflammatory response is elicited by *P. brasiliensis* in pulmonary infections. Neutrophilic abscesses may predominate in one area of tissue while another area contains mainly granulomas. In rapidly progressing lesions, necrosis is frequently observed. In long-standing disease, fibrosis is common and calcification may occasionally occur. In mucocutaneous infections, ulceration and pseudoepitheliomatous hyperplasia may be seen.

MORPHOLOGY OF ORGANISM: Yeast cells are round to oval and can become quite large (3–30 μm or more in diameter). The outstanding characteristic is the presence of multiple buds that are attached to the parent cell by narrow connections. Buds may be small and all are approximately the same size. A large parent cell surrounded by small buds creates the classic mariner's-wheel appearance; parent cells with fewer, but larger, buds are common, and single budding may also be seen.

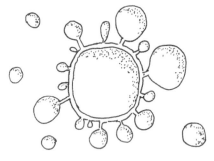

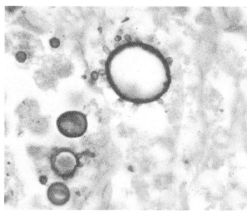

Courtesy of Ron C. Neafie.

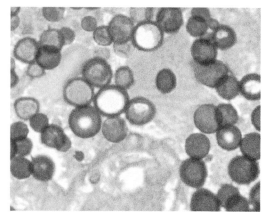

Courtesy of Douglas Flieder.

Lobomycosis

ETIOLOGIC AGENT: *Lacazia loboi* (does not grow in culture)

SITES OF INFECTION: Subcutis, predominantly of the auricles and limbs. Dolphins, in addition to humans, may be infected.

TISSUE REACTION: Clinically, these appear as a keloid-like lesion. Giant cells and numerous histocytes are typical of this infection with or without granuloma formation. Numerous fungal organisms are seen, which are best visualized with the GMS stain. Associated fibrosis is also seen in the longstanding lesions. The overlying skin may disclose areas of acanthosis with hyperkeratosis, spongiosis and infiltration by neutrophils.

MORPHOLOGY OF ORGANISM: The yeast organisms are round to oval (6 × 12 μm) and under polarized light exhibit a "Maltese cross" birefringence. The cells appear singly or in chains joined with isthmus (tubelike) connections. The chains have been likened to rosary or rosario beads.

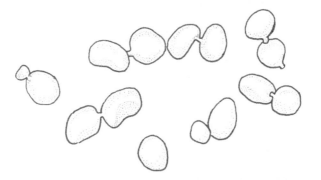

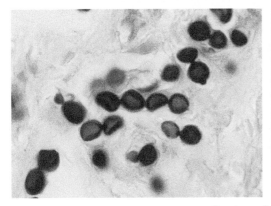
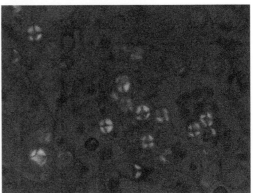

Courtesy of Bobbi Pritt.

For further information, see
Gonçalves et al., 2022

Candidiasis

ETIOLOGIC AGENTS: *Candida albicans*, *Candida glabrata*, *Candida parapsilosis*, *Candida tropicalis*, and other *Candida* spp.

SITES OF INFECTION: Blood, mucous membranes, skin, nails, multiple systemic sites (appearance in the urine can be an early indication of candidemia).

TISSUE REACTION: In systemic infections, *Candida* spp. most commonly elicit an acute suppurative inflammation, sometimes forming abscesses composed of polymorphonuclear as well as mononuclear cells. Coagulative necrosis replaces the suppurative reaction in neutropenic patients. Granulomas only rarely occur, generally in patients with chronic systemic candidiasis; the yeast forms of dimorphic fungi are more likely than *Candida* to form granulomas.

MORPHOLOGY OF ORGANISM: All species of *Candida* form round to oval budding yeast cells (blastoconidia, 3–6 µm in diameter) singly, in chains, or in small, loose clusters. Most species, when invading tissue, form both pseudohyphae and true hyphae. Pseudo-hyphae are actually chains of blastoconidia that have elongated and have not separated from one another. They can be recognized by the distinct constrictions at the septa; also, pseudohyphal branching will only occur at the site of a septation. Blastoconidia develop at the points of constriction in the pseudohyphae. True hyphae have no, or only slight, con-strictions at the septa, and there is often no septation at the initiation of a branch.

Candida glabrata is unique in that it is slightly smaller (2–5 µm in diameter) than the other species of *Candida* and it does not produce any hyphal forms. The small yeast cells often aggregate in clusters and may closely resemble *Histoplasma capsulatum*, but no halo or pseudocapsular effect is seen when the cells are stained with H&E. *Candida* tends to stain bluish or basophilic in H&E stained sections.

Culture is required to identify any *Candida* to species level.

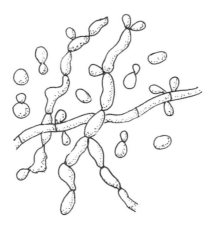

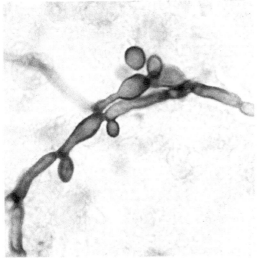

Candida albicans; courtesy of Joan Barenfanger.

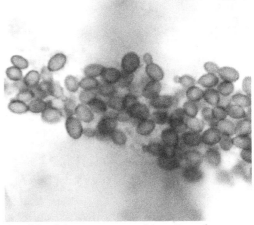

Candida glabrata; courtesy of Joan Barenfanger.

Trichosporonosis

ETIOLOGIC AGENTS: *Trichosporon asahii*, *Trichosporon asteroides*, *Trichosporon inkin*, *Trichosporon ovoides*, *Cutaneotrichosporon cutaneum*, and *Cutaneotrichosporon mucoides*.

SITES OF INFECTION: Lung, liver, spleen, kidney, gastrointestinal tract, bone marrow, heart, brain, eye, multiple systemic sites (most frequently *T. asahii* and, much less often, *C. mucoides* and *T. inkin*); hair (*T. ovoides* in white piedra on scalp hairs, *C. cutaneum* on axilla hair, *T. inkin* on pubic hair); very occasionally skin (*T. asteroides*, *C. cutaneum*, *T. inkin*, *T. ovoides*).

TISSUE REACTION: In systemic *Trichosporon* infections, acute inflammatory cells are generally absent due to the neutropenic state of the patient. Nodular infarcts are more regularly formed as a result of fungal occlusion of blood vessels. Abscesses and granulomatous inflammation are occasionally seen in nonneutropenic patients.

MORPHOLOGY OF ORGANISM: In systemic infections, the fungal elements of *Trichosporon* spp. commonly grow from a focal point in a parallel radiating fashion, similar to that of aspergillosis. They clearly differ from *Aspergillus* by characteristically forming (i) pleomorphic yeast cells (blastoconidia) 3–8 μm in diameter; (ii) pseudohyphae; (iii) septate true hyphae (without predominant dichotomous branching); and (iv) arthroconidia, formed by the fragmentation of the true hyphae. Although the yeast cells of *Trichosporon* are usually larger than those of *Candida*, it can be very difficult to differentiate *Trichosporon* spp. from *Candida* spp. if arthroconidia are not seen (it is fairly common for arthroconidia to be sparse or seemingly absent in *Trichosporon* spp. in tissue). To assist in such instances, diluted periodic acid methenamine silver stain exhibits a substantially more intense staining of *Trichosporon* than it does of *Candida* (Obana et al., 2010). In most cases, molecular or culture-based methods are required for definitive identification.

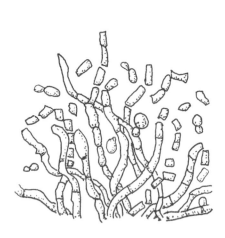 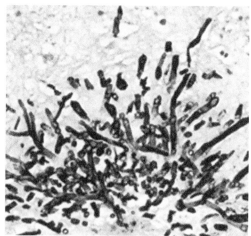

Courtesy of Thomas Walsh (from Walsh et al., 1992).

Cryptococcosis

ETIOLOGIC AGENTS: *Cryptococcus neoformans* and *Cryptococcus gattii*.

SITES OF INFECTION: Lung, meninges and cerebrospinal fluid, blood, skin, mucous membranes, multiple systemic sites.

TISSUE REACTION: In immunocompetent patients, a predominantly granulomatous reaction with various degrees of necrosis is seen. Chronic pulmonary infection results in the formation of residual granulomas with central caseous necrosis (cryptococcomas). These, with time and containment of the fungus result in fibrocaseous nodules like those seen with histoplasmosis (i.e., a histoplasmoma).

The inflammatory reaction may be minimal or absent in immunocompromised patients, particularly those with advanced HIV/AIDS. The yeasts, in this case, proliferate abundantly, creating mucoid "cystic" lesions packed with round, encapsulated cryptococci that resemble soap bubbles; these are seen most frequently in the brain, as *Cryptococcus* is highly neurotropic. The number of organisms present in the tissue is inversely proportional to the number of inflammatory cells.

Candidiasis differs from cryptococcosis by most commonly producing a purely suppurative reaction.

MORPHOLOGY OF ORGANISM: The yeast cells (i) are 2–20 μm in diameter (usually 4–10 μm); (ii) vary in size within the microscopic field; (iii) may be oval, but are more typically round with thin walls; (iv) budding is from a narrow base; and (v) characteristically produce thick capsules, but cells with reduced capsular material sometimes occur.

Capsules should be suspected when the yeast cells do not appear to touch one another (due to the surrounding mucopolysaccharide capsular material). In smeared specimens, capsules can be demonstrated with India ink. (Image Appendix Figure 33.) Tissues stained with mucicarmine show the capsule as bright carmine red, often with a spiny or scalloped appearance. (Image Appendix Figure 34.) The mucicarmine stain may slightly also highlight the cell walls of *Rhinosporidium seeberi* and *Blastomyces*. The cryptococcal yeast cell (but not the capsule) is stained by GMS. Because the cell walls of *C. neoformans* and *C. gattii* contain melaninlike substances, they become brown to black with the Fontana-Masson stain. Drying, fixing, and staining may cause the yeast cells to collapse or become crescent shaped.

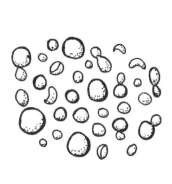

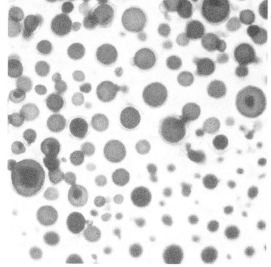

Courtesy of Joan Barenfanger.

Pneumocystosis

ETIOLOGIC AGENT: *Pneumocystis jirovecii* (formerly *Pneumocystis carinii*). *P. jirovecii* is the species found in humans, and *P. carinii* is the species found in rats. The acronym PCP, originally for *Pneumocystis carinii* pneumonia, is still used, but meaning *Pneumocystis* pneumonia.

SITE OF INFECTION: Lung.

TISSUE REACTION: The prominent characteristic in the lung is a foamy material in the alveolar spaces; this foam can be observed in lung biopsies as well as in specimens of bronchoalveolar lavage and, in many cases, induced sputum. This reaction is almost diagnostic of infection with *P. jirovecii*. The organisms are seen in the foamy exudate with histochemical or immunohistochemical/immunofluorescent stains. Granulomatous reaction has been reported on rare occasions, largely secondary to recovering immunity (i.e., immune reconstitution syndrome) or in individuals who are only moderately immunosuppressed.

MORPHOLOGY OF ORGANISM: The most commonly used stains for *Pneumocystis* (GMS, calcofluor white, and toluidine blue O) stain the cyst form, not the trophozoite. The cysts (4–7 μm in diameter) are nonbudding and are round, ovoid, or collapsed crescent forms. They characteristically have intracystic bodies that are focal thickenings in the wall that, when stained with GMS, appear as dark double commas or a set of parentheses. The organisms occur in small clusters on a thick, foamy background. (Image Appendix Figure 35.) Immunospecific stains are commercially available. *P. jirovecii* does not grow on routine culture.

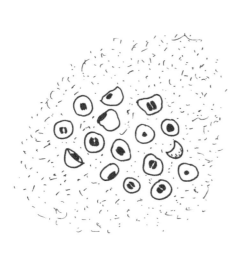
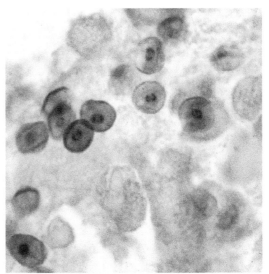

Courtesy of Joan Barenfanger.

Protothecosis

ETIOLOGIC AGENTS: *Prototheca wickerhamii* (the species more commonly encountered in human infections) and *Prototheca zopfii*. These are actually achlorophyllous algae.

SITES OF INFECTION: Skin and subcutaneous tissue, bursa of the elbow, very rarely systemic sites.

TISSUE REACTION: Skin biopsies show varying degrees of nonspecific changes, including hyperkeratosis, parakeratosis, and acanthosis. The inflammatory response may consist of a neutrophilic component with abundant neutrophilic debris. Mononuclear and/or granulomatous infiltrates may also be present. Bursitis of the elbow typically exhibits necrotizing granulomas.

MORPHOLOGY OF ORGANISM: Round or oval sporangia of *P. wickerhamii* vary from 3–15 μm in diameter, while those of *P. zopfii* are 7–30 μm in diameter. Each sporangium of *P. wickerhamii* contains 2–20 endospores; only 4–8 are usually visible in one plane, and they appear round, polyhedral, or wedge shaped in a radial arrangement. The endospores are densely basophilic, staining deep purplish blue with H&E. The organisms are best seen with the special stains for fungi. Hyaline, nonviable, ghostlike forms may also be present.

P. zopfii can be similar to *P. wickerhamii*, but it frequently forms oval, nonendosporulating cells, each having vacuolated cytoplasm and a single discrete, basophilic nucleus.

The size of the mother cells and differences in the number and morphology of endospores help differentiate *Prototheca* from *Coccidioides*.

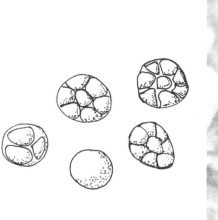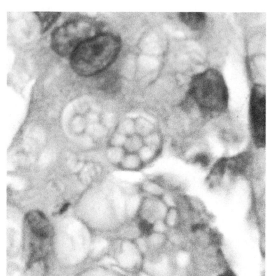

Courtesy of Evelyn Koestenblatt.

Coccidioidomycosis

ETIOLOGIC AGENTS: *Coccidioides immitis* and *Coccidioides posadasii.*

SITES OF INFECTION: Lung, skin, bone, meninges; dissemination to multiple systemic sites.

TISSUE REACTION: Necrotizing granulomas are the typical inflammatory response to *Coccidioides*. Intact, burst and immature spherules may be present in the necrosis or associated granulomatous reaction. Released endospores and "sterile" (i.e., empty) spherules may be mistaken for yeast forms, particularly if juxtaposed. When two immature spherules abut one another, they can give the impression of broad-based budding cells of *Blastomyces*. A minor subset (i.e., approximately 10%) of specimens will also demonstrate a noticeable eosinophilic infiltrate.

MORPHOLOGY OF ORGANISM: Immature and/or "sterile" spherules can be as small as 5 μm in diameter when immature (nonendosporulating) and grow to 30–100 μm or more in diameter upon maturity (endosporulating). Immature spherules and endospores stain well with PAS and GMS. Curiously, the wall of the mature spherules do not stain with GMS or PAS, presumably due to the high phospholipid content of the mature cell wall (1–2 μm in width). Endospores are round (2–5 μm in diameter) and uninucleate and have walls and cytoplasmic inclusions that are GMS and PAS positive. (Image Appendix Figure 36.) The spherules and endospores stain with H&E and are readily visible in sufficient numbers. Fragmented or empty ruptured spherules are common. Septate hyphae, barrel-shaped arthroconidia, and rarely small conidial forms singly (some budding) or in chains (Schuetz et al., 2012) have been observed in cavitary and necrotic lesions.

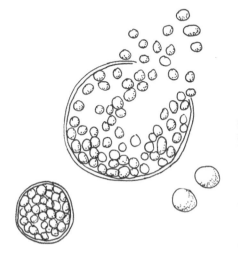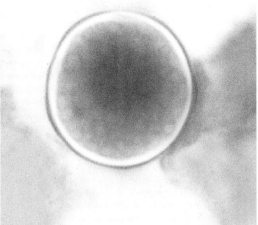

Courtesy of Joan Barenfanger.

Rhinosporidiosis

ETIOLOGIC AGENT: *Rhinosporidium seeberi* (does not grow on synthetic media). It is classified as a close relative to fungi rather than a fungus, but due to its similarities to fungi, it is commonly and traditionally regarded in mycology texts.

SITES OF INFECTION: Mucocutaneous tissue, primarily involving the nasal cavity, nasopharynx, and oral cavity; secondary skin infections and rarely limited systemic dissemination have been reported.

TISSUE REACTION: In the submucosa or dermis, a chronic inflammatory response (mostly lymphocytes, plasma cells, and various numbers of epithelioid cells and neutrophils) with granulation tissue is typically seen. If the sporangia rupture and endospores are released, a granulomatous reaction is likely, but in some instances a suppurative response may occur.

MORPHOLOGY OF ORGANISM: Mature sporangia are thick walled (~5 µm wide), round, large (100–350 µm in diameter; most commonly 100–200 µm), and contain numerous sporangiospores (endospores) that range from 1–10 µm in diameter. A zonal pattern of sporangiospore development is uniquely characteristic of this pathogen: small, young spores are seen peripherally along the inner wall or form a crescent-like mass at one pole of the sporangium; medium-size, enlarging spores are between the periphery and the center; and the larger, mature spores are centrally located. Mature sporangiospores appear lobulated due to globular eosinophilic inclusions and, when released into the tissue, can be suggestive of *Prototheca* (p. 162). The walls of the sporangiospores and the mature sporangia are GMS and PAS positive. Mucicarmine also will stain the walls of the spores and the inner surface of the sporangial wall. (Image Appendix Figure 37.) Special fungal stains are seldom necessary, as the organism is apparent in H&E stained sections.

Trophocytes (immature sporangia) are 10–100 µm in diameter with refractile eosinophilic walls ~2–3 µm thick. Trophocytes contain granular or flocculent cytoplasm and a round, pale nucleus with a prominent nucleolus or karyosome. They are readily seen with H&E but do not stain well with GMS.

The etiologic agent, *R. seeberi*, does not grow on synthetic media; diagnosis depends on direct examination of infected tissue.

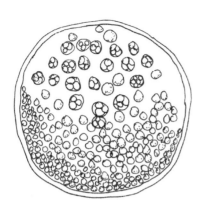
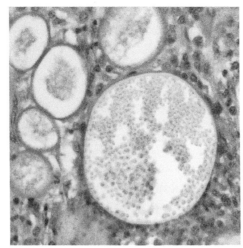

Courtesy of Douglas Flieder.

Adiaspiromycosis

ETIOLOGIC AGENT: *Emmonsia crescens*.

SITE OF INFECTION: Lung.

TISSUE REACTION: The typical inflammatory response is granulomatous and fibrotic. A granuloma forms around each adiaconidium (formerly adiaspore), which in turn is surrounded by dense fibrous connective tissue. Giant cells are often in contact with the outer spore wall. Polymorphonuclear leukocytes, especially eosinophils, may also be seen in the presence of small, immature adiaconidia. Necrosis or caseation is almost never seen. In some individuals, there is little, or no, host response (regardless of the level of immunocompetence).

MORPHOLOGY OF ORGANISM: Mature adiaconidia are round, large (200–400 µm in diameter), and thick walled (20–70 µm in width). The narrow outer layer of the adiaconidial wall is eosinophilic; a thin middle layer of the wall has irregular perforations that may appear as unstained spots; the inner layer of the wall is broad, hyaline, and composed predominantly of chitin. The walls can be readily seen with H&E and stain extremely well with GMS and PAS stains. The interior of the conidium usually appears empty, but small (1–3 µm in diameter), refractile, eosinophilic hyaline globules may be seen along the inner surface of the wall. There is no evidence of replication, i.e., no budding or endosporulation.

If starch granules of lentils and other legumes are aspirated into the lungs, a pneumonitis may develop that can somewhat resemble adiaspiromycosis, but the starch granules of the legumes will have thinner walls and contain loculated material that can be seen with PAS and other stains.

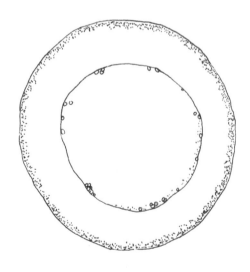 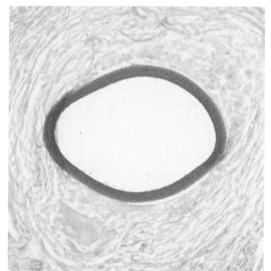

Courtesy of Ron C. Neafie.

PART II
Identification of Fungi in Culture

Larone's Medically Important Fungi: A Guide to Identification, 7th Edition.
Lars F. Westblade, Eileen M. Burd, Shawn R. Lockhart, and Gary W. Procop.
© 2023 American Society for Microbiology. DOI: 10.1128/9781683674436.pii

Guide to Identification
of Fungi in Culture

FILAMENTOUS BACTERIA

Very thin (1 μm or less in diameter), branching filaments*

Aerobic Actinomycetes

Nocardia (p. **111**)

Streptomyces (p. **114**)

Actinomadura (p. **116**)

Nocardiopsis dassonvillei (p. **117**)

*Growth characteristics and biochemical tests must be utilized for differentiation of genera; these are summarized in Table 2.1 (p. 110).

MONOMORPHIC YEASTS AND YEASTLIKE ORGANISMS

Yeastlike at 25–30°C and also at 35–37°C if growth occurs

All rapid growers except *Ustilago* spp.

All WHITE, CREAM, or TAN except *Rhodotorula*, *Cystobasidium*, and *Sporobolomyces* spp.

Microscopic morphology on cornmeal-Tween 80 agar (Dalmau plate)*

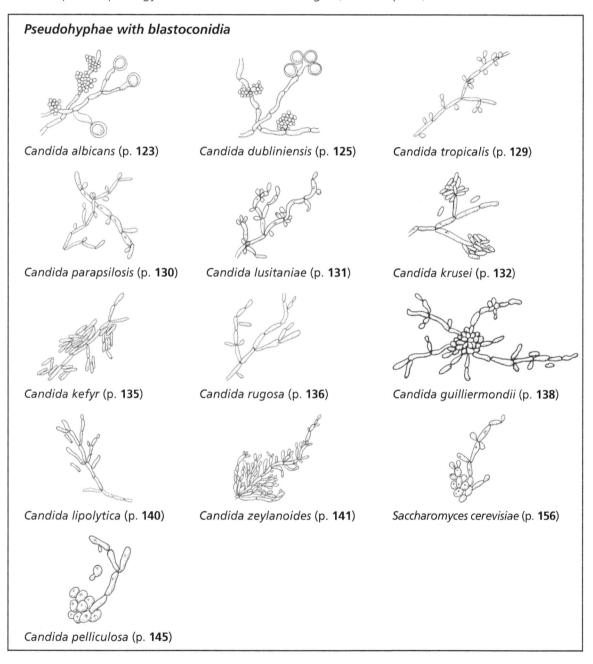

Pseudohyphae with blastoconidia

Candida albicans (p. **123**)

Candida dubliniensis (p. **125**)

Candida tropicalis (p. **129**)

Candida parapsilosis (p. **130**)

Candida lusitaniae (p. **131**)

Candida krusei (p. **132**)

Candida kefyr (p. **135**)

Candida rugosa (p. **136**)

Candida guilliermondii (p. **138**)

Candida lipolytica (p. **140**)

Candida zeylanoides (p. **141**)

Saccharomyces cerevisiae (p. **156**)

Candida pelliculosa (p. **145**)

MONOMORPHIC YEASTS AND YEASTLIKE ORGANISMS

Yeastlike at 25–30°C and also at 35–37°C if growth occurs (*continued*)

All rapid growers except *Ustilago* spp.

All WHITE, CREAM, or TAN except *Rhodotorula*, *Cystobasidium*, and *Sporobolomyces* spp.

Microscopic morphology on cornmeal-Tween 80 agar (Dalmau plate)*

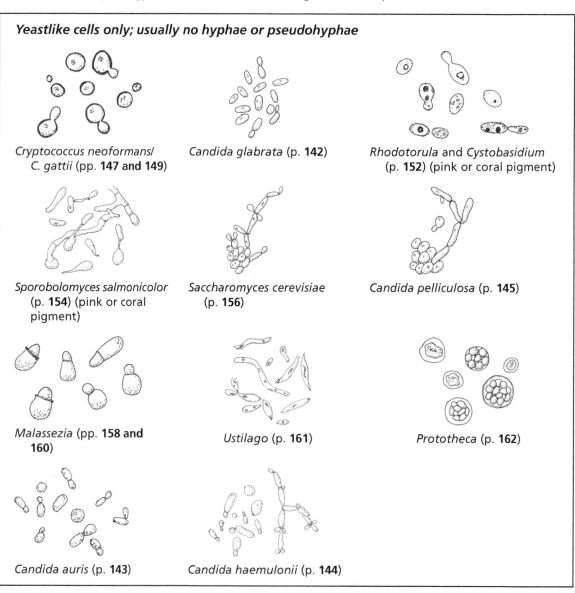

Yeastlike cells only; usually no hyphae or pseudohyphae

Cryptococcus neoformans/ C. gattii (pp. **147 and 149**)

Candida glabrata (p. **142**)

Rhodotorula and *Cystobasidium* (p. **152**) (pink or coral pigment)

Sporobolomyces salmonicolor (p. **154**) (pink or coral pigment)

Saccharomyces cerevisiae (p. **156**)

Candida pelliculosa (p. **145**)

Malassezia (pp. **158 and 160**)

Ustilago (p. **161**)

Prototheca (p. **162**)

Candida auris (p. **143**)

Candida haemulonii (p. **144**)

PART II Identification of Fungi in Culture

MONOMORPHIC YEASTS AND YEASTLIKE ORGANISMS

Yeastlike at 25–30°C and also at 35–37°C if growth occurs (*continued*)

All rapid growers except *Ustilago* spp.

All WHITE, CREAM, or TAN except *Rhodotorula*, *Cystobasidium*, and *Sporobolomyces* spp.

Microscopic morphology on cornmeal-Tween 80 agar (Dalmau plate)*

Hyphae and arthroconidia or annelloconidia

Trichosporon and
Cutaneotrichosporon
(p. **163**)

Magnusiomyces capitatus
(p. **166**)

Geotrichum candidum (p. **167**)

*Morphology alone cannot be relied upon for identification. Use procedure on p. 421 and Tables 2.2 through 2.9 (pp. 124, 126, 128, 134, 139, 150, and 151) for identification of genus and species.

THERMALLY DIMORPHIC AND/OR ENDEMIC FUNGI

Filamentous when cultured at 25–30°C; yeast when cultured at 35–37°C*

25°C mould phase on Sabouraud dextrose agar

	Sporothrix schenckii (p. 186)	Histoplasma capsulatum (p. 172)	Emergomyces (p. 175)	Blastomyces dermatitidis/ gilchristii (p. 177)	Paracoccidioi- des brasiliensis (p. 181)	Talaromyces marneffei (p. 183)	Coccidioides immitis/ posadasii** (p. 179)	Emmonsia crescens (p. 189)
MACROSCOPICALLY:	Wrinkled, waxy, some short aerial mycelium when old	Loose, cottony	Tufted, powdery	Smooth, then prickly, then cottony	Heaped; short mycelium	Flat, velvety	Loose, cottony	Heaped, velvety
	White, then tan or black	White or brownish	White to pale brown	White, then brownish	White, then brownish	Tan, then reddish yellow and bluish green; red, diffus- ing pigment	White, then gray or tan	White, then buff with tan center
MICROSCOPICALLY:	Fine, branched, septate hyphae; "floret" conidial form	Branched, septate hyphae; microco- nidia; tuberculate macroconidia in 3–4 weeks	Septate hyphae, conidiophores with 1–3 conidia	Branched, septate hyphae; single small conidia	Septate hyphae, chlamydoconidia, few microconidia	Septate hyphae, metulae, phialides, chains of conidia	Septate hyphae, barrel-shaped arthroconidia separated by empty cells	Septate hyphae, conidiophores with 2–3 conidia

37°C yeast phase on brain heart infusion agar

MACROSCOPICALLY: All cream or tan

MICROSCOPICALLY:

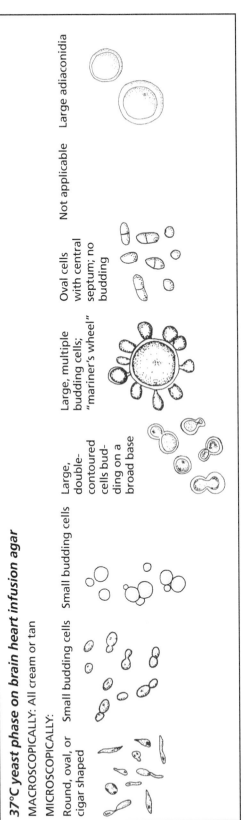

| Small budding cells | Small budding cells | Large, double-contoured cells budding on a broad base | Large, multiple budding cells; "mariner's wheel" | Oval cells with central septum; no budding | Not applicable | Large adiaconidia |

Round, oval, or cigar shaped

*See p. 427 for method of converting filamentous forms to yeast phase.

**Large spherules filled with endospores occur at 37°C in host tissue, yeast are not formed.

THERMALLY MONOMORPHIC MOULDS

Filamentous when cultured at 25–30°C and also at 35–37°C if growth occurs
SURFACE: WHITE, CREAM, OR LIGHT GRAY*
REVERSE: NONPIGMENTED

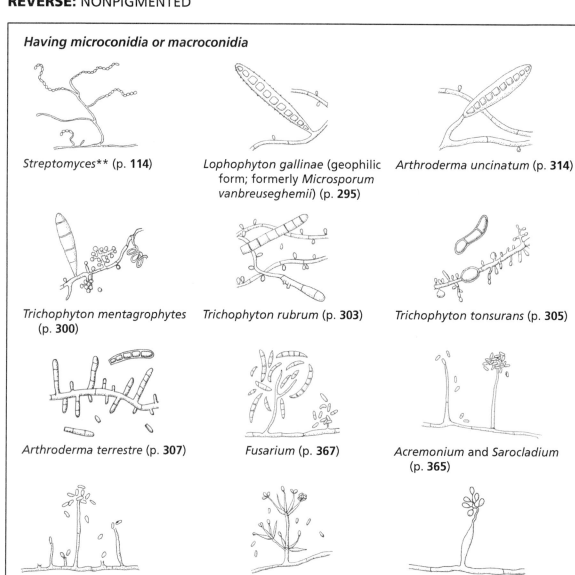

Having microconidia or macroconidia

Streptomyces** (p. **114**)

Lophophyton gallinae (geophilic form; formerly *Microsporum vanbreuseghemii*) (p. **295**)

Arthroderma uncinatum (p. **314**)

Trichophyton mentagrophytes (p. **300**)

Trichophyton rubrum (p. **303**)

Trichophyton tonsurans (p. **305**)

Arthroderma terrestre (p. **307**)

Fusarium (p. **367**)

Acremonium and Sarocladium (p. **365**)

Phialemonium (p. **228**)

Verticillium (p. **364**)

Beauveria bassiana (p. **363**)

THERMALLY MONOMORPHIC MOULDS

Filamentous when cultured at 25–30°C and also at 35–37°C if growth occurs

SURFACE: WHITE, CREAM, OR LIGHT GRAY*

REVERSE: NONPIGMENTED (*continued*)

Having microconidia or macroconidia (continued)

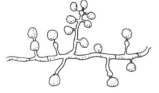

Emmonsia crescens*** (p. **189**)

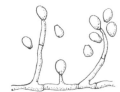

Scedosporium apiospermum
(p. **237**)

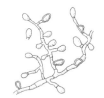

Chrysosporium (p. **371**)

Sporotrichum pruinosum (p. **374**)

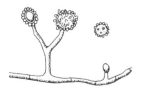

Sepedonium (p. **376**)

Stachybotrys chartarum (p. **262**)

Having sporangia or sporangiola

Rhizopus (p. **198**)

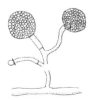

Mucor (p. **200**)

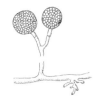

Rhizomucor (p. **201**)

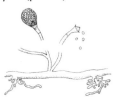

Lichtheimia corymbifera (p. **202**)

Apophysomyces elegans (p. **204**)

Saksenaea vasiformis (p. **206**)

Cunninghamella bertholletiae
(p. **209**)

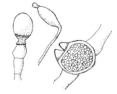

Basidiobolus (p. **212**)

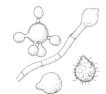

Conidiobolus coronatus (p. **213**)

THERMALLY MONOMORPHIC MOULDS

Filamentous when cultured at 25–30°C and also at 35–37°C if growth occurs
SURFACE: WHITE, CREAM, OR LIGHT GRAY*
REVERSE: NONPIGMENTED (*continued*)

Having arthroconidia

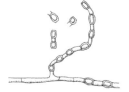

Coccidioides immitis/
posadasii**** (p. **179**)

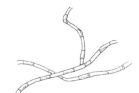

Malbranchea (p. **321**)

Hormographiella aspergillata
(p. **326**)

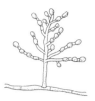

Pseudogymnoascus pannorum
(p. **323**)

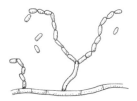

Arthrographis kalrae (p. **324**)

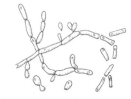

Trichosporon and
Cutaneotrichosporon (p. **163**)

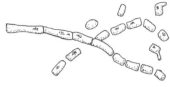

Geotrichum candidum (p. **167**)

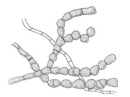

Neoscytalidium dimidiatum
(p. **259**)

Having only hyphae with chlamydoconidia

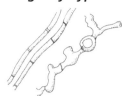

Microsporum ferrugineum
(p. **299**)

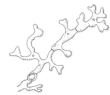

Trichophyton schoenleinii (p. **311**)

Trichophyton verrucosum (p. **312**)

THERMALLY MONOMORPHIC MOULDS

Filamentous when cultured at 25–30°C and also at 35–37°C if growth occurs

SURFACE: WHITE, CREAM, OR LIGHT GRAY*

REVERSE: NONPIGMENTED (*continued*)

Having only hyphae with chlamydoconidia (continued)

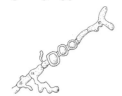

Trichophyton violaceum (p. **313**)

Having only septate hyphae on routine primary media*****

Septate hyphae

On malt extract agar

Aspergillus tanneri****** (p. **340**)

Penicillate

Schizophyllum commune (p. **378**)

---

*Also see p. 171, as several thermally dimorphic fungi may fit this description at 25–30°C.

**Streptomyces is a filamentous bacterium.

****E. crescens* is thermally dimorphic. Large adiaconidia form at 37°C.

****Large spherules filled with endospores occur at 37°C in host tissue.

*****Many moulds will produce only septate hyphae. An identification cannot be made based on this feature alone.

******On routine media, *A. tanneri* produces only hyphae. Conidial heads are seen only on Czapek agar or malt extract agar. See p. 340.

PART II Identification of Fungi in Culture

THERMALLY MONOMORPHIC MOULDS

SURFACE: WHITE, CREAM, BEIGE, OR LIGHT GRAY
REVERSE: YELLOW, ORANGE, OR REDDISH

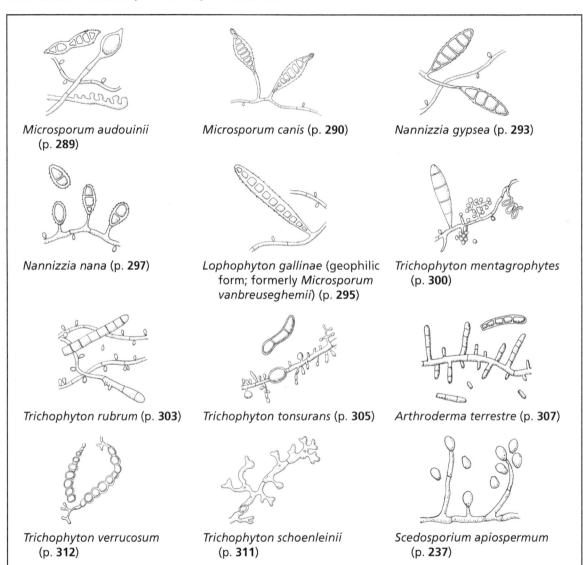

Microsporum audouinii (p. **289**)

Microsporum canis (p. **290**)

Nannizzia gypsea (p. **293**)

Nannizzia nana (p. **297**)

Lophophyton gallinae (geophilic form; formerly Microsporum vanbreuseghemii) (p. **295**)

Trichophyton mentagrophytes (p. **300**)

Trichophyton rubrum (p. **303**)

Trichophyton tonsurans (p. **305**)

Arthroderma terrestre (p. **307**)

Trichophyton verrucosum (p. **312**)

Trichophyton schoenleinii (p. **311**)

Scedosporium apiospermum (p. **237**)

THERMALLY MONOMORPHIC MOULDS

SURFACE: WHITE, CREAM, BEIGE, OR LIGHT GRAY

REVERSE: YELLOW, ORANGE, OR REDDISH (*continued*)

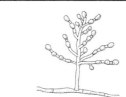

Pseudogymnoascus pannorum (p. **323**)

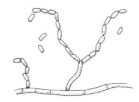

Arthrographis kalrae (p. **324**)

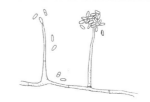

Acremonium and *Sarocladium* (p. **365**)

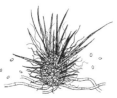

Chaetomium (p. **280**)

THERMALLY MONOMORPHIC MOULDS

SURFACE: WHITE, CREAM, BEIGE, OR LIGHT GRAY
REVERSE: DEEP RED TO PURPLE

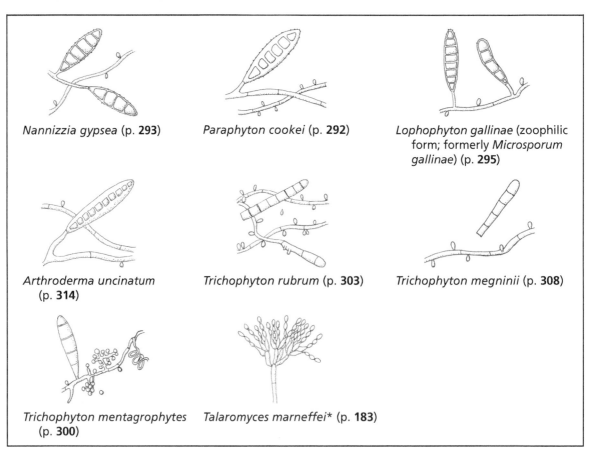

Nannizzia gypsea (p. **293**)

Paraphyton cookei (p. **292**)

Lophophyton gallinae (zoophilic form; formerly Microsporum gallinae) (p. **295**)

Arthroderma uncinatum (p. **314**)

Trichophyton rubrum (p. **303**)

Trichophyton megninii (p. **308**)

Trichophyton mentagrophytes (p. **300**)

Talaromyces marneffei* (p. **183**)

*T. marneffei is thermally dimorphic.

THERMALLY MONOMORPHIC MOULDS

SURFACE: WHITE, CREAM, BEIGE, OR LIGHT GRAY
REVERSE: BROWNISH

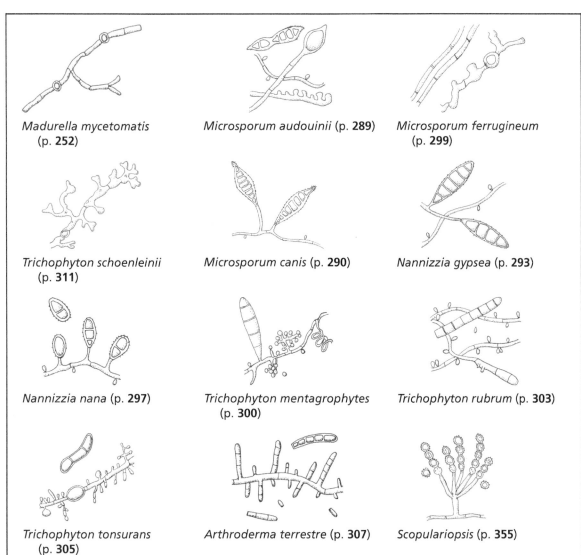

Madurella mycetomatis
(p. **252**)

Microsporum audouinii (p. **289**)

Microsporum ferrugineum
(p. **299**)

Trichophyton schoenleinii
(p. **311**)

Microsporum canis (p. **290**)

Nannizzia gypsea (p. **293**)

Nannizzia nana (p. **297**)

Trichophyton mentagrophytes
(p. **300**)

Trichophyton rubrum (p. **303**)

Trichophyton tonsurans
(p. **305**)

Arthroderma terrestre (p. **307**)

Scopulariopsis (p. **355**)

THERMALLY MONOMORPHIC MOULDS

SURFACE: WHITE, CREAM, BEIGE, OR LIGHT GRAY
REVERSE: BROWNISH (*continued*)

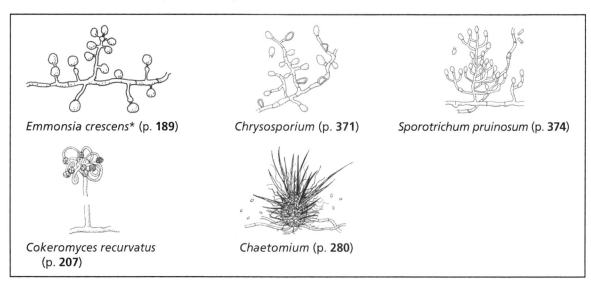

Emmonsia crescens* (p. **189**)   Chrysosporium (p. **371**)   Sporotrichum pruinosum (p. **374**)

Cokeromyces recurvatus
    (p. **207**)   Chaetomium (p. **280**)

*E. crescens is thermally dimorphic. Large adiaconidia form at 37°C.

THERMALLY MONOMORPHIC MOULDS

SURFACE: WHITE, CREAM, BEIGE, OR LIGHT GRAY
REVERSE: BLACKISH

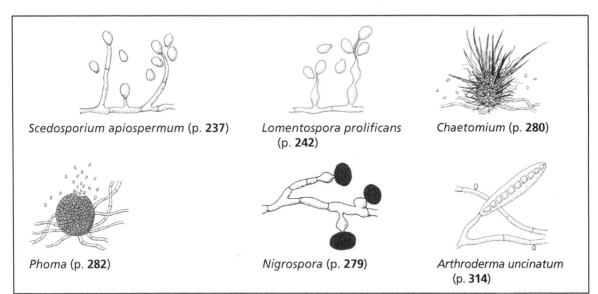

Scedosporium apiospermum (p. **237**)

Lomentospora prolificans (p. **242**)

Chaetomium (p. **280**)

Phoma (p. **282**)

Nigrospora (p. **279**)

Arthroderma uncinatum (p. **314**)

THERMALLY MONOMORPHIC MOULDS

SURFACE: TAN TO BROWN*

Having small conidia

Aspergillus versicolor (p. **336**)

Aspergillus ustus (p. **338**)

Aspergillus terreus (p. **345**)

Trichophyton tonsurans (p. **305**)

Cladophialophora carrionii (p. **233**)

Cladosporium (p. **230**)

Paecilomyces variotii (p. **350**)

Rasamsonia argillacea (p. **351**)

Scopulariopsis (p. **355**)

Verticillium (p. **364**)

Phaeoacremonium parasiticum (p. **226**)

Phialemonium (p. **228**)

Scedosporium apiospermum (p. **237**)

Emmonsia crescens** (p. **189**)

Chrysosporium (p. **371**)

THERMALLY MONOMORPHIC MOULDS

SURFACE: TAN TO BROWN* (*continued*)

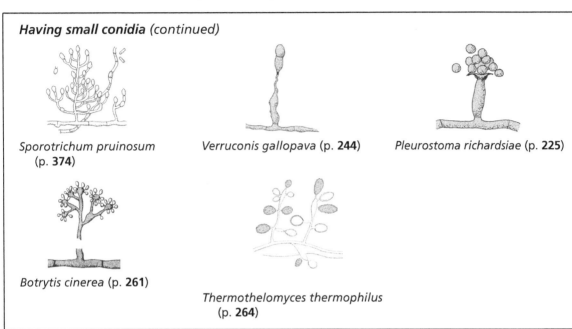

Having small conidia (*continued*)

Sporotrichum pruinosum (p. **374**)

Verruconis gallopava (p. **244**)

Pleurostoma richardsiae (p. **225**)

Botrytis cinerea (p. **261**)

Thermothelomyces thermophilus (p. **264**)

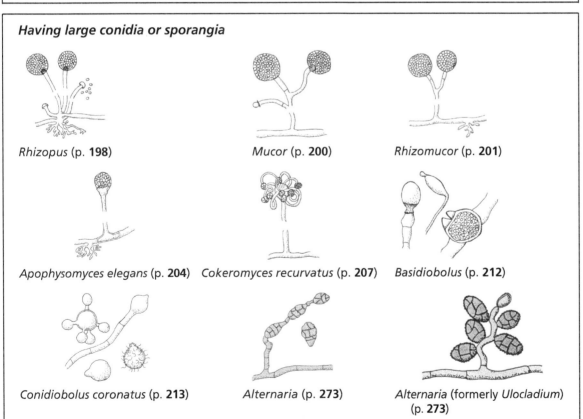

Having large conidia or sporangia

Rhizopus (p. **198**)

Mucor (p. **200**)

Rhizomucor (p. **201**)

Apophysomyces elegans (p. **204**)

Cokeromyces recurvatus (p. **207**)

Basidiobolus (p. **212**)

Conidiobolus coronatus (p. **213**)

Alternaria (p. **273**)

Alternaria (formerly *Ulocladium*) (p. **273**)

PART II Identification of Fungi in Culture

SURFACE: TAN TO BROWN* (*continued*)

Having large conidia or sporangia (continued)

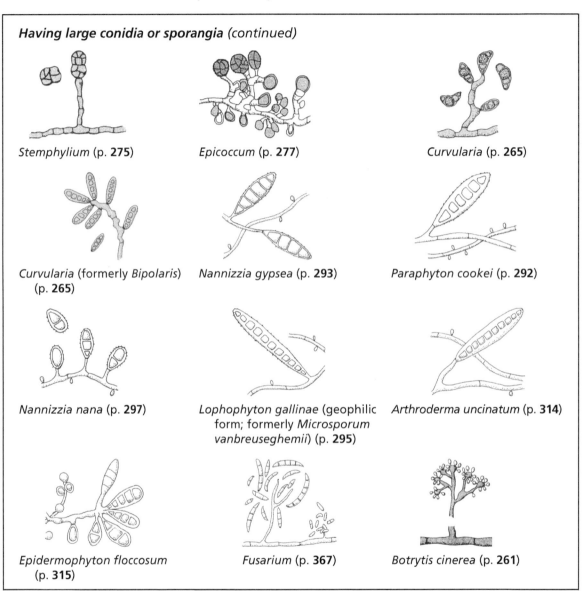

Stemphylium (p. **275**)

Epicoccum (p. **277**)

Curvularia (p. **265**)

Curvularia (formerly *Bipolaris*) (p. **265**)

Nannizzia gypsea (p. **293**)

Paraphyton cookei (p. **292**)

Nannizzia nana (p. **297**)

Lophophyton gallinae (geophilic form; formerly *Microsporum vanbreuseghemii*) (p. **295**)

Arthroderma uncinatum (p. **314**)

Epidermophyton floccosum (p. **315**)

Fusarium (p. **367**)

Botrytis cinerea (p. **261**)

PART II Identification of Fungi in Culture

THERMALLY MONOMORPHIC MOULDS

SURFACE: TAN TO BROWN* (*continued*)

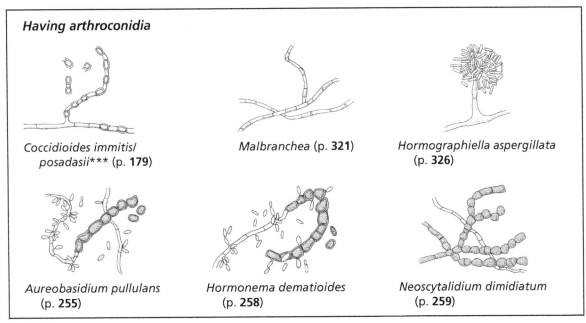

Having arthroconidia

*Coccidioides immitis/ posadasii*** (p. **179**)

Malbranchea (p. **321**)

Hormographiella aspergillata (p. **326**)

Aureobasidium pullulans (p. **255**)

Hormonema dematioides (p. **258**)

Neoscytalidium dimidiatum (p. **259**)

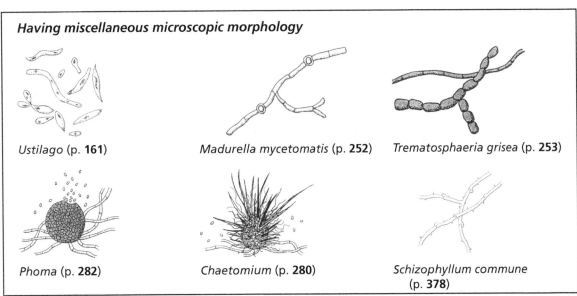

Having miscellaneous microscopic morphology

Ustilago (p. **161**)

Madurella mycetomatis (p. **252**)

Trematosphaeria grisea (p. **253**)

Phoma (p. **282**)

Chaetomium (p. **280**)

Schizophyllum commune (p. **378**)

*Also see p. 171, as several thermally dimorphic fungi may fit this description at 25–30°C.
**E. crescens* is thermally dimorphic. Large adiaconidia form at 37°C.
***Large spherules filled with endospores occur at 37°C in host tissue.

THERMALLY MONOMORPHIC MOULDS

SURFACE: YELLOW TO ORANGE

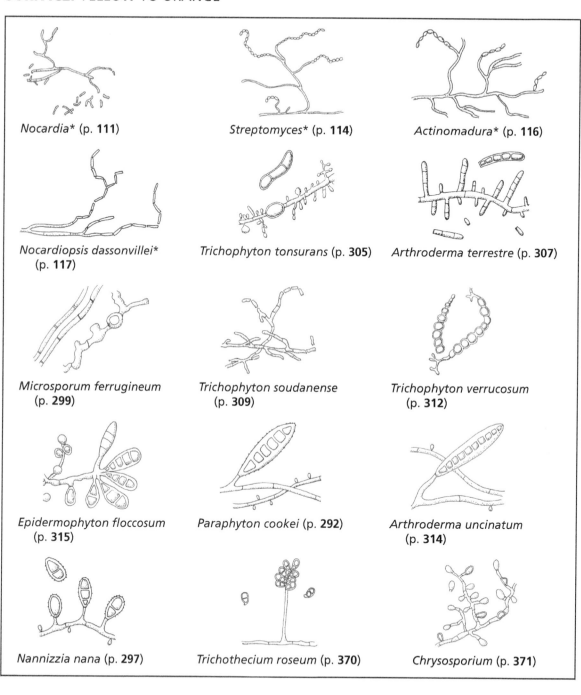

Nocardia* (p. 111)

Streptomyces* (p. 114)

Actinomadura* (p. 116)

Nocardiopsis dassonvillei*
(p. 117)

Trichophyton tonsurans (p. 305)

Arthroderma terrestre (p. 307)

Microsporum ferrugineum
(p. 299)

Trichophyton soudanense
(p. 309)

Trichophyton verrucosum
(p. 312)

Epidermophyton floccosum
(p. 315)

Paraphyton cookei (p. 292)

Arthroderma uncinatum
(p. 314)

Nannizzia nana (p. 297)

Trichothecium roseum (p. 370)

Chrysosporium (p. 371)

SURFACE: YELLOW TO ORANGE (*continued*)

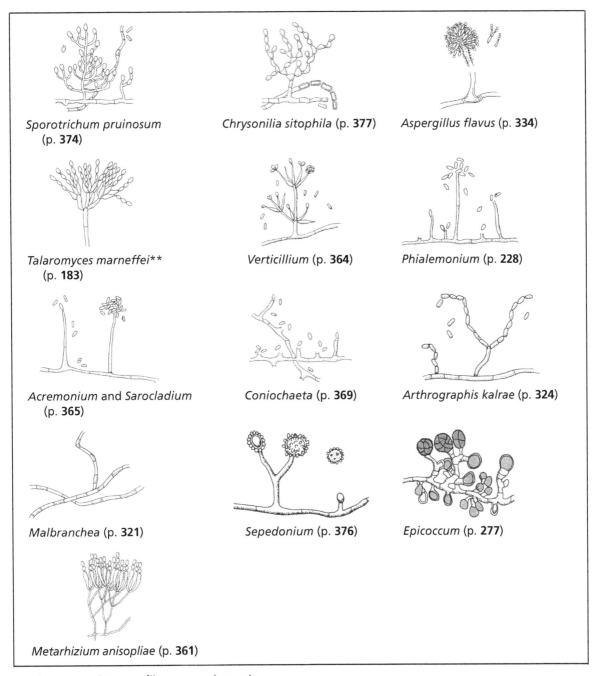

Sporotrichum pruinosum (p. **374**)

Chrysonilia sitophila (p. **377**)

Aspergillus flavus (p. **334**)

Talaromyces marneffei** (p. **183**)

Verticillium (p. **364**)

Phialemonium (p. **228**)

Acremonium and Sarocladium (p. **365**)

Coniochaeta (p. **369**)

Arthrographis kalrae (p. **324**)

Malbranchea (p. **321**)

Sepedonium (p. **376**)

Epicoccum (p. **277**)

Metarhizium anisopliae (p. **361**)

*These organisms are filamentous bacteria.
**T. marneffei* is thermally dimorphic.

THERMALLY MONOMORPHIC MOULDS

SURFACE: PINK TO VIOLET

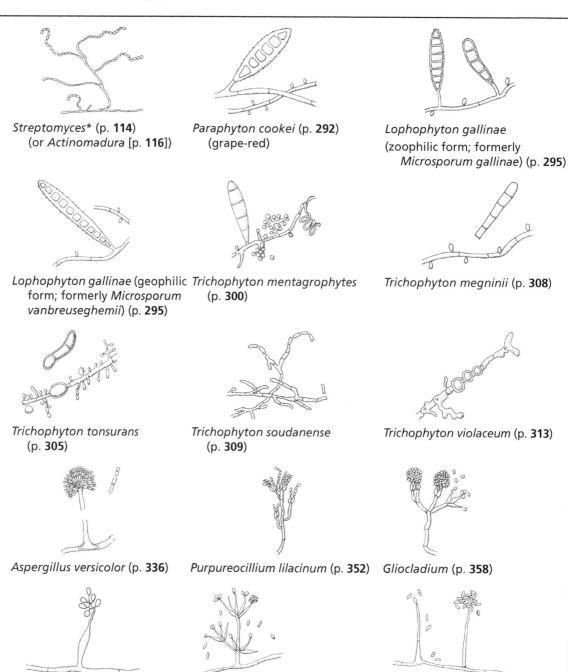

Streptomyces* (p. **114**)
    (or Actinomadura [p. **116**])

Paraphyton cookei (p. **292**)
    (grape-red)

Lophophyton gallinae
(zoophilic form; formerly
    Microsporum gallinae) (p. **295**)

Lophophyton gallinae (geophilic
form; formerly Microsporum
vanbreuseghemii) (p. **295**)

Trichophyton mentagrophytes
(p. **300**)

Trichophyton megninii (p. **308**)

Trichophyton tonsurans
(p. **305**)

Trichophyton soudanense
(p. **309**)

Trichophyton violaceum (p. **313**)

Aspergillus versicolor (p. **336**)

Purpureocillium lilacinum (p. **352**)

Gliocladium (p. **358**)

Beauveria bassiana (p. **363**)

Verticillium (p. **364**)

Acremonium and Sarocladium
(p. **365**)

PART II Identification of Fungi in Culture

SURFACE: PINK TO VIOLET (*continued*)

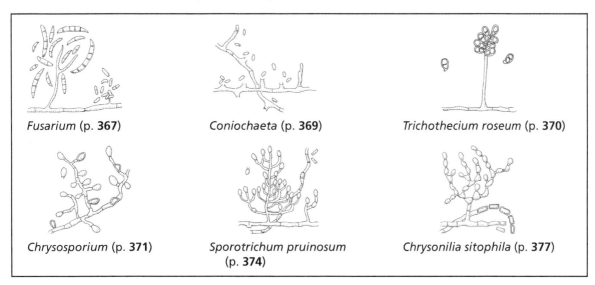

Fusarium (p. **367**) Coniochaeta (p. **369**) *Trichothecium roseum* (p. **370**)

Chrysosporium (p. **371**) *Sporotrichum pruinosum* (p. **374**) Chrysonilia sitophila (p. **377**)

Streptomyces and *Actinomadura* are filamentous bacteria.

THERMALLY MONOMORPHIC MOULDS

SURFACE: GREEN
REVERSE: LIGHT

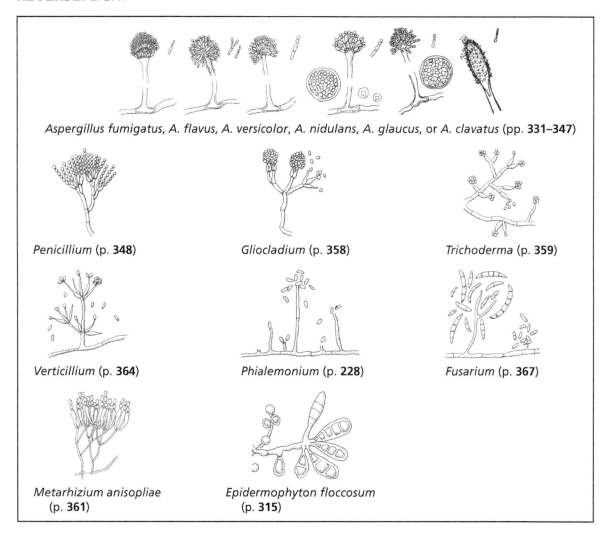

Aspergillus fumigatus, A. flavus, A. versicolor, A. nidulans, A. glaucus, or *A. clavatus* (pp. **331–347**)

Penicillium (p. **348**)

Gliocladium (p. **358**)

Trichoderma (p. **359**)

Verticillium (p. **364**)

Phialemonium (p. **228**)

Fusarium (p. **367**)

Metarhizium anisopliae
(p. **361**)

Epidermophyton floccosum
(p. **315**)

THERMALLY MONOMORPHIC MOULDS

SURFACE: DARK GRAY OR BLACK
REVERSE: LIGHT

Syncephalastrum racemosum (p. **211**)

Aspergillus niger (p. **333**)

THERMALLY MONOMORPHIC MOULDS

SURFACE: GREENISH, DARK GRAY, OR BLACK
REVERSE: DARK

Having small conidia*

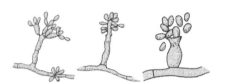

Fonsecaea (p. **218**)

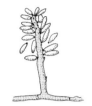

Myrmecridium schulzeri (p. **221**)

Rhinocladiella
mackenziei (p. **222**)

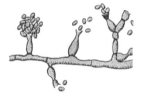

Phialophora verrucosa (p. **223**)

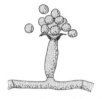

Pleurostoma richardsiae (p. **225**)

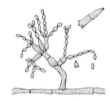

Cladosporium (p. **230**)

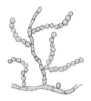

Cladophialophora boppii (p. **235**)

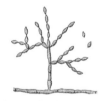

Cladophialophora carrionii
(p. **233**)

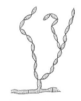

Cladophialophora
bantiana (p. **236**)

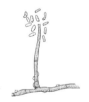

Phaeoacremonium parasiticum
(p. **226**)

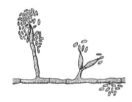

Exophiala jeanselmei (p. **247**)

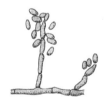

Exophiala dermatitidis
(p. **249**)

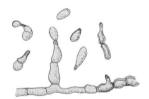

Hortaea werneckii (p. **251**)

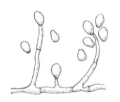

Scedosporium apiospermum
(p. **237**)

Lomentospora prolificans
(p. **242**)

THERMALLY MONOMORPHIC MOULDS

SURFACE: GREENISH, DARK GRAY, OR BLACK
REVERSE: DARK (*continued*)

Having small conidia* (continued)

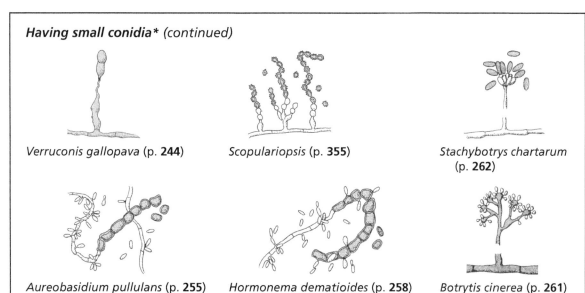

Verruconis gallopava (p. **244**)

Scopulariopsis (p. **355**)

Stachybotrys chartarum (p. **262**)

Aureobasidium pullulans (p. **255**)

Hormonema dematioides (p. **258**)

Botrytis cinerea (p. **261**)

Having large conidia

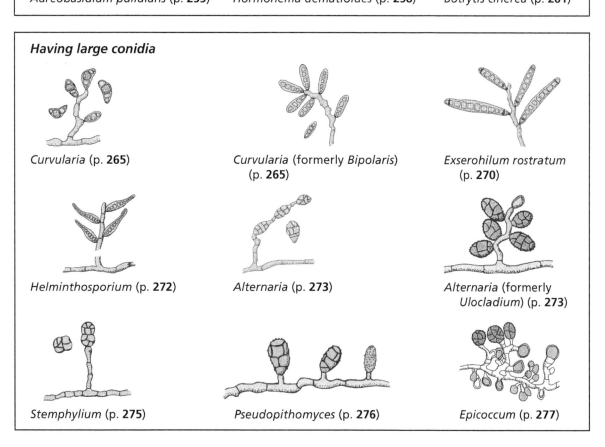

Curvularia (p. **265**)

Curvularia (formerly *Bipolaris*) (p. **265**)

Exserohilum rostratum (p. **270**)

Helminthosporium (p. **272**)

Alternaria (p. **273**)

Alternaria (formerly *Ulocladium*) (p. **273**)

Stemphylium (p. **275**)

Pseudopithomyces (p. **276**)

Epicoccum (p. **277**)

THERMALLY MONOMORPHIC MOULDS

SURFACE: GREENISH, DARK GRAY, OR BLACK
REVERSE: DARK (*continued*)

Having large conidia (continued)

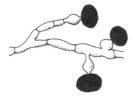

Nigrospora (p. **279**)

Having arthroconidia

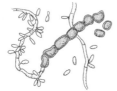 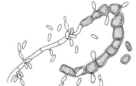 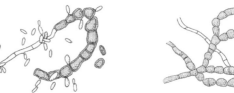

Aureobasidium pullulans (p. **255**)   *Hormonema dematioides* (p. **258**)   *Neoscytalidium dimidiatum* (p. **259**)

Having only hyphae (with or without chlamydoconidia)

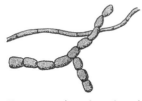 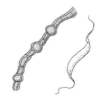

Trematosphaeria grisea (p. **253**)   *Piedraia hortae* (p. **254**)

Having large fruiting bodies

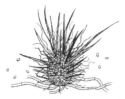 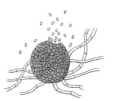

Chaetomium (p. **280**)   *Phoma* (p. **282**)

*Also see p. 186, as *Sporothrix schenckii* may fit this description at 25–30°C.

Detailed Descriptions

PART II Identification of Fungi in Culture

Filamentous Bacteria

Introduction to Filamentous Bacteria

Some of the aerobic actinomycetes resemble fungi in that they form filaments that are well developed and branched (commonly referred to as hyphae). However, the results of cell wall analysis, lack of a membrane-bound nucleus, lack of mitochondria, small size, and susceptibility to antibacterial agents have long defined these organisms as bacteria rather than fungi.

The aerobic actinomycetes are Gram positive and have filaments that are 1 µm or less in diameter. Some may be partially acid-fast when stained by a modified Kinyoun method (p. 432). These organisms grow on routine bacteriology and mycology media without some particular antibacterial additives and on routine mycobacteriology media. In order to isolate these organisms from contaminated specimens, it is often imperative to utilize selective media (see p. 441), along with nonselective media, to enhance their recovery. The colonies are usually glabrous and often become covered with aerial hyphae, forming a chalky or powdery coat. Visualization of aerial hyphae can be enhanced by examining the colony with a dissecting microscope. The microscopic morphology is best observed by slide culture on minimal medium, such as cornmeal-Tween 80 agar or 2% plain agar prepared with tap water.

In addition to morphology and staining characteristics, a battery of traditional observations and biochemical tests can be useful for preliminary differentiation of the organisms in this group (see Table 2.1, p. 110). However, nucleic acid-based molecular methods are often essential for accurate species identification, and are strongly recommended. These procedures are performed in many reference laboratories.

The most commonly encountered pathogenic aerobic actinomycetes belong to the genus *Nocardia*; they cause pulmonary, systemic, central nervous system, and cutaneous diseases, including actinomycotic mycetomas (swollen tumor-like subcutaneous lesions that yield granular pus through draining sinuses). Members of the other genera are etiologic agents of actinomycotic mycetoma and occasionally other infections. Many *Streptomyces* spp. are considered nonpathogenic saprobes.

For further information, see
Brown-Elliott et al., 2023
Mochon et al., 2016

FILAMENTOUS BACTERIA

PART II Identification of Fungi in Culture

TABLE 2.1 Differentiation of filamentous aerobic actinomycetes encountered in clinical specimens[a,b]

Organism	Colony on Sabouraud dextrose agar	Aerial hyphae	Fragmentation of hyphae[c]	Acid-fast (partially)[d]	Growth with lysozyme	Hydrolysis of starch
Nocardia spp.	White to pink or orange; glabrous or powdery; wrinkled	+	+	+	+	0[V]
Nocardiopsis dassonvillei	Yellowish; heaped; wrinkled; chalky or velvety	+	+	0	0	+
Actinomadura madurae	White, tan, pink, red, or orange; glabrous; wrinkled; hard; adherent; slow growing	0[V]	0	0	0	+
Actinomadura pelletieri	Bright red; heaped; glabrous	0[V]	0	0	0	0
Streptomyces somaliensis	Cream to brown or black; slow growing; leathery; folded	+	0	0	0	V
Streptomyces spp.	Variety of colors; glabrous, chalky, or velvety	+	0	0 (spores often +)	V	+[V]

[a] Molecular methods are highly recommended, and often essential, for definitive identification. Abbreviations: +, positive; 0, negative; V, variable.

[b] Other clinically encountered aerobic actinomycetes are not filamentous and are more likely handled in the bacteriology laboratory.

[c] Smears must be made with care to detect spontaneous fragmentation rather than that caused by trauma; slide culture may be best for evaluation of hyphal fragmentation.

[d] Stained by modified acid-fast method (p. 432).

Nocardia spp.

TAXONOMY NOTES: The genus contains over 100 validly named species and about half have been isolated from humans. The taxonomic history of *Nocardia* is complicated, as exemplified by *Nocardia asteroides*, the type species of the genus, and probably considered the most commonly isolated pathogenic *Nocardia* spp. from humans. Based on molecular analyses, *N. asteroides sensu stricto* is seldom isolated from humans and is rarely considered pathogenic. The term "*N. asteroides* complex" has been used for organisms that phenotypically resemble the *N. asteroides* type strain. However, clinical isolates formerly identified as *N. asteroides* complex are now separated based on molecular studies into *N. abscessus*, *N. brevicatena*/*N. paucivorans*, *N. cyriacigeorgica*, *N. farcinica*, *N. nova* complex, and *N. transvalensis* complex. As such, the term "*N. asteroides* complex" is no longer valid.

PATHOGENICITY: Cause nocardiosis, which symptomatically may be similar to tuberculosis or actinomycosis. The disease, especially in immunocompromised hosts, most frequently begins as a pulmonary infection and disseminates to the brain, kidneys, and other organs. Traumatic inoculation is usually the source of infection in immunocompetent hosts, and skin lesions or subcutaneous abscesses occur. Mycetomas, which typically involve the subcutaneous tissues, muscle, tendon, and bone, usually develop in the extremities. *Nocardia* spp. are the most common cause of actinomycotic mycetoma (mycetomas caused by aerobic actinomycetes), and actinomycotic mycetomas due to *Nocardia* spp. occur mostly in regions of higher humidity. The organisms are ubiquitous in nature and may therefore be encountered as colonizers or specimen contaminants.

RATE OF GROWTH: Moderate; usually mature within 6–10 days, but should be incubated for at least 2–3 weeks in case growth is delayed. Optimal growth is at 35–37°C. Grow on Sabouraud dextrose agar (SDA) without antibiotics and on Lowenstein-Jensen and Middlebrook 7H11 media (frequently survive decontamination procedures used for isolation of acid-fast bacilli when exposure to the reagents does not exceed 15 minutes). Excellent recovery occurs on nonselective and selective buffered charcoal-yeast extract agar (the formulation containing vancomycin rather than cefamandole is preferred) and on other selective media such as colistin-nalidixic acid agar and modified Thayer-Martin agar (containing vancomycin, colistin, and nystatin). Inclusion of a selective medium is usually essential for inhibition of faster-growing organisms and recovery of *Nocardia* spp. from nonsterile sites. Media containing chloramphenicol or gentamicin are not recommended, as they may prevent growth of *Nocardia* spp.

COLONY MORPHOLOGY: Grow aerobically on SDA without antibiotics, forming raised, irregular, folded colonies varying from white to orange, depending on the species. Color may be best observed on the reverse when grown on translucent media such as SDA. May be glabrous, velvety, or develop a white chalky coating of short aerial mycelia. If aerial hyphae are sparse, they may be best observed with a dissecting microscope.

Nocardia spp. *(continued)*

MICROSCOPIC MORPHOLOGY: Delicate, branching, often beaded, intertwining filaments that fragment into bacillary and coccoid forms; best exhibited on slide culture using a minimal medium, such as cornmeal-Tween 80 agar or tap water agar. They are Gram positive and often, but not always, partially acid-fast (use a modified Kinyoun method [p. 432]). Young primary cultures may be the most acid-fast; or acid-fastness may be enhanced on Middlebrook 7H11 medium or by growing cultures for 3–4 weeks in a proteinaceous medium, such as litmus milk or bromocresol purple milk.

See Table 2.1 (p. 110) for differentiation of filamentous aerobic actinomycetes.

Matrix-assisted laser desorption ionization–time of flight mass spectrometry (MALDI-TOF MS) for identification of *Nocardia* spp. shows promise; however, at present molecular nucleic acid-based methods for definitive identification of all etiologically significant *Nocardia* isolates is recommended and often essential.

In vitro antimicrobial susceptibility testing is recommended in cases of disseminated or refractory infection or if the patient cannot tolerate sulfonamides (the usual agent of choice for treating nocardiosis). Susceptibility profiles may assist in the phenotypic identification of *Nocardia* species; conversely, accurate identification may predict the isolate's probable susceptibility profile. Only laboratories having extensive experience and expertise in performing susceptibility tests on *Nocardia* ought to do so; all others are advised to send their isolates to a qualified reference laboratory.

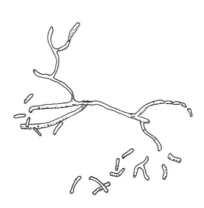
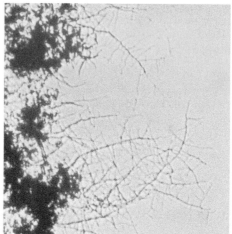

From Joseph Staneck. *Aerobic actinomycetes: Nocardia* and related organisms. ASM Teleconference of August 9, 1994.

Nocardia spp. *(continued)*

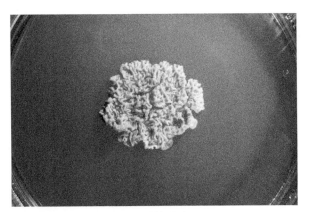

Nocardia brasiliensis. SDA, 30°C, 9 days.

For further information, see

Brown-Elliott et al., 2006
Conville et al., 2017
Girard et al., 2017
Schlaberg et al., 2014

Streptomyces spp.

TAXONOMY NOTES: The genus contains more than 950 named species and subspecies. The taxonomy of this group remains problematic.

PATHOGENICITY: Most *Streptomyces* spp. are considered nonpathogenic contaminants or colonizers. The major exception is *S. somaliensis*, which causes actinomycotic mycetomas and occasionally invasive infections. It prefers arid regions with sandy soil and is found predominantly, but not entirely, in Africa, Mexico, and portions of South America. Isolates are usually identified only to genus level (molecular testing is required for even a presumptive species identification); more studies are needed to improve identification.

RATE OF GROWTH: Rapid (mature within 5 days) or moderate (mature within 6–10 days). Optimum growth usually occurs at 25–30°C.

COLONY MORPHOLOGY: Surface is slightly folded, hard, leathery; may develop a fine chalky or powdery aerial mycelium. Many strains have various pigments of gray, black, brown, tan, orange, rose, red, or occasionally green. Culture often produces the characteristic odor of freshly tilled soil.

MICROSCOPIC MORPHOLOGY: Filaments are long, thin (1 μm or less in diameter), and abundantly branching. Filaments may be straight, wavy, or spiral. Small, oblong conidia (also referred to as spores) are produced at distinct points on the filament, often in chains; this is best observed on slide culture. Spores may stain partially acid-fast; some species do not form spores readily.

See Table 2.1 (p. 110) for differentiation of filamentous aerobic actinomycetes.

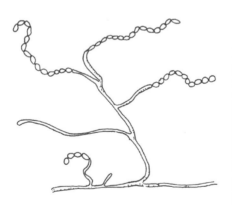 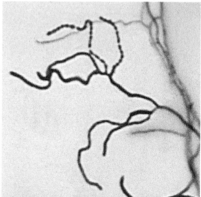

Courtesy of Morris Gordon.

Streptomyces **spp.** *(continued)*

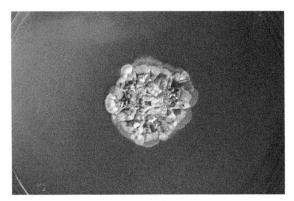

Streptomyces sp. SDA, 30°C, 9 days.

For further information, see
Kapadia et al., 2007

Actinomadura spp.

PATHOGENICITY: A frequent cause of actinomycotic mycetoma. Although there are many species, *A. madurae* and *A. pelletieri* are the two species most commonly considered of clinical importance. They are closely related, but *A. madurae* is the more commonly encountered and has on rare occasion caused severe, deeply invasive infections (e.g., pneumonia, peritonitis, and bacteremia) in immunocompromised patients. It has also been isolated as a saprobic contaminant from a variety of body sites.

RATE OF GROWTH: Usually rapid on Lowenstein-Jensen (LJ) medium; slower on Sabouraud dextrose agar. Optimum growth is at 35–37°C.

COLONY MORPHOLOGY: Waxy, folded, membranous, or mucoid. May be white, tan, pink, orange, or red. White aerial hyphae may develop after 2 weeks of incubation; best seen on LJ medium.

MICROSCOPIC MORPHOLOGY: Narrow, abundantly branched filaments (0.5–1 μm in diameter) that are Gram positive, non-acid-fast, and nonfragmenting. Short chains of round spores may be produced from limited portions of the aerial hyphae; this is best observed on slide culture. The microscopic and colonial morphologies of members of the genus are very similar to *Streptomyces*. Nucleic acid-based molecular methods are the only procedures that permit species-level identification.

See Table 2.1 (p. 110) for differentiation of filamentous aerobic actinomycetes.

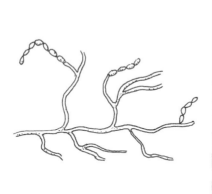

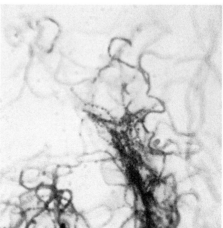

Nocardiopsis dassonvillei

PATHOGENICITY: Occasional etiologic agent of actinomycotic mycetoma; also considered a rare potential cause of cutaneous, pulmonary, conjunctival, and blood infections. There have been relatively few reports of clinical disease.

RATE OF GROWTH: Rapid (mature within 5 days) or moderate (mature within 6–10 days).

COLONY MORPHOLOGY: Yellowish, heaped, irregularly wrinkled. Aerial hyphae may develop to form a velvety coating. *N. synnemataformans* forms a deep pimento-red colony.

MICROSCOPIC MORPHOLOGY: Narrow filaments (1 μm or less in diameter) that are long, extensive, and sometimes branched; they are Gram positive and non-acid-fast. The filaments fragment into chains of arthroconidia-like structures, giving a characteristic zig-zag appearance. The total length of the aerial hyphae turns into conidial chains, in contrast to *Actinomadura* spp. and *Streptomyces* spp., which produce conidial chains only at distinct parts of the hyphae.

See Table 2.1 (p. 110) for differentiation of filamentous aerobic actinomycetes.

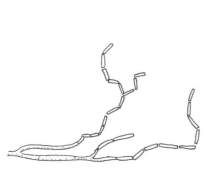
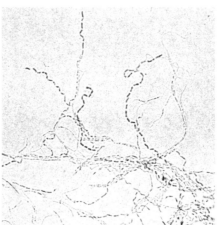

From McNeil and Brown, 1994.

For further information, see
Yassin et al., 1997

Yeasts and Yeastlike Organisms

Introduction to Yeasts and Yeastlike Organisms

In this guide, the terms "yeast" and "yeastlike" refer to unicellular organisms that generally reproduce by budding. If the buds (blastoconidia) elongate and remain attached to the parent cell, they form chains known as pseudohyphae. Some of the organisms included here produce true septate hyphae, while others form no hyphal elements of any sort. A few are capable of producing ascospores (the sexual state). Organisms that are actually algae but that grow in a yeastlike manner are traditional members of this group.

Colonies are smooth and glabrous and may be moist or dry; they are usually white to cream colored, but some are tan, pinkish, or orangey.

The ability to produce pseudohyphae, true hyphae, and/or terminal chlamydospores and the shape and arrangement of blastoconidia are used along with other morphologic characteristics and biochemical tests to identify the yeasts to the genus and species levels. A number of commercial systems are available for biochemical testing (see pp. 422–423). Microscopic morphology is studied on agar, such as cornmeal-Tween 80 agar, by using the Dalmau method (p. 454), which ensures the decreased oxygen environment required for the production of structures upon which identification depends. Isolates of *Candida* spp. from patients being treated with antimicrobial agents occasionally exhibit atypical microscopic morphologies, most often exceptionally large yeast cells. Identification of *Candida* spp. and other yeasts is achieved biochemically on a wide range of systems characterizing differential assimilation properties. Identification of *Candida* spp. and other yeasts is being increasingly performed by proteomics using MALDI-TOF MS technology (see p. 389).

Yeasts are the most common fungi isolated in the clinical laboratory. They are ubiquitous in our environment and also live as normal inhabitants in and on our bodies. Thus, it is often difficult to determine the clinical significance of an isolate. Implication of the yeast as the etiologic agent of infection often requires repeated recovery from the site and direct microscopic demonstration of the yeast in infected tissue. The yeasts and yeastlike organisms are considered opportunistic pathogens, causing disease in patients (i) with an impairment of the body's immune system; (ii) receiving prolonged treatment with antibiotics, corticosteroids, or cytotoxic drugs; (iii) with intravascular catheters; (iv) with diabetes mellitus; or (v) who are intravenous illicit drug users.

Candidiasis (also called candidosis) is by far the most common fungal infection (other than ringworm) seen in humans. Mucocutaneous infections are seen in individuals with defects in cell-mediated immunity, while systemic infections are primarily seen in neutropenic patients. Although *Candida* spp. are often isolated from lower respiratory specimens, they are seldom of clinical significance; definitive diagnosis of lower respiratory infection due to *Candida* requires histologic confirmation.

Many taxonomic revisions related to clinically relevant yeast have occurred recently, and more are likely over the coming years. For those *Candida* spp. whose names have been changed it is recommended at this time to use the *Candida* spp.

name (e.g., *Candida krusei*) that is more widely recognized and used by health care workers, rather than the revised name (e.g., *Pichia kudriavzevii*). To develop familiarity, a note indicating the revised name can be added to the clinical report.

For further information, see
Anaissie et al. (ed.), 2009
Borman and Johnson, 2021
Borman and Johnson, 2023
de Hoog et al., 2020
Kidd et al., 2023a
Kidd et al., 2023b
Kurtzman et al. (ed.), 2011
McCarty et al., 2021
Pappas et al., 2018
Patel, 2019
St-Germain and Summerbell, 2011
Warnock, 2017

Candida albicans

PATHOGENICITY: Most common cause of candidiasis (candidosis) (see p. 62), which is an acute, subacute, or chronic infection involving any part of the body. This organism is found as part of the normal microbiota in the skin, mouth, vaginal tract, and gastrointestinal tract (therefore, it is often present in stools without significance).

RATE OF GROWTH: Rapid; mature within 5 days.

COLONY MORPHOLOGY: Cream colored, pasty, smooth. On enriched media (e.g., blood agar or chocolate agar), extensions commonly called "feet" develop at the border of the colony. Colonies are green on CHROMagar Candida. (Image Appendix Figure 38.)

MICROSCOPIC MORPHOLOGY: On routine primary media, yeast cells are round to oval (3.5–7 × 4–8 μm). On cornmeal-Tween 80 agar (Dalmau plate [p. 454]) at 25°C for 72 h, pseudohyphae (and some true hyphae) form with clusters of round blastoconidia at the septa. Large, thick-walled, usually single terminal chlamydospores are characteristically formed; they are most likely to be seen near the edge of the coverslip. Chlamydospore formation is inhibited at 30–37°C. *C. albicans* yields a positive reaction on the germ tube test (p. 425), as does *Candida dubliniensis*; to differentiate the two species, see Table 2.4 (p. 128).

See Table 2.2 (p. 124) for differentiation of yeasts and yeastlike genera and Table 2.3 (p. 126) for characteristics of the most commonly encountered species of *Candida*.

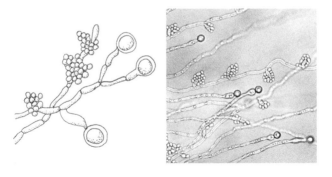

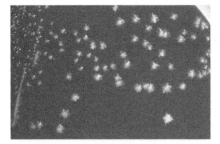

Candida albicans. Colonies with "feet" on sheep blood agar, 35°C, 2 days.

For further information, see
Barnes and Vale, 2005
Odds and Bernaerts, 1994

TABLE 2.2 Characteristics of the genera of clinically encountered yeasts and yeastlike organisms[a]

Organism	On cornmeal-Tween 80 agar at 25°C							Capsule	Urease	Growth:		
	Pseudo-hyphae	True hyphae	Blasto-conidia along hyphae	Arthro-conidia	Annello-conidia	Asco-spores	Sporangia			With cyclo-heximide at 25°C	On SDA at 37°C	In Sabouraud broth
Candida	+	Few	+	0	0	0	0	0	0^v	V	$+^v$	Some species show surface growth
Rhodotorula and Cystobasidium	0^R	0		0	0	0	0	V	+	0^v	$+^v$	NSG
Cryptococcus	0^R	0		0	0	0	0	+	+	0	V	NSG
Saccharomyces	V	0		0	0	+	0	0	0	0	+	NSG
Malassezia	0^R	0^R		0	0	0	0	0	+	$+^{w,v}$	$+^v$	NSG
Prototheca	0	0	0	0	0	0	+	0^v	0	0	$+^v$	Surface growth
Geotrichum	0	+	0	+	0	0	0	0	0	0	0^w	Pellicle forms
Trichosporon and Cutaneotri-chosporon	+	+	+	+	0	0	0	0	+	$+^v$	$+^v$	Pellicle forms
Magnusiomyces capitatus (formerly *Blas-toschizomyces capitatus*)	+	+	+	0^v	+	0	0	0	0	+	+	Pellicle forms

[a] Abbreviations: SDA, Sabouraud dextrose agar; +, positive; 0, negative; V, species or strain variation; W, weak; R, rarely few rudimentary forms; NSG, no surface growth.

Candida dubliniensis

PATHOGENICITY: Appears in bloodstream and other infections. The organism is widespread throughout the world and has been recovered from a variety of clinical specimens.

RATE OF GROWTH: Rapid; mature within 5 days.

COLONY MORPHOLOGY: Cream colored, pasty, smooth. On enriched media (e.g., blood agar or chocolate agar), extensions commonly called "feet" develop at the border of the colony, as occurs with *Candida albicans* (p. 123) but not as well when incubated in 5% CO_2.

MICROSCOPIC MORPHOLOGY: Very similar to that of *C. albicans*. On cornmeal-Tween 80 agar (Dalmau plate [p. 454]) at 25°C for 72 h, forms pseudohyphae, and some true hyphae, with clusters of round blastoconidia at the septa. Large, thick-walled terminal chlamydospores characteristically form in pairs or small clusters (as opposed to *C. albicans*, which usually produces terminal chlamydospores singly). *C. dubliniensis* (like *C. albicans*) yields a positive reaction with the germ tube test (p. 425); to differentiate the two species, see Table 2.4 (p. 128).

See Table 2.2 (p. 124) for differentiation of yeasts and yeastlike genera and Table 2.3 (p. 126) for characteristics of the most commonly encountered species of *Candida*.

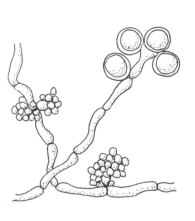 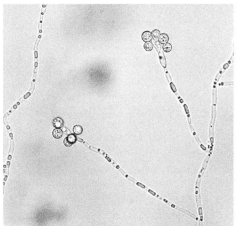

For further information, see
Sullivan and Coleman, 1998
Sullivan et al., 2005

TABLE 2.3 Characteristics of *Candida* spp. most commonly encountered in the clinical laboratory[a]

Organism	Microscopic morphology on cornmeal-Tween 80 agar at 25°C	Growth:				Urease (25°C)	Assimilation of:		
		In Sabouraud broth	With cyclohexi-mide at 25°C	On SDA at 37°C	Germ tubes		Glucose	Maltose	Sucrose
C. albicans, *C. dubliniensis*	Pseudohyphae with terminal chlamydospores; clusters of blastoconidia at septa	NSG	+	+	+	0	+	+	V
C. tropicalis	Blastoconidia anywhere along pseudohyphae	Narrow surface film with bubbles	0^v	+	0	0	+	+	+^v
C. parapsilosis	Blastoconidia along curved pseudohyphae; giant mycelial cells	NSG	0	+	0	0	+	+	+
C. lusitaniae	Short chains of elongate blastoconidia along curved pseudohyphae	NSG	0	+	0	0	+	+	+
C. guilliermondii	Fairly short, fine pseudohyphae; clusters of blastoconidia at septa	NSG	+	+	0	0	+	+	+
C. kefyr	Elongated blastoconidia resembling logs in a stream along pseudohyphae	NSG	+	+	0	0	+	0	+
C. rugosa	Pseudohyphae with elongated blastoconidia, some in chains	NSG	0	+	0	0	+	0	0
C. zeylanoides	Pseudohyphae give featherlike appearance at low power	Pellicle (delayed)	+	0^v	0	0	+	0	0
C. glabrata	No pseudohyphae; cells small; terminal budding	NSG	0	+	0	0	+	0	0
C. krusei	Pseudohyphae with cross-matchsticks or treelike blastoconidia	Wide surface film up sides of tube	0	+	0	+^v	+	0	0
C. lipolytica	Elongated blastoconidia in short chains along pseudohyphae	Pellicle (delayed)	+	+	0	+	+	0	0
C. auris	May form short, undeveloped pseudohyphae	NSG	0	+	0	0	+	+	+
C. pelliculosa[c]	May form pseudohyphae	NSG	0	V	0	0	+	+	+

[a] Abbreviations: SDA, Sabouraud dextrose agar; +, positive; 0, negative; W, reaction may be weak; V, strain variation; NSG, no surface growth; ND, not determined.

[b] Fermentation is demonstrated by production of gas (acid does not indicate fermentation).

[c] Ascospores are formed when the organism is grown on ascospore medium (p. 443) and stained with Kinyon stain (p. 432) or ascospore stain (p. 433).

Lactose	Galactose	Melibiose	Cellobiose	Inositol	Xylose	Raffinose	Trehalose	Dulcitol	KNO₃	Fermentation of:[b]						
										Glucose	Maltose	Sucrose	Lactose	Galactose	Trehalose	Cellobiose
0	+	0	0	0	+^{v} 0^v	0	+ 0^v	0	0	+	+	0	0	V	V	0
0	+	0	+^{v}	0	+	0	+	0	0	+	+	+^{v}	0	+^{v}	+^{v}	0
0	+	0	0	0	+	0	+	0	0	+	0	0	0	V	0	0
0	+	0	+	0	+	0	+	0	0	+	0^v	V	0	+^{v}	V	+
0	+	+	+	0	+	+	+	+	0	+	0	+^{w}	0	+^{w}	+^{w}	0
+^{v}	+	0	+^{v}	0	+^{v}	+	0	0	0	+	0	+	+^{v}	+	0	0
0	+	0	0	0	V	0	0	0	0	0	0	0	0	0	0	0
0	0^v	0	0^v	0	0	0	+	0	0	0^w	0	0	0	0	0^v	0
0	0	0	0	0	0	0	+	0	0	+	0	0	0	0	+^{v}	0
0	0	0	0	0	0	0	0	0	0	+	0	0	0	0	0	0
0	V	0	0	0	0	0	0	0	0	0	0	0	0	0	0	0
0	0	0	0	0	0	+	+	+	0	+	0	+^{w}	0	0	+^{w}	ND
0	+^{v}	0	+	0	+^{v}	+^{v}	+	0	+	+	+	+^{v}	+	0	+^{v}	0^v	V

TABLE 2.4 Characteristics that assist in differentiating *Candida dubliniensis* from *Candida albicans*[a]

Organism	Growth at 42–45°C at 48 h[b]	Chlamydospores on appropriate agar[c]	Colonies on Staib agar[d]	Assimilation at ≤48 h[e]		
				XYL	MDG	TRE
C. dubliniensis	0 or poor	Usually abundant and in pairs or small clusters	Rough; may have hyphal fringe	0	0	0[v]
C. albicans	+[v]	Usually single, very occasionally in pairs or small clusters	Smooth, shiny	+[v]	+[v]	+

[a] Variability has been reported in all of the above tests; there is no single phenotypic test that can reliably discriminate *C. dubliniensis* from *C. albicans*. It is advisable to perform several of the tests simultaneously. Abbreviations: XYL, xylose; MDG, α-methyl-D-glucoside; TRE, trehalose; +, positive; 0, negative; V, variable.

[b] Inoculate isolate onto two Sabouraud dextrose agar slants or plates; incubate one at 42–45°C and the other at 37°C (as a comparative growth control). *C. albicans* grows well at the higher temperatures, but often at a slower rate. It is essential that the temperature of the incubator be carefully controlled to ensure accuracy.

[c] Media used for the production of chlamydospores (room temperature): cornmeal-Tween 80 agar, Tween 80-oxgall-caffeic acid agar, rice agar Tween. Clusters of chlamydospores are best seen on primary isolates; storage of isolate may diminish chlamydospore production.

[d] Inoculate a Staib agar (p. 448) plate for isolated colonies and incubate at 30°C for 48–72 h; see Al Mosaid et al., 2001.

[e] The assimilation results refer only to commercial rapid miniature systems, not to the conventional Wickerham tube method. Commercial databases may not be updated; therefore, the individual significant substrate reactions must be examined. For further information on the various commercial systems and their ability to identify *C. dubliniensis*, see Pincus et al., 1999.

Candida tropicalis

PATHOGENICITY: As is true of many species of *Candida* and other yeasts, *C. tropicalis* is known to cause infection, especially in immunocompromised, predisposed patients, as discussed on pp. 121–122. It is especially virulent in neutropenic patients with leukemia or other hematological malignancies. It is also recovered from mucosal sites without evidence of disease.

RATE OF GROWTH: Rapid; mature within 5 days.

COLONY MORPHOLOGY: Creamy; near the edge it may be wrinkled or have a slight mycelial fringe. Colonies are metallic blue on CHROMagar Candida. (Image Appendix Figure 38.)

MICROSCOPIC MORPHOLOGY: On routine primary media, yeast cells are round to oval (3.5–7 × 5.5–10 μm). On cornmeal-Tween 80 agar at 25°C for 72 h, *C. tropicalis* forms blastoconidia singly or in very small groups along long pseudohyphae. True hyphae may also be present. A few teardrop-shaped chlamydospores may rarely be produced.

See Table 2.2 (p. 124) for differentiation of yeasts and yeastlike genera and Table 2.3 (p. 126) for characteristics of the most commonly encountered species of *Candida*.

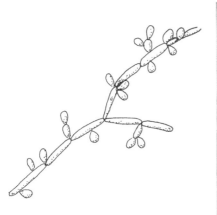 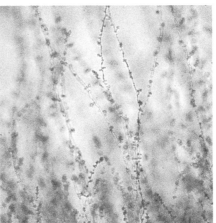

For further information, see
Odds and Bernaerts, 1994
Zuza-Alves et al., 2017

Candida parapsilosis species complex

TAXONOMY NOTES: The species complex includes *Candida metapsilosis*, *C. orthopsilosis*, and *C. parapsilosis sensu stricto*. These species are difficult to differentiate phenotypically. *Lodderomyces elongisporus* is a closely related species that can be misidentified as *C. parapsilosis* using phenotypic methods; however, *L. elongisporus* exhibits a unique turquoise color on CHROMagar Candida medium.

PATHOGENICITY: Known to cause infections in particularly susceptible individuals, as discussed on pp. 121–122. It is the second most common agent of fungal endocarditis (*Candida albicans* being the most common). It is also frequently responsible for invasive fungal infections in neonates. The MICs of echinocandins are elevated in *C. parapsilosis* compared to other *Candida* species, although no clinical studies have demonstrated superiority of fluconazole over echinocandins for treatment of *C. parapsilosis* infections. Additionally, observational data demonstrate no difference in outcome among patients with *C. parapsilosis* candidemia who received initial treatment with an echinocandin compared to those who received other regimens.

RATE OF GROWTH: Rapid; mature within 5 days.

COLONY MORPHOLOGY: Creamy, sometimes developing a lacy appearance.

MICROSCOPIC MORPHOLOGY: On routine primary media, yeast cells are ovoid (2.5–4 × 3–8 μm). On cornmeal-Tween 80 agar at 25°C for 72 h, blastoconidia, singly or in small clusters, are seen along the pseudohyphae. Outstanding characteristics are the crooked or curved appearance of relatively short pseudohyphae (compared to those of *Candida tropicalis*) and the occasional presence of large hyphal elements called giant cells.

See Table 2.2 (p. 124) for differentiation of yeasts and yeastlike genera and Table 2.3 (p. 126) for characteristics of the most commonly encountered species of *Candida*.

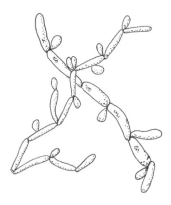 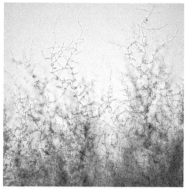

For further information, see
Al-Obaid et al., 2018
Baddley et al., 2008
Pammi et al., 2013
Pappas et al., 2016
Tavanti et al., 2005

Candida lusitaniae

TAXONOMY NOTES: *Candida lusitaniae* (anamorph) is currently recognized as *Clavispora lusitaniae* (teleomorph). It is recommended *Candida lusitianiae* is reported.

PATHOGENICITY: Encountered as an opportunistic pathogen in immunocompromised patients. *C. lusitaniae* does not appear to exhibit intrinsic resistance to antifungals, including amphotericin B, but can readily develop multidrug resistance to different antifungal classes (polyenes, azoles, and echinocandins) upon treatment.

RATE OF GROWTH: Rapid; mature within 5 days.

COLONY MORPHOLOGY: Cream colored, smooth, glistening.

MICROSCOPIC MORPHOLOGY: On routine primary media, yeast cells are round to oval (2–6 × 3–10 μm). On cornmeal-Tween 80 agar at 25°C for 72 h, pseudohyphae are slender, branched, and curved with short chains of elongate blastoconidia. Morphologically *C. lusitaniae* resembles *Candida tropicalis* and *Candida parapsilosis* but differs in its ability to ferment cellobiose and usually to assimilate rhamnose.

See Table 2.2 (p. 124) for differentiation of yeasts and yeastlike genera and Table 2.3 (p. 126) for characteristics of the most commonly encountered species of *Candida*.

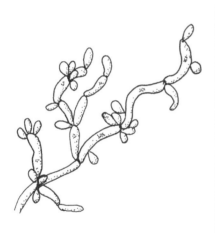
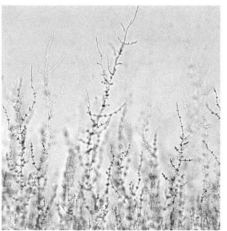

For further information, see
Asner et al., 2015
Borman et al., 2020
Kannan et al., 2019
Rodrigues de Miranda, 1979

Candida krusei

TAXONOMY NOTES: *Candida krusei* (anamorph) is currently recognized as *Pichia kudriavzevii* (teleomorph). It is recommended *C. krusei* is reported. *Issatchenkia orientalis* is a former name.

PATHOGENICITY: Known to cause infections in particularly susceptible individuals, as discussed on pp. 121–122. It is considered to be innately resistant to fluconazole.

RATE OF GROWTH: Rapid; mature within 5 days.

COLONY MORPHOLOGY: Flat, dry, dull, developing a mycelial fringe. Cream colored. On CHROMagar Candida agar, colonies are rough with a pink center and white border. (Image Appendix Figure 38.)

MICROSCOPIC MORPHOLOGY: On routine primary media, yeast cells are round to oval or elongate (2–6 × 4–10 µm). On cornmeal-Tween 80 agar at 25°C for 72 h, *C. krusei* forms pseudohyphae with elongate blastoconidia forming a cross-matchsticks or treelike appearance. The formations may be confused with the annellides of *Magnusiomyces capitatus* (formerly *Blastoschizomyces capitatus* [p. 166]); see Table 2.5 (p. 134) for the differentiation of these two yeasts.

Although the biochemical profiles of *Candida inconspicua* and *Candida norvegensis* are extremely similar to that of *C. krusei*, they can be distinguished by the characteristics in Table 2.6 (p. 134).

See Table 2.2 (p. 124) for differentiation of yeasts and yeastlike genera and Table 2.3 (p. 126) for characteristics of the most commonly encountered species of *Candida*.

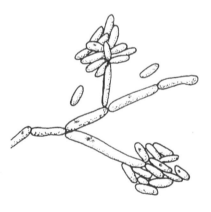
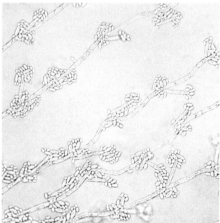

Candida krusei (continued)

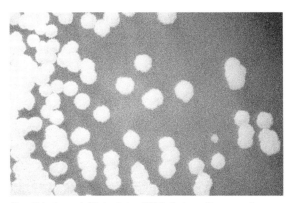

Candida krusei. SDA plate, 30°C, 2 days. Dry, rough colonies.

For further information, see
Borman et al., 2020
Odds and Bernaerts, 1994

TABLE 2.5 Differentiating characteristics of *Magnusiomyces capitatus* (formerly *Blastoschizomyces capitatus*) versus *Candida krusei*[a]

Organism	Growth with cycloheximide	Galactose assimilation	Glucose fermentation	Urease	Conidia
M. capitatus (formerly *B. capitatus*)	+	+	0	0	Annelloconidia
C. krusei	0	0	+	+[V]	Blastoconidia

[a] Abbreviations: +, positive; 0, negative; V, variable.

TABLE 2.6 Differentiating characteristics of *Candida krusei*, *Candida inconspicua*, and *Candida norvegensis*[a]

Organism	Colonies on CHROMagar Candida	Pseudohyphae on cornmeal-Tween 80 agar	Growth on Trichophyton agar #1[b]	Fermentation of glucose	Assimilation of cellobiose	Esculin hydrolysis
C. krusei	Rough; pink center with white border	+	+	+	0	0
C. inconspicua	May resemble *C. krusei*	0 Short chains of oval cells may form	0[c]	0	0	0
C. norvegensis	May resemble *C. krusei*	0[V] Pseudohyphae may form	0	+[D]	+	+

[a] All three of these species show resistance to fluconazole. If definitive identification of *C. inconspicua* versus *C. norvegensis* is required, molecular analysis is recommended. Abbreviations: +, positive; 0, negative; V, variable; D, delayed/slow.

[b] Casein agar, vitamin free (p. 451).

[c] May grow after an initial lag period.

Candida kefyr

TAXONOMY NOTES: *Candida kefyr* (anamorph) is currently recognized as *Kluyveromyces marxianus* (teleomorph). It is recommended *Candida kefyr* is reported. *Candida pseudotropicalis* is a former name.

PATHOGENICITY: Occasionally causes infection in particularly susceptible individuals, as discussed on pp. 121–122.

RATE OF GROWTH: Rapid; mature within 5 days.

COLONY MORPHOLOGY: Smooth, white to cream colored.

MICROSCOPIC MORPHOLOGY: On routine primary media, yeast cells are round to oval (3–8 × 5–12 μm). On cornmeal-Tween 80 agar at 25°C for 72 h, *C. kefyr* forms pseudohyphae with elongate blastoconidia that characteristically line up in parallel, giving the appearance of logs in a stream.

See Table 2.2 (p. 124) for differentiation of yeasts and yeastlike genera and Table 2.3 (p. 126) for characteristics of the most commonly encountered species of *Candida*.

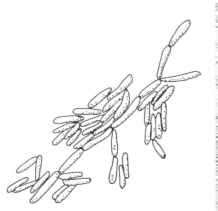
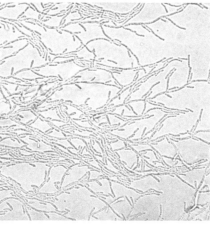

Candida rugosa species complex

TAXONOMY NOTES: The species complex includes *Candida mesorugosa*, *C. neorugosa*, *C. pararugosa*, *C. pseudorugosa*, and *C. rugosa sensu stricto*. With the exception of *C. pararugosa* (which has been reclassified as *Wickerhamiella pararugosa*), members are currently recognized as *Diutina mesorugosa*, *D. neorugosa*, *D. pseudorugosa*, and *D. rugosa sensu stricto*. Despite transfer to these genera, it is recommended the ana-morph *Candida* name is reported. While *C. pseudorugosa* and *C. rugosa* may be differentiated biochemically, the other species are not using conventional culture-based biochemical methods.

PATHOGENICITY: Initially known as a major cause of mastitis in cattle. Now consid-ered an emerging fungal pathogen in humans; occasionally reported in individual cases as well as in outbreaks of central venous catheter-related candidemia and urinary tract infections, especially in burn and trauma centers. Variable *in vitro* antifungal suscepti-bility results have been described in the literature, and appear to be related to differ-ences between members of the complex and possibly geographic variations. Therefore, antifungal susceptibility testing of clinically significant isolates is usually necessary.

RATE OF GROWTH: Rapid; mature within 5 days.

COLONY MORPHOLOGY: White to cream colored, dry, often wrinkled, may have myce-lial fringe. Unique in forming dry, fairly rough, blue-green colonies with a white border when grown on CHROMagar Candida agar.

MICROSCOPIC MORPHOLOGY: On routine primary media, budding yeast cells are oval to almost cylindrical (2.0–3.5 × 6–12 µm). On cornmeal-Tween 80 agar at 25°C for 72 h, *C. rugosa* forms pseudohyphae (sometimes short) with elongate blastoconidia, some in chains.

See Table 2.2 (p. 124) for differentiation of yeasts and yeastlike genera and Table 2.3 (p. 126) for characteristics of the most commonly encountered species of *Candida*.

Candida rugosa species complex (continued)

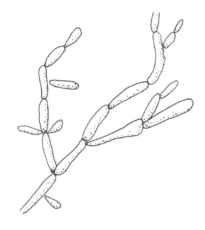 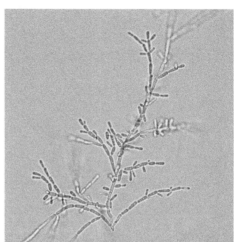

For further information, see

Colombo et al., 2007
Hospenthal et al., 2006
Khunnamwong et al., 2015
Padovan et al., 2013
Pérez-Hansen et al., 2019
Pfaller et al., 2006

Candida guilliermondii species complex

TAXONOMY NOTES: The species complex includes *Candida carpophila, C. guilliermondii sensu stricto,* and *C. fermentati. C. carpophila* and *C. guilliermondii sensu stricto* have been transferred to the genus *Meyerozyma* (teleomorph), and are currently recognized as *Meyerozyma carpophila* and *M. guilliermondii,* respectively. Despite transfer to the genus *Meyerozyma,* it is recommended the anamorph *Candida* name is reported. These species are difficult to differentiate phenotypically.

PATHOGENICITY: Has occasionally been reported to cause endocarditis, osteomyelitis, cutaneous and urinary tract infections, and disseminated disease. Infections can be fatal in immunocompromised patients. Infects particularly susceptible individuals, as described on pp. 121–122.

RATE OF GROWTH: Rapid; mature within 5 days.

COLONY MORPHOLOGY: Flat, glossy, smooth edged, and usually cream colored but may become tan or pinkish with age.

MICROSCOPIC MORPHOLOGY: On routine primary media, yeast cells are ovoid to elongate (2–5 × 3–7 μm). On cornmeal-Tween 80 agar at 25°C for 72 h, *C. guilliermondii* forms clusters of yeast cells with relatively few, short pseudohyphae often having small groups of blastoconidia at the septa. True hyphae are not produced.

See Table 2.2 (p. 124) for differentiation of yeasts and yeastlike genera, Table 2.3 (p. 126) for characteristics of the most commonly encountered species of *Candida,* and Table 2.7 (p. 139) for distinguishing *C. guilliermondii* from *Candida famata.*

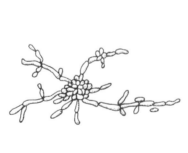 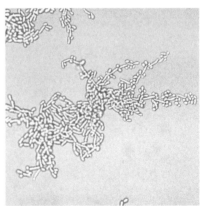

For further information, see
Borman and Johnson, 2021
Girmenia et al., 2006
Kurtzman and Suzuki, 2010
Savini et al., 2011
Vaughan-Martini et al., 2005

TABLE 2.7 Differentiating characteristics of *Candida guilliermondii* versus *Candida famata*[a]

Organism	Shape of cell	Growth at 37°C	Growth at 42°C	Pseudohyphae on cornmeal-Tween 80 agar	Glucose fermentation
C. guilliermondii	Ovoid or elongate	+	V	V (often short, primitive)	+
C. famata	Round	V	0	0	0^w

[a] Commercial identification systems often show results with low discrimination between these species. Abbreviations: +, positive; 0, negative; V, variable; W, weak.

Candida lipolytica

TAXONOMY NOTES: *Candida lipolytica* (anamorph) is currently recognized as *Yarrowia lipolytica* (teleomorph). It is recommended *C. lipolytica* is reported.

PATHOGENICITY: A rarely encountered emerging opportunistic pathogen; may cause candidemia and other disease in immunocompromised patients, as discussed on pp. 121–122.

RATE OF GROWTH: Moderate; mature within 6–10 days.

COLONY MORPHOLOGY: Smooth, may be delicately wrinkled, white to cream colored.

MICROSCOPIC MORPHOLOGY: On routine primary media, yeast cells are round to oval or elongate (3–6 × 4–16 µm). On cornmeal-Tween 80 agar at 25°C for 72 h, pseudohyphae and septate true hyphae bearing elongate blastoconidia in short chains form and produce a stark, branching appearance. Arthroconidia may be present. *C. lipolytica* physiologically resembles *Candida krusei* but clearly differs by growing in the presence of cycloheximide and not fermenting glucose (in addition to the morphologic differences).

The teleomorph (sexual state) may appear on culture. It produces round to oval asci (5–8 × 6–15 µm) near the septa of the hyphae; the asci usually contain two ascospores, 3–4 × 3.5–6 µm.

See Table 2.2 (p. 124) for differentiation of yeasts and yeastlike genera and Table 2.3 (p. 126) for characteristics of the most commonly encountered species of *Candida*.

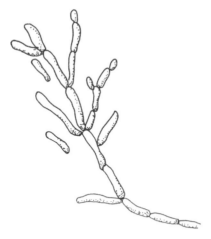
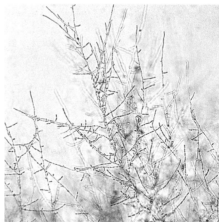

For further information, see
D'Antonio et al., 2002
Liu et al., 2013

Candida zeylanoides

PATHOGENICITY: Rarely reported as cause of fungemia, *Candida* arthritis, and skin and nail infections.

RATE OF GROWTH: Rapid; mature within 5 days at 25–30°C; variable growth at 35–37°C.

COLONY MORPHOLOGY: Smooth, dull, cream colored to yellowish.

MICROSCOPIC MORPHOLOGY: On routine primary media, yeast cells are oval to elongate (3–5 × 6–11 μm). On cornmeal-Tween 80 agar at 25°C for 72 h, pseudohyphae consist of cells that are frequently curved and bear oval or elongate blastoconidia singly and in small clusters and short chains. More blastoconidia are formed at the beginnings of the pseudohyphae than at the distal ends, creating a featherlike appearance at low power.

See Table 2.2 (p. 124) for differentiation of yeasts and yeastlike genera and Table 2.3 (p. 126) for characteristics of the most commonly encountered species of *Candida*.

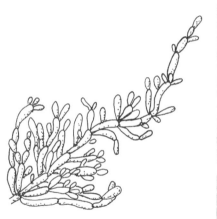 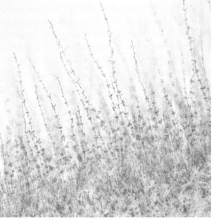

For further information, see
Levenson et al., 1991

Candida glabrata species complex

TAXONOMY NOTES: The species complex includes *Candida bracarensis*, *C. glabrata sensu stricto*, and *C. nivariensis*. These species are difficult to differentiate phenotypically. The genus name has been changed to *Nakaseomyces* (teleomorph). Despite this change, it is recommended the anamorph *Candida* name is reported. *Torulopsis glabrata* is a former name.

PATHOGENICITY: Causes infections of the bloodstream or urogenital tract and occasionally disseminated disease. A significant number of clinical isolates have shown reduced susceptibility to fluconazole (and other azoles). There are reports of increasing frequency of resistance to echinocandins.

RATE OF GROWTH: Rapid; mature within 5 days; grows a bit more slowly than the other species of *Candida*.

COLONY MORPHOLOGY: Small colonies; pasty, smooth, white to cream.

MICROSCOPIC MORPHOLOGY: On cornmeal-Tween 80 agar at 25°C for 72 h, only small (2–3 × 3–4 μm), oval yeast cells with single terminal budding are seen. No pseudohyphae are formed; on rare occasion a few short chains of ovoid cells may be seen.

See Table 2.2 (p. 124) for differentiation of yeasts and yeastlike genera and Table 2.3 (p. 126) for characteristics of the most commonly encountered species of *Candida*. *C. glabrata* can be quickly identified by the rapid assimilation of trehalose (RAT) test (p. 460). (Image Appendix Figure 39.)

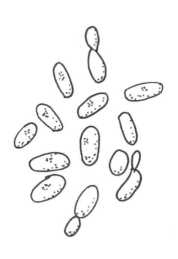
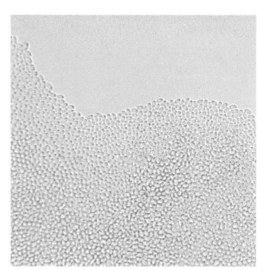

For further information, see
Angoulvant et al., 2016
Colombo et al., 2017
Frías-De-León et al., 2021
Hassan et al., 2021

Candida auris

PATHOGENICITY: Initially recovered from the external ear canal of a patient in a Japanese hospital. Since its initial description in 2009, *C. auris* has emerged globally as a multidrug-resistant pathogen causing candidemia and other forms of deeply invasive candidiasis. It has the propensity to form biofilms and to persist in the hospital environment. Skin colonization allows spread and can lead to invasive infections in colonized patients. Isolates are typically resistant to fluconazole and may have elevated MICs to amphotericin B; some isolates also may be resistant to echinocandins. Infection control measures are important in infected and colonized cases for prevention of nosocomial transmission.

RATE OF GROWTH: Rapid; mature within 5 days. Grows at 25–37°C. Isolates can grow at 40°C, and most strains grow at 42°C, which is a useful differential characteristic. Growth is inhibited by cycloheximide; therefore, it does not grow on Mycosel agar.

COLONY MORPHOLOGY: Cream colored, smooth on Sabouraud dextrose agar and on enriched media. The colonies of isolates on CHROMagar Candida are undistinctive and have a pink to purple color and may become red with extended incubation. A recently formulated chromogenic agar, CHROMgar Candida Plus, permits differentiation of *C. auris* from common clinical *Candida* spp. On this medium, *C. auris* colonies are colored light blue with a light blue halo. There are other rare *Candida* spp. that have the same phenotype. Therefore, results are considered preliminary and should be confirmed.

MICROSCOPIC MORPHOLOGY: In nutrient broth, small, budding, ovoid, elongated, or ellipsoid yeasts measuring ~2–3 by 2.5–5 µm. The budding yeasts may grow as singlets, doublets, or in small clusters. Pseudohyphae and hyphae are not usually formed; however, rudimentary pseudohyphae occasionally may be observed. On cornmeal-Tween 80 agar at 30°C for 72 h, usually yeast cells only are seen, but isolates may very occasionally form short, undeveloped pseudohyphae.

There are no morphological or biochemical features that are sufficiently specific to identify *C. auris*. Instead, the organism may be initially misidentified as *Candida haemulonii*, *Candida duobushaemulonii*, *Candida famata*, *Saccharomyces cerevisiae*, or *Rhodotorula glutinis*. Isolates of *C. haemulonii*, *C. duobushaemulonii*, and suspicious isolates that are not obviously *S. cerevisiae* or *R. glutinis* should be further evaluated by MALDI-TOF MS or DNA sequencing for definitive identification. See Table 2.2 (p. 124) for differentiation of yeasts and yeastlike genera and Table 2.3 (p. 126) for characteristics of the most commonly encountered species of *Candida*.

For further information, see
Colombo et al., 2017
de Jong et al., 2021
Du et al., 2021
González-Durán et al., 2022
Jeffery-Smith et al., 2017
Kathuria et al., 2015
Lyman et al., 2021
McCarthy and Walsh, 2017

Mulet Bayona et al., 2022
Satoh et al., 2009
Southwick et al., 2018

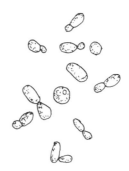

Candida haemulonii species complex

TAXONOMY NOTES: The species complex includes *Candida duobushaemulonii*, *C. haemulonii sensu stricto*, and *C. haemulonii* var. *vulnera*. These species are difficult to differentiate phenotypically.

PATHOGENICITY: Increasingly recognized cause of fungemia and deeply invasive candidiasis. Isolates have elevated fluconazole MICs and can have high amphotericin B MICs.

RATE OF GROWTH: Rapid; mature within 5 days. Isolates can grow at 35°C but not at 42°C, and are not inhibited by cycloheximide and therefore grow on Mycosel agar.

COLONY MORPHOLOGY: On routine primary media, colonies are white to cream colored, smooth, and glabrous. Colonies on CHROMagar Candida are pink at 24 h and develop a darker violet center at 72 h. This is not unique to *C. haemulonii*, *C. glabrata* may also become violet after 3–4 days' incubation, and *C. auris* can be somewhat similar.

MICROSCOPIC MORPHOLOGY: On routine primary media, budding yeast cells are round to oval (3–5 × 3–6.5 μm). On cornmeal-Tween 80 agar at 25°C for 72 h, yeast cells are seen; true hyphae are absent; pseudohyphae are usually absent but may appear in fragmentary forms. Any clinically significant isolate of a member of the *C. haemulonii* species complex identified using biochemical methods should be confirmed by MALDI-TOF MS or DNA sequencing.

For further information, see
Cendejas-Bueno et al., 2012
Colombo et al., 2017
Kathuria et al., 2015

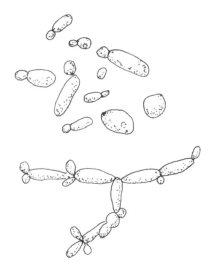

Candida pelliculosa

TAXONOMY NOTES: *Candida pelliculosa* (anamorph) is currently recognized as *Wickerhamomyces anomalus* (teleomorph). It is recommended *C. pelliculosa* is reported. *Hansenula anomala* and *Pichia anomala* are former names.

PATHOGENICITY: Occasionally causes infection in predisposed patients. Commonly encountered as a saprobe.

RATE OF GROWTH: Rapid; mature within 5 days.

COLONY MORPHOLOGY: Smooth, moist, cream colored.

MICROSCOPIC MORPHOLOGY: On cornmeal-Tween 80 agar at 25°C for 72 h, budding yeast cells are seen (2–4 × 2–6 µm). Pseudohyphae form in some isolates. In the sexual state, when cultured on ascospore medium (p. 443) and stained with Kinyoun (p. 432) or ascospore (p. 433) stain, one to four ascospores per ascus are seen. There is a brim that turns downward around each ascospore, giving the impression of a helmet or hat.

See Tables 2.2 (p. 124) and 2.9 (p. 151) for identification of yeasts and yeastlike fungi.

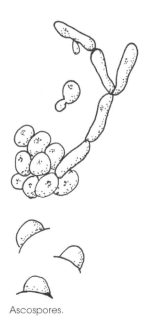

Ascospores.

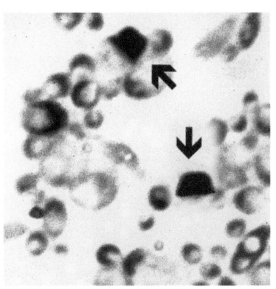

Arrows point to ascospores.

Candida pelliculosa (continued)

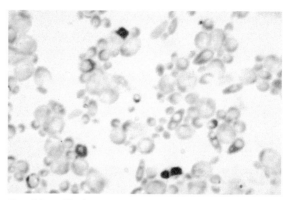

Candida pelliculosa. Kinyoun stain of ascospores (red) after growth on ascospore agar. Note brimmed-hat shape of ascospores.

Cryptococcus neoformans species complex

TAXONOMY NOTES: The species complex includes *Cryptococcus neoformans sensu stricto* (formerly *C. neoformans* var. *grubii* [serotype A]) and *C. deneoformans* (formerly *C. neoformans* var. *neoformans* [serotype D]). These species are difficult to differentiate phenotypically.

PATHOGENICITY: Causes cryptococcosis, a subacute or chronic infection most frequently involving the tissue of the central nervous system but occasionally producing lesions in the skin, bones, lungs, or other internal organs. Meningitis due to *C. neoformans* is extremely common in HIV/AIDS patients. With the exception of *C. gattii* (p. 149), the other species of this genus (or former members of the genus) are commonly considered nonpathogenic and only occasionally cause disease in severely immunosuppressed patients. The most common environmental source of *C. neoformans* is pigeon droppings. *C. neoformans* is intrinsically resistant to echinocandins but susceptible to amphotericin B, triazoles, and flucytosine.

RATE OF GROWTH: Rapid; mature within 5 days.

COLONY MORPHOLOGY: Colonies are flat or slightly heaped, shiny, moist, and usually mucoid, with smooth edges. Color is cream at first, later becoming tannish. Usually grows equally well at 25 and 37°C, whereas other members, or former members, of the genus will not grow well, if at all, at 37°C. Produces brown colonies on birdseed (or similar) agar (p. 448).

MICROSCOPIC MORPHOLOGY: On cornmeal-Tween 80 agar at 25°C for 72 h, cells (4–8 µm in diameter) are round, dark walled, and budding. Usually no hyphae are seen. Capsules are often discernible on cornmeal-Tween 80 by the spaces (due to capsular material) between the yeast cells. The capsules are best demonstrated with an India ink preparation (p. 414). Production of capsular material may be increased by growth in 1% peptone solution. Some strains of *C. neoformans*, as well as other cryptococci, may not produce apparent capsules *in vitro*.

See Table 2.2 (p. 124) for differentiation of yeasts and yeastlike genera and Table 2.8 (p. 150) for characteristics of *Cryptococcus* spp. and former members of the genus. *C. neoformans* and *C. gattii* can be rapidly differentiated from other species of *Cryptococcus* by the caffeic acid test (p. 426). (Image Appendix Figure 40.) *C. neoformans* can be differentiated from *C. gattii* with the use of canavanine glycine bromothymol blue (CGB) agar (p. 450).

Cryptococcus neoformans species complex *(continued)*

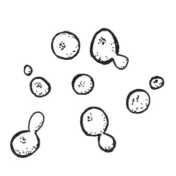

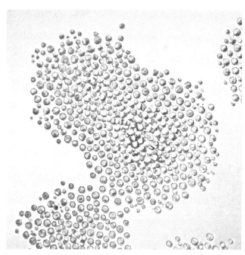

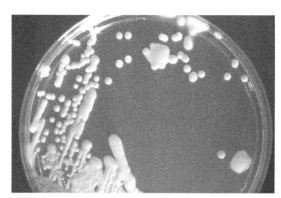

Cryptococcus neoformans. SDA plate, 30°C, 3 days. Note mucoid nature of colonies.

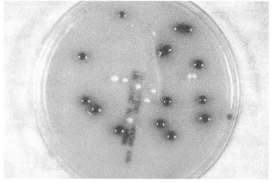

Birdseed agar. Room temperature, 3 days. The brown colonies could be *C. neoformans* or *C. gattii* (see p. 448).

For further information, see
Borman et al., 2020
Fera et al., 2009
Gushiken et al., 2021
Hagen et al., 2015
Klein et al., 2009
Kwon-Chung et al., 2017
Morales-López and Garcia-Effron, 2021

Cryptococcus gattii species complex

TAXONOMY NOTES: The species complex includes *Cryptococcus bacillisporus*, *C. deca-gattii*, *C. deuterogattii*, *C. gattii sensu stricto*, and *C. tetragattii*. The complex encompasses serotypes B and C. These species are difficult to differentiate phenotypically.

PATHOGENICITY: Similar to that of *C. neoformans* (p. 147). Infection in immunocompetent persons and development of cryptococcomas (mass lesions) in lung and brain are far more commonly associated with *C. gattii* than with *C. neoformans*. Infections occur most commonly in tropical, subtropical, and temperate regions; have been most numerous in Australia, Papua New Guinea, British Columbia, and the Pacific Northwest region of the United States. However, a wider geographic range of infections caused by *C. gattii* is increasingly recognized. Its preferred ecologic niche is decayed hollows and surfaces of a variety of trees throughout the world; it has been recovered from wood products, soil, water, air, various mammals, and other sources. *C. gattii* is intrinsically resistant to echinocandins.

RATE OF GROWTH: Rapid; mature within 5 days.

COLONY MORPHOLOGY: Same as that of *C. neoformans* (p. 147).

MICROSCOPIC MORPHOLOGY: Similar to *C. neoformans* (p. 147), but in addition to round yeast cells, some more oval ones commonly form.

The major phenotypic method for differentiation of *C. gattii* from *C. neoformans* is the use of CGB agar (p. 450). *C. gattii* grows on CGB medium and turns the agar blue; *C. neoformans* does not grow on the medium, and the color of the agar remains unchanged (yellow). As treatment for both species is essentially the same, differentiation is often not required.

See Table 2.2 (p. 124) for differentiation of yeasts and yeastlike genera and Table 2.8 (p. 150) for characteristics of *Cryptococcus* spp. and former members of the genus. *C. neoformans* and *C. gattii* can be rapidly differentiated from other species of *Cryptococcus* by the caffeic acid test (p. 426). (Image Appendix Figure 40.)

As *C. gattii* is considered morphologically indistinguishable from *C. neoformans*, see images on p. 148.

For further information, see

Chen et al., 2014
Gushiken et al., 2021
Hagen et al., 2015
Klein et al., 2009
Kwon-Chung et al., 2017
Trilles et al., 2004

TABLE 2.8 Characteristics of *Cryptococcus* spp. and former members of the genus[a]

Organism	Phenol oxidase production[b]	Growth at 37°C on SDA	Growth with cyclo-heximide at 25°C	Pseudo-hyphae (short)	Urease (25°C; 4 days)	Assimilation of:													Fermentation
						Glucose	Maltose	Sucrose	Lactose	Galactose	Melibiose	Cellobiose	Inositol	Xylose	Raffinose	Trehalose	Dulcitol	KNO₃	
C. neoformans and *C. gattii*	+	+	0	0^R	+	+	+	+	0	+	0	+^v	+	+	+^v	+	+	0	All species lack fermentative ability
C. uniguttulatus[c]	0	0	0	0	+	+	+	+	0	0^v	0	0^v	+	+	+^v	+^v	0	0	
Naganishia albida (formerly *C. albidus* var. *albidus*)	0	0^v	0	+^v	+	+	+	+	+^v	0^v	0^v	+	+	+	+^w	+^v	+^v	+	
Naganishia diffluens (formerly *C. albidus* var. *diffluens*)	0	0^v	0	0^v	+	+	+	+	0	0^v	+^v	+	+	+	+^w	+	+^v	+	
Papiliotrema laurentii (formerly *C. laurentii*)	0	0	0^v	0	+	+	+	+	+	+	+^v	+	+	+	+^v	+^v	+	0	
Hannaella luteola (formerly *C. luteolus*)	0	0	0	0	+	+	+	+	0^v	+	+	+	+	+	+	+	+^v	0	
Solicoccozyma terrea (formerly *C. terreus*)	0	V	0	0^v	+	+	+^v	0^v	V	+^v	+^w	+	+	+	0	+^v	V	+	
Goffeauzyma gastrica (formerly *C. gastricus*)	0	0	0	0	+	+	+	0^v	0^v	+	0	+	+	+	0	+	0	0	

[a] Abbreviations: SDA, Sabouraud dextrose agar; +, positive; 0, negative; V, strain variation; R, occur rarely; W, reaction may be weak.

[b] The caffeic acid disk test (p. 426) is the preferred method for rapid and sensitive detection of phenoloxidase production. Birdseed agar (p. 448) is an alternative method, but results are significantly delayed.

[c] *Cryptococcus uniguttulatus* is currently recognized as *Cryptococcus neoformans* var. *uniguttulatus*, but *Cryptococcus uniguttulatus* will be used in this text.

TABLE 2.9 Characteristics of yeasts and yeastlike organisms other than *Candida* spp. and *Cryptococcus* spp.[a]

Organism	Microscopic morphology on cornmeal-Tween 80 agar at 25°C	Growth at 37°C	Ascospores	Urease (25°C; 4 days)	Assimilation of: Glucose	Maltose	Sucrose	Lactose	Galactose	Melibiose	Cellobiose	Inositol	Xylose	Raffinose	Trehalose	Dulcitol	KNO₃	Fermentation of: Glucose	Maltose	Sucrose	Lactose	Galactose	Trehalose	Cellobiose
Saccharomyces cerevisiae	Occasional short pseudohyphae	V	+	0	+	$+^v$	+	0	$+^v$	V	0	0	0	+	$+^v$	0	0	+	V	+	0	V	$+^v$	0
Geotrichum candidum	True hyphae, arthroconidia; no blastoconidia	0^v	0	0	+	0	0	0	+	0	0	0	+	0	0	0	0	0	0	0	0	0	0	0
Magnusiomyces capitatus (formerly *Blastoschizomyces capitatus*)[b]	Pseudohyphae and true hyphae; annelloconidia; few arthroconidia	+	0	0	+	0	0	0	+	0	0	0	0	0	0	0	0	0	0	0	0	0	0	0
Trichosporon spp. and *Cutaneotrichosporon* spp. (see Table 2.10 [p. 165])	Pseudohyphae and true hyphae; arthroconidia; blastoconidia	$+^v$	0	+	+	$+^v$	$+^v$	+	$+^v$	$+^v$	$+^v$	$+^v$	+	$+^v$	$+^v$	$+^v$	0	0	0	0	0	0	0	0
Rhodotorula mucilaginosa	Usually no pseudohyphae	+	0	+	+	V	+	0	V	0	V	0	+	+	+	0	0	0	0	0	0	0	0	0
Rhodotorula glutinis	Usually no pseudohyphae	V	0	+	+	+	+	0	V	0	V	0	V	$+^v$	+	+	+	0	0	0	0	0	0	0
Cystobasidium minutum (formerly *Rhodotorula minuta*)	No pseudohyphae	V	0	+	+	0	+	V	V	0	V	0	+	0	+	0	0	0	0	0	0	0	0	0
Sporobolomyces salmonicolor	Ballistoconidia; various amounts of true and pseudohyphae	V	0	+	+	V	+	0	V	0	V	0	$+^w$	V	+	0	+	0	0	0	0	0	0	0
Malassezia pachydermatis	Usually no hyphae	+	0	+	+	0	0	0	0	0	0	0	0	0	0	0	0	0	0	0	0	0	0	0
Prototheca wickerhamii	Sporangia; no hyphae	$+^v$	0	0	+	0	0	0	$+^v$	0	0	0	0	0	+	0	0	0	0	0	0	0	0	0
Prototheca zopfii		$+^v$	0	0	+	0	0	0	0^v	0	0	0	0	0	0	0	0	0	0	0	0	0	0	0
Prototheca stagnora		0	0	0	+	0	V	0	+	0	0	0	0	0	0	0	0	0	0	0	0	0	0	0

[a] Abbreviations: SDA, Sabouraud dextrose agar; +, positive; 0, negative; V, strain variation; W, reaction may be weak.

[b] Annelloconidia forming clusters at the ends of hyphae of *Magnusiomyces capitatus* (formerly *Blastoschizomyces capitatus*) may resemble the elongated blastoconidia of *Candida krusei*.

PART II Identification of Fungi in Culture

YEASTS AND YEASTLIKE ORGANISMS

Rhodotorula and *Cystobasidium* spp.

TAXONOMY NOTES: *Rhodotorula mucilaginosa*, *R. glutinis*, and *R. minuta* are the major clinically relevant species. *R. mucilaginosa* and *R. glutinis* are retained in the genus *Rhodotorula*, while *R. minuta* is currently recognized as *Cystobasidium minutum*.

PATHOGENICITY: Commonly known as contaminants, but they have increasingly been agents of severe infections, mostly fungemia in immunosuppressed patients with central venous catheters. Endocarditis, peritonitis, meningitis, endophthalmitis, and other infections have been reported to a lesser extent. They are intrinsically resistant to echinocandins and fluconazole.

RATE OF GROWTH: Rapid; mature within 5 days.

COLONY MORPHOLOGY: Usually pink to coral, but can also be more orange to red. Colony is soft, smooth, moist, and sometimes mucoid.

MICROSCOPIC MORPHOLOGY: On cornmeal-Tween 80 agar at 25°C for 72 h, budding cells are round to oval or elongate (2.5–5 × 3–10 μm); occasionally a few rudimentary pseudohyphae are seen. A capsule is sometimes formed.

See Tables 2.2 (p. 124) and 2.9 (p. 151) for differentiation of yeast and yeastlike fungi.

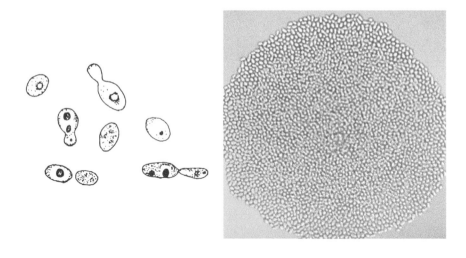

Rhodotorula and *Cystobasidium* spp. *(continued)*

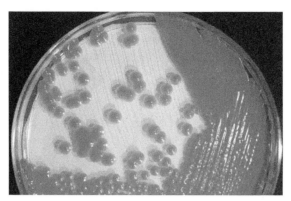

Rhodotorula sp. SDA, 30°C, 3 days.

For further information, see

Borman et al., 2020
Chen et al., 2021b
Diekema et al., 2005
Ioannou et al., 2019
Fera et al., 2009
Wang et al., 2015

Sporobolomyces salmonicolor

PATHOGENICITY: Most commonly isolated from environmental sources. Seldom reported as the cause of fungemia in immunocompromised patients.

RATE OF GROWTH: Rapid; mature within 5 days. Best growth is at 25–30°C; may not grow well at 35–37°C.

COLONY MORPHOLOGY: Smooth to slightly rough; characteristic salmon pink/coral color resembles that of *Rhodotorula* spp. (p. 152). Satellite colonies eventually form around the original colonies due to production of ballistoconidia. Ballistoconidia can be best demonstrated by taping an inoculated cornmeal agar plate face to face to an uninoculated cornmeal plate. After extended incubation at 25°C, with the inoculated plate on top, the ballistoconidia that are shot off the inoculated plate will form a mirror image of the colonies on the other plate.

MICROSCOPIC MORPHOLOGY: On cornmeal-Tween 80 agar at 25°C, oval to elongate yeast cells (2–12 × 3–35 μm) are seen; pseudohyphae and true hyphae may be absent or abundant. Kidney-shaped ballistoconidia (3–5 × 5–12 μm) are produced on denticles; they are forcibly discharged, forming the satellite colonies.

See Tables 2.2 (p. 124) and 2.9 (p. 151) for differentiation of yeasts and yeastlike fungi.

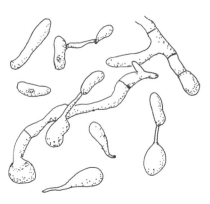
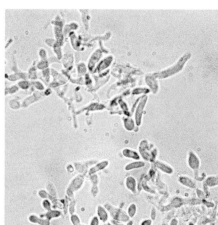

Sporobolomyces salmonicolor (continued)

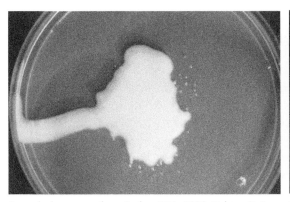

Sporobolomyces salmonicolor. SDA, 30°C, 5 days. Note small satelliting colonies (due to ballistoconidia).

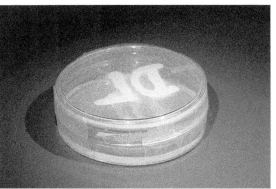

SDA plates taped together to best demonstrate ballistoconidia formation.

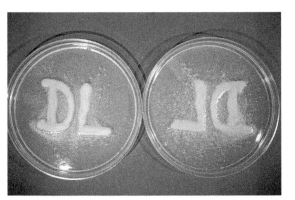

SDA plates separated after being taped together for 5 days at room temperature. Note mirror-image colonies of *S. salmonicolor* formed by ballistoconidia.

For further information, see
Chen et al., 2021b
Wang et al., 2015

Saccharomyces cerevisiae

PATHOGENICITY: Previously seldom known to cause disease, but it is increasingly reported as an agent of invasive infection in a wide range of body sites; most significant is fungemia in immunocompromised or critically ill patients, as well as some relatively healthy patients. Many patients with infection caused by *Saccharomyces cerevisiae* have a history of receiving the probiotic *Saccharomyces cerevisiae* subtype *boulardii* for prophylaxis or treatment of antibiotic-associated diarrhea. Nosocomial spread of this organism to patients not being administered the probiotic also occurs; this appears to be due to the organism entering the environment when capsules or packets of the yeast are opened for deposit into the nasogastric tube of a patient being treated. The organism has been shown to persist in the environment; subsequent central vascular catheter hub or insertion-site contamination is the likely route of entry into the bloodstream of patients in the affected locale.

RATE OF GROWTH: Rapid; mature within 5 days.

COLONY MORPHOLOGY: Smooth colonies, moist, white to cream colored.

MICROSCOPIC MORPHOLOGY: On cornmeal-Tween 80 agar at 25°C for 72 h, round to oval yeast cells (3–8 × 5–10 μm) with multilateral budding are seen. A few very short pseudohyphae may form.

Note: Characteristic roundish ascospores (one to four per ascus) are best demonstrated when the organism is grown on a special medium, such as V-8 medium, acetate ascospore agar, or Gorodkowa medium (p. 443), and stained with ascospore stain (p. 433) or Kinyoun stain (p. 432). Additionally, ascospores are Gram negative, while vegetative cells are Gram positive.

See Tables 2.2 (p. 124) and 2.9 (p. 151) for differentiation of yeasts and yeastlike organisms.

Saccharomyces cerevisiae (continued)

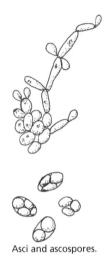

Asci and ascospores.

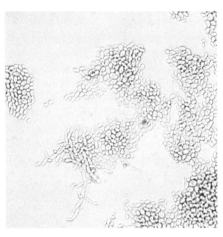

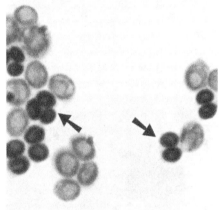

Arrows point to ascospores.

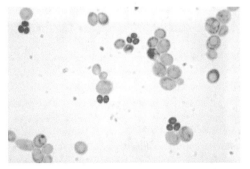

Saccharomyces cerevisiae. Kinyoun stain of
ascospores (red) after growth on ascospore agar.

For further information, see

Chen et al., 2021b

Enache-Angoulvant and Hennequin, 2005

Thygesen et al., 2012

Malassezia spp.

TAXONOMY NOTES: Lipid-dependent *Malassezia* spp. associated with humans include *M. dermatis*, *M. furfur*, *M. globosa*, *M. japonica*, *M. obtusa*, *M. restricta*, *M. slooffiae*, *M. sympodialis*, and *M. yamatoensis*.

PATHOGENICITY: Part of the normal skin microbiota in >90% of adults. Several of the species found on healthy skin are etiologic agents of pityriasis (tinea) versicolor, a superficial infection characterized by pale or dark patches of skin, especially that of the chest, shoulders, and back. They have also been associated with folliculitis, resembling acne, and seborrheic dermatitis, characterized by red, scaly lesions. Catheter-associated sepsis due to *Malassezia* is seen in neonates and adults receiving prolonged intravenous lipids; pulmonary infection may develop in these patients, with respiratory failure in neonates related to propagation of the organism in subendothelial deposits of lipid. The organisms have been isolated from infected areas in a variety of body sites, but their etiologic role is uncertain.

RATE OF GROWTH: Rapid; mature within 5 days at 30–35°C. Grow poorly at 25°C, and some species do not grow well at 37°C; they grow on media containing cycloheximide. The organisms require long-chain fatty acids for growth (*M. pachydermatis* [p. 160] is the exception); solid medium overlaid with a thin film of sterile olive oil is the most common method used (sterile olive oil-saturated disks [p. 426] can be used in place of the overlay method), but more-complex media, such as Leeming-Notman agar (p. 458), are required for growth of some of the clinically significant species (*M. restricta* is the most difficult to cultivate). Blood for culture must be taken through the lipid infusion catheter for best recovery of the organism.

COLONY MORPHOLOGY: Smooth, cream to yellowish brown; often becomes dry, dull, brittle, and wrinkled with age.

MICROSCOPIC MORPHOLOGY: Cells (1.5–4.5 × 3–7 μm) are actually phialides with small collarettes; the collarettes are very difficult to discern with a routine light microscope. The cells of this genus are unique in being round at one end and bluntly cut off at the other, where wide budlike structures form singly; the buds are usually on a broad base, but narrow in some species. Staining with safranin and examining under oil immersion is a simple and effective way to observe the shape of the organism; also, calcofluor white allows for very clear delineation of the cell wall and distinctive outline. Hyphal elements are usually absent, but sparse rudimentary forms may occasionally develop.

Identification to species level is not routinely required but may be useful in cases of fungemia. Phenotypic identification can be achieved, but requires unique media not currently commercially available. If required, referral to a laboratory specializing in medical mycology and/or performing molecular analyses is suggested.

Malassezia spp. *(continued)*

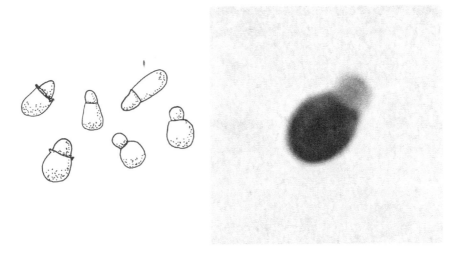

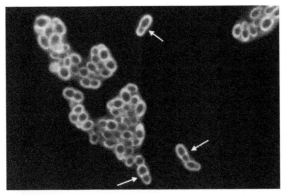

Malassezia sp. Calcofluor white stain of organism from culture. Arrows indicate bluntly cut-off neck at point of conidiation.

For further information, see

Cabañes, 2014
Gaitanis et al., 2012
Velegraki et al., 2015

Malassezia pachydermatis

PATHOGENICITY: More often found in lower animals than in humans, it has been associated with inflammation of the ears of dogs. Occasionally reported to cause human infection, particularly in premature neonates receiving intravenous lipid emulsions. Isolates from patients' cases have been found as colonizers in participant health care workers and their pets.

RATE OF GROWTH: Rapid; mature within 5 days. Best growth is at 35–37°C; weak growth is seen at 25°C. Not inhibited by cycloheximide.

COLONY MORPHOLOGY: Creamy, dull, smooth; at first it is cream colored, becoming buff to orange-beige with age. Addition of fatty acids to the medium is not required for growth.

MICROSCOPIC MORPHOLOGY: Yeast cells are similar to other *Malassezia* spp. (p. 158); they are round to oval (2.5–5.5 × 3.0–6.5 µm); conidia are produced on a broad base at one pole, which develops a collarette. Pseudohyphae and true hyphae are usually absent, occasionally sparsely present. Commercial biochemical yeast identification systems may misidentify this organism as *Candida lipolytica*; examination of microscopic morphology is essential.

See Tables 2.2 (p. 124) and 2.9 (p. 151) for differentiation of yeastlike fungi.

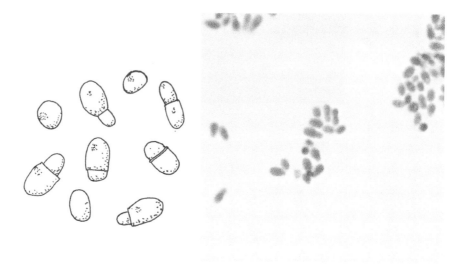

For further information, see

Cabañes, 2014
Gaitanis, 2012
Morris et al., 2005
Velegraki et al., 2015

Ustilago spp.

PATHOGENICITY: Parasitic on seeds and flowers of many cereals and grasses. May cause contamination in cultures. It has seldom been implicated in human disease but may be inhaled and subsequently isolated from sputum specimens.

RATE OF GROWTH: Varies; rapid (mature within 5 days) to slow (mature after 10 days).

COLONY MORPHOLOGY: At first white, moist, pasty, and yeastlike; later it becomes tan to brown, wrinkled, raised, membranous, or velvety. Reverse is light in color.

MICROSCOPIC MORPHOLOGY: Elongate (2–3 × 9–30 μm), irregular, spindle-shaped or beanpod-shaped yeastlike cells. Short hyphae with clamp connections are sometimes observed.

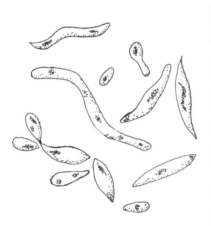 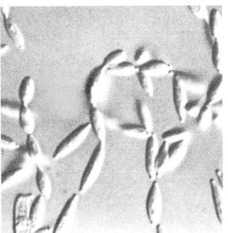

Courtesy of Michael McGinnis.

For further information, see
McGinnis, 1980

Prototheca spp.

TAXONOMY NOTES: *Prototheca* spp. are achlorophyllous algae and included in this guide because they cause mycosis-like infections and are often mistaken for yeasts.

PATHOGENICITY: Can cause protothecosis, which may be cutaneous, subcutaneous, or systemic. Infection may arise through traumatic implantation into subcutaneous tissue. The olecranon bursa has been especially associated with subcutaneous traumatic injury. Trauma to the cornea may result in *Prototheca* keratitis. Only *P. wickerhamii* and *P. zopfii* have been involved in human disease, *P. wickerhamii* being the more commonly encountered. The organisms have also been isolated from clinical specimens in the absence of disease. *P. zopfii* is a common cause of bovine fungal mastitis.

RATE OF GROWTH: Rapid; mature within 5 days. Optimum growth is at 30°C; *P. wickerhamii* and *P. zopfii* grow at 37°C, but *P. stagnora* does not. They are inhibited by cycloheximide.

COLONY MORPHOLOGY: Dull white to cream colored; yeastlike in consistency.

MICROSCOPIC MORPHOLOGY: Sporangia of various sizes (7–25 μm in diameter) containing sporangiospores (endospores). Budding does not occur and no hyphae are produced. The sporangia of *P. wickerhamii* are somewhat smaller (4–11 μm in diameter) than those of *P. zopfii* (9–28 μm in diameter), but the size may depend on the substrate and environmental conditions. Endospores are formed by cleavage and are often arranged in a symmetrical, daisylike pattern. *P. stagnora* cells are 7–14 μm in diameter and produce capsules.

See Tables 2.2 (p. 124) and 2.9 (p. 151) for identification of yeastlike organisms.

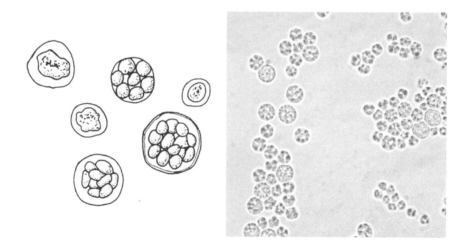

For further information, see
Kano, 2020
Lass-Flörl and Mayr, 2007

Trichosporon and *Cutaneotrichosporon* spp.

TAXONOMY NOTES: *Trichosporon asahii*, *T. asteroides*, *T. inkin*, and *T. ovoides* have been retained in the genus *Trichosporon*, while *T. cutaneum* and *T. mucoides* are currently recognized as *Cutaneotrichosporon cutaneum* and *C. mucoides*, respectively. *T. mycotoxinivorans* is currently recognized as *Apiotrichum mycotoxinovorans*.

PATHOGENICITY: *Trichosporon* is increasingly involved in invasive localized and disseminated disease, including of the kidney, lung, skin, eye, heart, and other tissue sites. Immunocompromised patients with neutropenia are especially susceptible. Some species cause white piedra, a superficial infection of the hair characterized by relatively soft, white nodules located along the shafts of hair. (Black piedra is caused by *Piedraia hortae* [p. 254].) The type and site of infection are somewhat predictive of the involved species (Table 2.10 [p. 165]). *A. mycotoxinivorans* is capable of colonization and infection in patients with cystic fibrosis. The organisms are also found as normal microbiota in the skin, nails, and mouth. *Trichosporon asahii* is the cause of summer-type hypersensitivity in Japan. *Trichosporon* spp. are resistant to echinocandins. *T. asahii* is inhibited by amphotericin B but resistant to its fungicidal effect. The cell wall of *T. asahii* shares antigenicity with the capsular polysaccharide of *Cryptococcus neoformans*; this may yield a positive cryptococcal antigen assay on serum of some patients with disseminated *Trichosporon* disease.

RATE OF GROWTH: Rapid (mature within 5 days) to moderate (mature within 6–10 days).

COLONY MORPHOLOGY: At first cream colored, moist, and soft. The surface may become irregularly wrinkled, rather powdery or crumblike; the center may become heaped, and the colony may adhere to, and crack, the agar. The color often darkens to yellowish gray.

MICROSCOPIC MORPHOLOGY: On cornmeal-Tween 80 agar at 25°C for 72 h, true hyphae and pseudohyphae with blastoconidia singly or in short chains are seen. Arthroconidia (2–4 × 3–9 μm) form on older cultures. The presence of pseudohyphae and blastoconidia differentiates *Trichosporon* spp. from *Geotrichum* spp.

See Table 2.2 (p. 124) and 2.9 (p. 151) for further differentiation of yeasts and yeastlike organisms.

See Table 2.10 (p. 165) for key characteristics of clinically encountered *Trichosporon* and *Cutaneotrichosporon* spp.

See Table 2.21 (p. 320) for differential characteristics of fungi in which arthroconidia predominate.

Trichosporon and *Cutaneotrichosporon* spp. *(continued)*

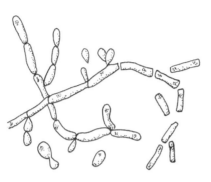
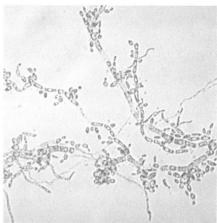

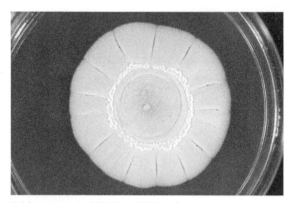

Trichosporon asahii. PDA, 30°C, 8 days.

For further information, see
Borman et al., 2020
Chen et al., 2021b
Colombo et al., 2011
de Almeida et al., 2016
Fera et al., 2009
Hickey et al., 2009
Liu et al., 2015
Mehta et al., 2021
Walsh et al., 1992

TABLE 2.10 Key characteristics of the most common clinically encountered *Trichosporon* spp. and *Cutaneotrichosporon* spp.[a]

Species	Infections	Urease	Growth at 37°C	Assimilation of:		
				Inos	Arab	Sorb
T. asahii[b]	Systemic with predilection for hematogenous dissemination	+	+	0	+	0
C. mucoides (formerly *T. mucoides*)	Systemic with preference for central nervous system; also infects hair and nails	+	+	+	+	+
C. cutaneum (formerly *T. cutaneum*)	Rarely skin lesions and white piedra of underarm hairs	+	0	+	+	+
T. inkin	Mostly white piedra of pubic hairs; occasionally systemic	+	+	+	0	0
T. ovoides	White piedra of head hairs; occasional skin lesions	+	V	0	V	0

[a] As the species of *Trichosporon* have rather distinct antifungal susceptibility profiles, molecular identification and/or susceptibility testing are essential for isolates from invasive infections. Abbreviations: +, positive; 0, negative; V, strain variation; Inos, inositol; Arab, L-arabinose; Sorb, sorbitol.

[b] *Trichosporon asteroides*, a rare cause of superficial and systemic infection, is physiologically indistinguishable from *T. asahii* and is therefore regularly misidentified, but its microscopic morphology is unique in producing hyphae that swell and develop large, multiseptate cells that separate into packets of smaller cells. See de Hoog et al., 2020.

Magnusiomyces capitatus

TAXONOMY NOTES: *Magnusiomyces capitatus* is the currently recognized name for this fungus. Former names include *Blastoschizomyces capitatus*, *Geotrichum capitatum*, *Saprochaete capitata*, and *Trichosporon capitatum*.

PATHOGENICITY: Infrequent cause of fungemia and disseminated infection in immunocompromised hosts, most commonly in neutropenic leukemia patients. Mortality is high in neutropenic patients. Lesions have occurred in the lung, kidney, liver, spleen, brain, and other organs; it has also caused endocarditis. The organism is distributed in nature and may be found as normal microbiota of the skin, respiratory tract, and gastrointestinal tract.

RATE OF GROWTH: Rapid; mature within 5 days.

COLONY MORPHOLOGY: Smooth to wrinkled, radiating edges, developing short aerial hyphae with age; white to cream colored.

MICROSCOPIC MORPHOLOGY: On cornmeal-Tween 80 agar, round to oval budding yeastlike cells, hyphae, and pseudohyphae; few arthroconidia and many annelloconidia are seen. Annellides form along the hyphae or at the ends of hyphal branches; annelloconidia are elongate (2.5–3.5 × 7–10 µm) and flattened at the base and accumulate in clusters at the tips of the annellides. It is difficult to determine that the conidia are annelloconidia and not arthroconidia or blastoconidia; this may account for its confusion with (and sometimes misidentification as) *Trichosporon* or *Candida krusei*. Careful attention to a few biochemical test results is required to differentiate these organisms.

See Tables 2.2 (p. 124) and 2.9 (p. 151) for differentiation of yeastlike fungi.

See Table 2.5 (p. 134) for comparison with *C. krusei*.

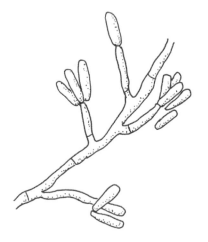 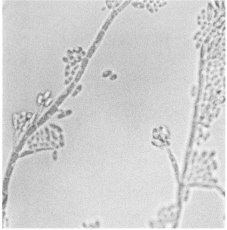

For further information, see
Chen et al., 2021b
de Hoog and Smith, 2004
Mazzocato et al., 2015

Geotrichum candidum

PATHOGENICITY: Has been isolated from a variety of specimens (lungs, blood, mouth, intestines, vagina, and skin), but its role in infection is uncertain. It is found as normal microbiota in humans and seems to cause disease (primarily of the lungs) only in severely compromised hosts. Dissemination has been reported, but only rarely.

RATE OF GROWTH: Rapid; mature within 5 days.

COLONY MORPHOLOGY: At 25°C, young colonies are white, moist, yeastlike, and easily picked up. Submerged hyphae are later seen at the periphery, giving the appearance of ground glass. Some strains develop a short, white, cottony aerial mycelium. Many strains do not grow at 37°C, but some may have a small amount of surface growth and extensive subsurface growth at this temperature.

MICROSCOPIC MORPHOLOGY: Coarse true hyphae (no pseudohyphae) that segment into rectangular arthroconidia that vary in length (most are 4–10 µm) and in the roundness of their ends. Some may become quite round. The rectangular cells characteristically germinate from one corner. The biochemical characteristics and the absence of blastoconidia along the hyphae differentiate this organism from *Trichosporon* spp. (p. 163); the consecutive formation of the arthroconidia (not alternating with empty cells) serves to separate it from *Coccidioides* spp. (p. 179), *Malbranchea* (p. 321), and *Pseudogymnoascus* (formerly *Geomyces*) (p. 323); and the absence of conidiophores distinguishes it from *Arthrographis* (p. 324).

See Tables 2.2 (p. 124) and 2.9 (p. 151) for differentiation of yeasts and yeastlike organisms.

See Table 2.21 (p. 320) for differential characteristics of fungi with predominating arthroconidia.

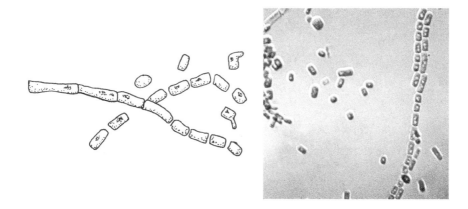

Geotrichum candidum (continued)

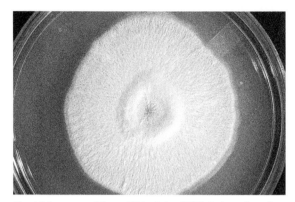

Geotrichum candidum. SDA plate, 30°C, 3 days. Powdery to cottony strain.

For further information, see
Chen et al., 2021b

Thermally Dimorphic and/or Endemic Fungi

PART II   Identification of Fungi in Culture

THERMALLY DIMORPHIC AND/OR ENDEMIC FUNGI

Introduction to Thermally Dimorphic and/or Endemic Fungi

The fungi included here are unique in that they grow as moulds in the environment or when cultured on routine mycology agar (e.g., Sabouraud dextrose agar, inhibitory mould agar, and similar primary media) at 25–30°C and grow as yeast or other nonfilamentous forms in tissue or when cultured on an enriched medium (e.g., brain heart infusion [BHI] agar) at 37°C. All of the fungi in this section are known to be primary pathogens and must be handled with caution. For laboratory safety, isolates suspected of being *Blastomyces* spp., *Coccidioides* spp., or *Histoplasma capsulatum* should be grown on slants rather than on petri plates, and slide cultures should not be performed. Their identifying characteristics are observable on well-prepared lactophenol cotton (aniline) blue preparations, and conversion of the mycelial form to the yeast phase is typically not required for most organisms.

Many of the thermally dimorphic genera are endemic in specific regions of the world. However, our understanding of the geographic distribution of endemic mycoses is constantly changing. When mentioned in this text, the geographic distribution of these fungi is described to the best of our current knowledge. Nonetheless, due to expanding endemic regions, coupled with increasing global travel, these organisms may be recovered outside of recognized endemic regions.

Cokeromyces recurvatus is thermally dimorphic, but because it is a mucormycete, it has been placed within that class (p. 207).

For further information, see
Anaissie et al. (ed.), 2009
Ashraf et al., 2020
Chen et al., 2023
de Hoog et al., 2020
Guarro et al., 2023
Kidd et al., 2023b
Lockhart et al., 2021
St-Germain and Summerbell, 2011
Thompson and Gomez, 2023

Histoplasma capsulatum

TAXONOMY NOTES: There are three recognized species of *Histoplasma* (although in some texts they are referred to as varieties of *H. capsulatum*): *H. capsulatum*, *H. duboisii*, and *H. farciminosum*. Other species of *Histoplasma* have been proposed, but are not currently taxonomically valid.

PATHOGENICITY: Histoplasmosis most commonly develops as an asymptomatic or mildly symptomatic infection in immunocompetent patients. The infection may reactivate years later or may develop as a primary infection that manifests as an acute, benign pulmonary disease or may be chronic or progressive and fatal. It may be localized or cause a disseminated, life-threatening infection (primarily of the reticuloendothelial system) and involve various tissues and organs of the body, particularly in immunocompromised patients with impairments of cellular immunity (resulting from, e.g., transplantation or HIV/AIDS). The organism is most often found associated with bird and bat droppings. It is endemic over much of the United States east of the Rocky Mountains and in other regions of the world, both temperate and tropical. Clusters of histoplasmosis have been classically reported in spelunkers exploring bat dwelling caves or in construction workers dismantling old buildings occupied with birds or bats.

H. duboisii is endemic only in central and western Africa (most commonly reported in Nigeria). It differs from *H. capsulatum* by producing thick-walled, larger yeast cells (8–15 μm in diameter) in infected tissue; when recovered in culture the two species are similar.

H. capsulatum produces a galactomannan carbohydrate antigen that can be detected in urine for diagnosis of pulmonary and disseminated histoplasmosis.

RATE OF GROWTH: Slow; mycelial forms usually mature after 10 days (typically within 15–20 days, but may take up to 8 weeks). The organism does not survive well in clinical specimens; therefore, when histoplasmosis is suspected, the specimen should be processed immediately.

COLONY MORPHOLOGY: Thermally dimorphic. At 25–30°C, mould colonies are white to brown, or pinkish, with a fine, dense cottony texture. The reverse is white, sometimes yellow or orange-tan. An enriched agar is recommended for initial isolation, but characteristic morphology of the mould phase can be seen on most routine media. The mould phase will grow on agar containing cycloheximide.

Upon direct culture of the patient's specimen at 37°C on brain heart infusion (BHI) or other enriched agar, colonies are moist, white, and yeastlike. The yeast phase is inhibited by cycloheximide.

Histoplasma capsulatum (continued)

MICROSCOPIC MORPHOLOGY: Slide cultures should not be performed on isolates suspected of being *Histoplasma*; the identifying characteristics will be observable on well-prepared wet mounts.

At 25–30°C in young cultures, septate hyphae are seen bearing round to pear-shaped, smooth or occasionally spiny microconidia (2–5 μm in diameter) on short branches or directly on the sides of the hyphae. At this early stage, *H. capsulatum* might be confused with a rare small form of *Blastomyces* spp. (p. 177). After several weeks, large, thick-walled, round macroconidia (7–15 μm in diameter) form; they are tuberculate, knobby, or have short, cylindrical projections; occasionally they may be smooth. The macroconidia greatly resemble those of *Sepedonium* spp. (p. 376), but *Sepedonium* spp. does not produce microconidia and grows poorly or not at all at 37°C. *Chrysosporium tuberculatum* can also produce large tuberculate macroconidia but does not produce microconidia.

At 37°C, small, round or oval budding cells (2–3 × 3–5 μm) and occasional abortive hyphae are formed. The yeast phase can be confused with *Emergomyces* spp. Conversion from the mould to the yeast phase often requires many generations at 37°C. The conversion of the mycelial form to the yeast phase, although required in the past for morphologic identification (see p. 427), is seldom possible *in vitro* in a reasonable amount of time. Instead, conversion is usually used in a research or educational setting. Identification can be achieved through DNA sequencing or MALDI-TOF MS analysis.

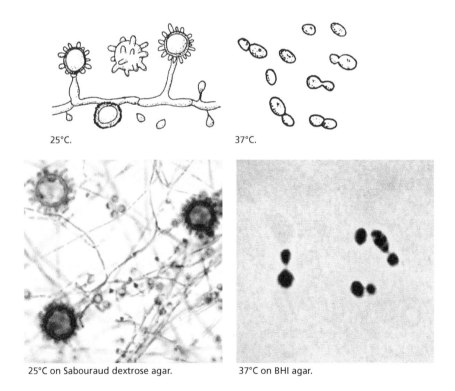

25°C.

37°C.

25°C on Sabouraud dextrose agar.

37°C on BHI agar.

Histoplasma capsulatum (continued)

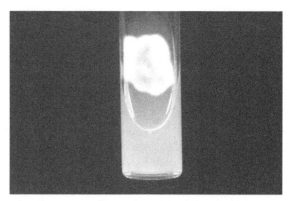

Histoplasma capsulatum slant. SDA, 30°C, 18 days.

For further information, see
Develoux et al., 2021
Kauffman, 2007

Emergomyces spp.

TAXONOMY NOTES: *Emergomyces pasteurianus* is the predominant species and was formerly known as *Emmonsia pasteuriana*. Other medically important species include *Emergomyces africanus*, *E. canadensis*, *E. europaeus*, and *E. orientalis*.

PATHOGENICITY: *Emergomyces* spp. cause emergomycosis and primarily infect immunocompromised patients including those with advanced HIV disease, transplant recipients, and those individuals on immunosuppressive therapy. Cutaneous lesions are the most frequent manifestation, and can appear as papules, nodules, or ulcers. Lesions are widespread throughout the skin surface. Pulmonary disease is common but is mainly a manifestation of widespread dissemination. *E. pasteurianus* has been recovered from Africa, Asia, Europe, and India; *E. africanus* from South Africa; *E. canadensis* from North America; *E. orientalis* from India and China; and *E. europaeus* from Europe.

RATE OF GROWTH: Slow; mycelial forms mature after 10 days at 25–30°C on most solid media including Sabouraud dextrose agar, potato dextrose agar, and malt extract agar. Growth on cycloheximide is variable.

COLONY MORPHOLOGY: Thermally dimorphic. At 25–30°C, colonies are yellowish white to tan and powdery. Reverse is tan.

MICROSCOPIC MORPHOLOGY: At 25–30°C, septate hyphae with short unbranched conidiophores at right angles. Conidiophores bear 1–3 (can be as many as 8) conidia on short pedicels that resemble florets. Conidia are spherical, 2–3 μm in diameter, and 3–4 μm in length. Conversion to the yeast phase can be achieved on enriched media (e.g., brain heart infusion, potato dextrose or malt extract agars at 35–40°C), and small ellipsoidal yeast cells (usually 2–4 μm in diameter) with narrow-based budding are formed. *Emergomyces* is differentiated from *Emmonsia* and *Blastomyces* by the presence of small narrow-based budding yeast cells, but cannot be distinguished from *Histoplasma* in the yeast phase. Superficial resemblance to *Scedosporium* in the mould phase, but the presence of multiple conidia on a single conidiophore should aid in the identification of *Emergomyces* spp.

Emergomyces spp. *(continued)*

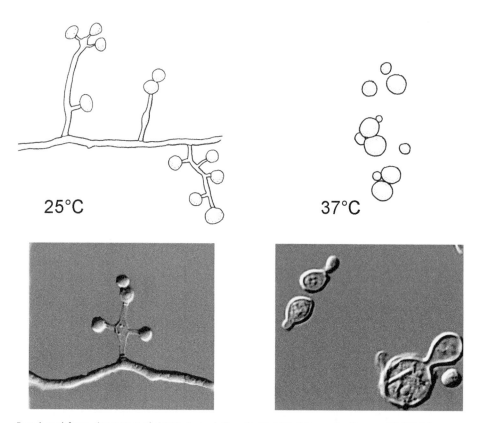

25°C   37°C

Reprinted from Jiang Y et al. 2018. *Fungal Diversity* 90:245–291, under license CC BY 4.0.

For further information, see
Dukik et al., 2017
Kenyon et al., 2013
Schwartz et al., 2018
Schwartz et al., 2019a

Blastomyces dermatitidis/gilchristii

TAXONOMY NOTES: *Blastomyces dermatitidis* and *B. gilchristii* are morphologically indistinguishable. *Emmonsia parva* has been renamed *B. parvus*. Two new species, *B. helicus* (endemic to the western United States and Canada) and *B. percursus* (recovered from specimens in Africa and Asia), have been described.

PATHOGENICITY: *Blastomyces dermatitidis/gilchristii* cause blastomycosis, which may range from a transient pulmonary infection to a chronic infection characterized by suppurative and granulomatous lesions of the lungs, bone, and skin, but potentially of any part of the body; it most commonly begins in the lungs and is disseminated to the skin and bones. The disease occurs throughout the United States east of the Mississippi River and northward into Canada (Ontario, Quebec, Manitoba, and Saskatchewan). There may be differences in the geographic distribution of these species in North America, with *B. dermatitidis* found more frequently to the south and *B. gilchristii* found more frequently to the north. *B. dermatitidis* is also found across much of eastern and southern Africa. There are no known differences in disease caused by either *B. dermatitidis* or *B. gilchristii*; therefore, differentiating the two species for reasons other than epidemiological purposes is unnecessary.

RATE OF GROWTH: Slow; mycelial forms mature after 10 days. Some strains are slower; cultures should be held for 8 weeks if blastomycosis is suspected. Organism does not survive well in specimens and should therefore be cultured immediately.

COLONY MORPHOLOGY: Thermally dimorphic. At 25–30°C, it is at first yeastlike, then prickly, and finally very cottony with a white aerial mycelium that turns tan or brown with age. Reverse is tan. The mould phase will grow on agar containing cycloheximide.

At 35–37°C, it is cream to tan in color, heaped or wrinkled, and waxy in appearance; it grows best on brain heart infusion (BHI) or other enriched agar. Yeast phase is inhibited by cycloheximide.

MICROSCOPIC MORPHOLOGY: Slide cultures should not be performed on isolates suspected of being *Blastomyces*; the identifying characteristics will be observable on well-prepared lactophenol cotton blue preparations.

At 25–30°C, septate hyphae form with short or long stalks; round or pear-shaped conidia (2–10 μm in diameter) develop at the apex of the stalk (causing a lollipop-like appearance) or directly on the hyphae. It may resemble *Scedosporium* spp. (p. 237) or *Chrysosporium* spp. (p. 371). Older cultures have thick-walled chlamydoconidia (7–18 μm in diameter). At 37°C on BHI or other enriched agar, forms yeast cells (usually 8–15 μm in diameter) that bud on a broad base (4–5 μm wide) and appear to be thick walled and double contoured; the bud often remains attached until it becomes the same size as the parent cell.

Identification can be achieved through DNA sequencing or MALDI-TOF MS analysis. *B. dermatitidis* and *B. gilchristii* are only differentiated by DNA sequencing.

Blastomyces dermatitidis/gilchristii *(continued)*

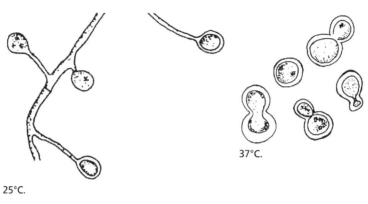

25°C.

37°C.

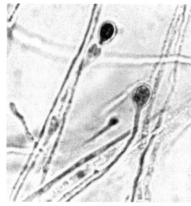

25°C on Sabouraud dextrose agar.

37°C on BHI agar.

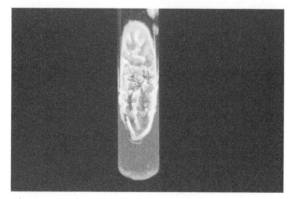

Blastomyces dermatitidis slant. SDA, 30°C, 18 days.

For further information, see
Castillo et al., 2016
Dukik et al., 2017
Jiang et al., 2018
Schwartz et al., 2019b

Coccidioides immitis/posadasii

PATHOGENICITY: *Coccidioides immitis/posadasii* cause coccidioidomycosis, which is a highly infectious process that may be an acute but benign self-limiting respiratory disease or a chronic, malignant, sometimes fatal infection involving the skin, bone, joints, lymph nodes, adrenals, and central nervous system. It is endemic in the arid southwestern United States and in dry regions of Mexico, Central America, and South America. These areas are known as the Sonoran life zones, which are characterized by arid climate punctuated by occasional rainfall; this type of climate allows for the life cycle of *Coccidioides* spp. to be completed between a hyphal stage in the soil, acquisition of arthroconidia by a host, and transformation to spherules in mammalian tissue. *C. immitis* is primarily located in the San Joaquin Valley of southern California and has occasionally been recovered in Mexico; it has been shown to be endemic in a small region of Washington state near the Oregon border. *C. posadasii* is more widespread, found in Utah, Texas, New Mexico, and Arizona and in other endemic regions throughout the Americas. There are no known differences in the infections caused by *C. immitis* or *C. posadasii* and they are morphologically indistinguishable; therefore, differentiating the two species for reasons other than epidemiological purposes is unnecessary.

RATE OF GROWTH: Moderate; mature within 6–10 days. Growth occurs in 3–5 days, but production of arthroconidia may take 1–2 weeks.

COLONY MORPHOLOGY: There may be great variation in colony morphology. On Sabouraud dextrose agar at 25 or 37°C, the colony often is at first moist, grayish, and membranous and soon develops a white, cottony aerial mycelium, which becomes gray or tan to brown with age; may also be pinkish or yellow. Reverse is white to gray, sometimes yellow or brownish. The spherule, or tissue phase, can only be formed *in vitro* under very special conditions and conversion is not generally performed in clinical laboratories.

MICROSCOPIC MORPHOLOGY: Cultures exhibit coarse, septate, branched hyphae that produce thick-walled, barrel-shaped arthroconidia (3–4 × 3–6 μm) that alternate with empty cells (disjunctor cells). The walls of the empty cells break and are characteristically present on either end of the freed arthroconidia. Racquet hyphae are formed in young colonies and can serve as a sign, before development of arthroconidia, that *Coccidioides* may be present. Careful microscopic examination should prevent confusion with *Geotrichum candidum* (p. 167). *Coccidioides* is more likely to be confused with *Malbranchea* (p. 321), which also forms alternating arthroconidia along the hyphae but has a more narrow, delicate appearance.

See Table 2.21 (p. 320) for differential characteristics of fungi in which arthroconidia predominate.

To confirm the identity of *Coccidioides* and definitively differentiate it from organisms that it may closely resemble, it is necessary to perform molecular testing either by DNA sequencing or MALDI-TOF MS analysis.

Coccidioides immitis/posadasii (continued)

In tissues or body fluids, *Coccidioides* exists as large, round, thick-walled spherules (10–80 μm in diameter), which contain endospores (2–5 μm in diameter). Immature nonendosporulating cells may resemble nonbudding forms of *B. dermatitidis/gilchristii* (p. 177). When cultured on routine media, whether incubated at 25, 30, or 37°C, the organism is filamentous.

Because the arthroconidia are highly infectious, the cultures must be handled with great care and grown in tubes only, not petri plates, if suspected or upon initial identification. Slide cultures should not be made. The characteristic arthroconidia can be readily seen with a wet preparation.

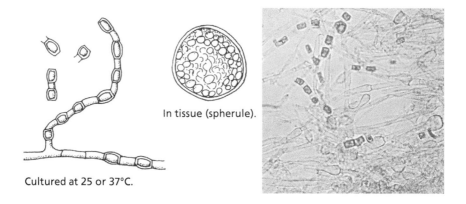

In tissue (spherule).

Cultured at 25 or 37°C.

For further information, see
Bays and Thompson, 2021

Paracoccidioides brasiliensis

TAXONOMY NOTES: *Paracoccidioides lutzii* is another medically important species. Other *Paracoccidioides* spp. have been proposed but they are currently not taxonomically valid.

PATHOGENICITY: *Paracoccidioides* spp. cause paracoccidioidomycosis (South American blastomycosis), a chronic granulomatous disease characteristically beginning in the lungs and spreading to the mucous membranes of the nose, mouth, and occasionally the gastro-intestinal tract. Dissemination to skin, lymph nodes, and other internal organs is common. It is endemic in areas from Mexico to Argentina, but is most prevalent in South America, especially northern Brazil, Colombia, and Venezuela. It causes disease predominantly in males due to the role of estrogen in preventing dimorphic transformation in females.

RATE OF GROWTH: Very slow; mycelial forms mature after 10 days (within 21 days).

COLONY MORPHOLOGY: Thermally dimorphic. At 25–30°C, colony is white, heaped, compact, usually folded, and almost glabrous or with a short nap of white aerial mycelium that often turns brown with age. Reverse is light or brownish.

At 37°C on brain heart infusion (BHI) or other enriched agar, colony is heaped, cream to tan, moist, and soft, becoming waxy and yeastlike.

MICROSCOPIC MORPHOLOGY: The most useful identifying characteristics will be observable on a wet preparation of the yeast form at 37°C.

At 25–30°C, usually forms only septate, branched hyphae with some intercalary and terminal chlamydospores; a few microconidia are sometimes observed along the hyphae.

At 35–37°C on BHI or other enriched agar, the characteristic large, round, fairly thick-walled cells (5–50 μm in diameter) with single and multiple buds (2–10 μm in diameter) are seen. The buds are attached to the mother cell by narrow connections and may almost completely surround the cell, giving the characteristic mariner's-wheel appearance. When single-budding cells occur, the narrow necks of attachment should prevent confusion with *Blastomyces dermatitidis/gilchristii*.

Conversion of the mould form to the yeast phase is definitive for identification (see p. 427). Identification can be achieved through DNA sequencing or MALDI-TOF MS analysis.

Paracoccidioides brasiliensis (continued)

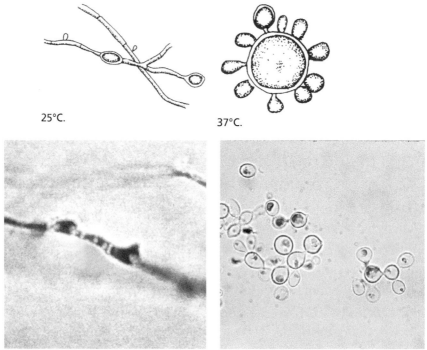

25°C.

37°C.

25°C on potato dextrose agar.

37°C on BHI agar.

For further information, see
Marques, 2012
Pinheiro et al., 2020

Talaromyces marneffei

TAXONOMY NOTES: This species was formerly known as *Penicillium marneffei*.

PATHOGENICITY: Causes deep-seated infection that can be focal or disseminated, predominantly in immunocompromised patients (those with HIV/AIDS, lymphoma, or autoimmune disorders) and occasionally in seemingly immunocompetent individuals who live in, or have traveled in, areas of Southeast Asia where *T. marneffei* is endemic. The organism has been isolated from blood, bone marrow, skin, lung, mucosa, lymph nodes, urine, stool, cerebrospinal fluid, and various internal organs.

RATE OF GROWTH: Rapid; mature within 5 days at 25–30°C. Yeast forms develop more slowly at 35–37°C. Sabouraud dextrose agar (SDA) supports growth at 25–37°C. Cycloheximide inhibits growth.

COLONY MORPHOLOGY: Thermally dimorphic. At 25–30°C on SDA, colony is flat, powdery to velvety, and tan, later becoming reddish yellow with a yellow or white edge; it is often bluish gray-green in the center. A deep-reddish soluble pigment diffuses into the medium after 3–7 days; this is best seen on potato dextrose agar. Some other *Talaromyces* and *Penicillium* species may also produce a red pigment but will not convert to a yeast form at 35–37°C. Reverse is brownish red.

At 35–37°C on SDA, inhibitory mould agar, or brain heart infusion (BHI) or other enriched agar, colony is soft, white to tan, and dry. Conversion from the mould to yeast form may take up to 14 days; it is most rapidly accomplished (in ~4 days) by culturing in BHI broth on a shaker; the next-best method is on 5% sheep blood agar.

MICROSCOPIC MORPHOLOGY: Distinction between *T. marneffei* and members of the genus *Penicillium* is important. The identifying characteristics will be observable on well-prepared wet mounts of the mould at 30°C and the yeast form at 37°C.

At 25–30°C, structures typical of the genus *Penicillium* (p. 348) develop, i.e., smooth conidiophores with four or five terminal metulae, each metula bearing four to six phialides. Conidia are smooth or slightly rough and round to oval (2–3 × 2.5–4 μm) and form chains; short, narrow extensions connect the conidia. It is generally biverticilliate (conidiophore once branched, each branch bearing a whorl of phialides) but can be monoverticilliate (whorl of phialides directly on the conidiophore).

Further distinguishing *T. marneffei* from members of the genus *Penicillium*, when conidia are incubated at 35–37°C, they form hyphal elements that eventually fragment at the septa, producing single-celled, round to oval arthroconidia (3–5 μm in diameter); buds are not produced. The yeast cells of *T. marneffei* continue to reproduce by fission and in so doing may elongate to 8–9 μm.

Talaromyces marneffei (continued)

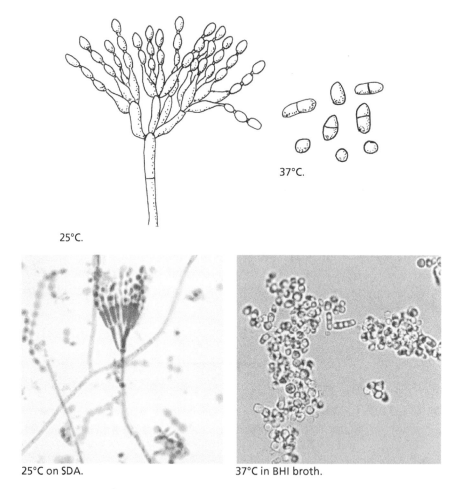

37°C.

25°C.

25°C on SDA.

37°C in BHI broth.

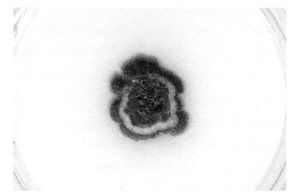

Talaromyces marneffei. PDA, 30°C, 3 days. Surface of colony. Note pale red diffusing pigment of stock culture.

Talaromyces marneffei (continued)

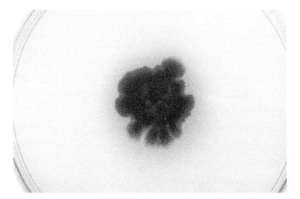

Talaromyces marneffei. PDA, 30°C, 3 days. Reverse of colony. Note pale red diffusing pigment of stock culture.

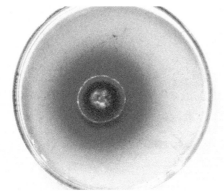

Talaromyces marneffei. SDA, 30°C, 4 days. Surface of colony. Note strong red diffusing pigment of primary isolate. (Courtesy of William Merz.)

For further information, see

Cooper and Haycocks, 2000
Narayanasamy et al., 2021
Samson et al., 2011

Sporothrix schenckii species complex

TAXONOMY NOTES: The species complex includes *S. brasiliensis*, *S. globosa*, *S. luriei*, *S. mexicana*, and *S. schenckii sensu stricto*.

PATHOGENICITY: *Sporothrix schenkii* species complex members cause sporotrichosis, a chronic infection that frequently begins as a lesion of the skin and subcutaneous tissue and then involves the lymphatic channels and lymph nodes draining the area. The lymphocutaneous form of nocardiosis can mimic sporotrichosis, and for this reason is often referred to as sporotrichoid nocardiosis. Initial introduction into the body is usually due to a puncture by contaminated plant material (e.g., wood splinters, thorns, sphagnum moss, or hay). Primary pulmonary sporotrichosis may develop in predisposed individuals after inhaling the fungus. On rare occasions the infection has disseminated with fatal outcome in immunocompromised patients.

By comparison, *S. brasiliensis* predominantly infects cats and causes ulcerative lesions that serve as a source for infecting owners and those who have contact with the animals. These lesions in humans also may be ulcerative and behave aggressively with loss of skin and subcutaneous tissue.

RATE OF GROWTH: Moderate; mature within 6–10 days.

COLONY MORPHOLOGY: Thermally dimorphic. At 25–30°C, the colonies are at first small and white or pale orange to orange-gray with no cottony aerial hyphae. Later, the colonies become moist, wrinkled, leathery, or velvety and often darken to a salt-and-peppery brown or black with a narrow white border. Some isolates are black from the beginning; stock cultures may become, and remain, nonpigmented. Colonies with a dark surface have a reverse that is commonly dark in the center and light at the periphery.

At 35–37°C, colonies are cream or tan, smooth, and waxy. It is best to use brain heart infusion (BHI) agar and transfer several generations to obtain a good yeast phase (pp. 427 and 449).

MICROSCOPIC MORPHOLOGY: At 25–30°C, hyphae are very narrow (1–2 μm in diameter), septate, and branching, with slender, tapering conidiophores rising at right angles. The apex of the conidiophore is often slightly swollen and bears many small, tear-shaped or almost round hyaline conidia (2–3 × 2–6 μm) on delicate threadlike denticles, forming a "rosette" or "daisy" cluster in young cultures; sessile conidia (usually thick walled and brown) can form singly along the hyphae. Occasionally conidiophores lined with sympodial conidia and conidia associated through hydrophobicity, forming a sleevelike pattern, are observed. Microscopic features may be best observed on cornmeal agar.

At 35–37°C, round, oval, and fusiform budding cells of various sizes (1–3 × 3–10 μm), commonly called cigar bodies, are seen. The cigar shape is more typical of cells that are actively budding.

The conversion of the mycelial form to the yeast form is confirmatory for identification of the genus (see p. 427).

Sporothrix schenckii species complex *(continued)*

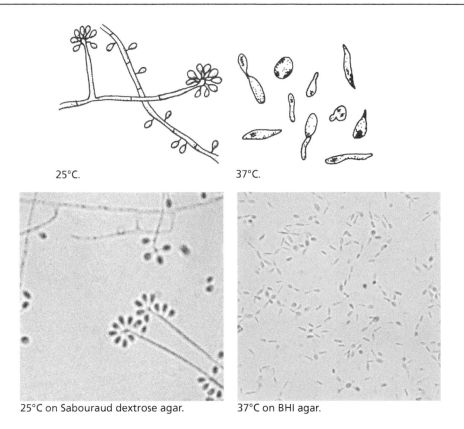

25°C.

37°C.

25°C on Sabouraud dextrose agar.

37°C on BHI agar.

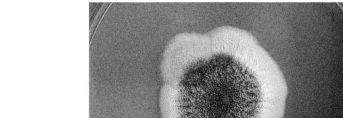

Sporothrix schenckii. Mould phase, SDA, 30°C, 6 days.
Surface of colony.

Sporothrix schenckii **species complex** *(continued)*

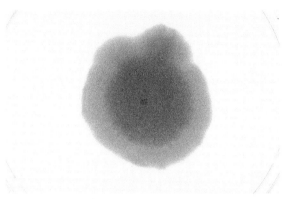

Sporothrix schenckii. Mould phase, SDA, 30°C, 6 days.
Reverse of colony.

For further information, see

Barros et al., 2011
Chakrabarti et al., 2015
Marimon et al., 2007

Emmonsia crescens

TAXONOMY NOTES: *Emmonsia crescens* is the only species in the genus capable of causing human infection. *E. parva* is now recognized as *Blastomyces parvus*, and *E. pasteuriana* is now recognized as *Emergomyces pasteurianus* (p. 175).

PATHOGENICITY: *Emmonsia* causes adiaspiromycosis, a pulmonary disease seen mainly in rodents and small animals living in soil; only occasionally in humans. This mycosis is characterized by the *in vivo* enlargement, without multiplication, of inhaled conidia. The mycosis is usually self-limited, benign, localized, and relatively asymptomatic but may be more severe; disseminated infection has been reported in patients with AIDS. Lung biopsy is usually required for diagnosis; sputum or bronchoalveolar lavage will not suffice. *E. crescens* is the main etiologic agent in animals and the only agent of the disease in humans.

RATE OF GROWTH: Moderate (mature within 6–10 days) to slow (mature after 10 days). For primary isolation, minced lung tissue should be cultured on routine mycology agar at 25°C; *E. crescens* grows best at 20–25°C. *E. crescens* is somewhat inhibited by growth on cycloheximide.

COLONY MORPHOLOGY: Surface is white, occasionally buff to pale brown in the center; some areas may be glabrous, while others will have tufts of matted mycelia; slight radial grooves may form. Reverse is cream to pale brown.

MICROSCOPIC MORPHOLOGY: Hyphae are septate (1–2.5 μm wide); conidiophores are at right angles to the vegetative hyphae and produce conidia that are round or almost so (2–4.5 μm in diameter) and may become finely roughened with age. The conidiophores may swell at the apex and produce two or three conidia on short, narrow denticles. The conidia also form directly on short stalks along the sides of the hyphae.

When the hyphae and conidia are incubated at their maximum temperatures on enriched medium, the hyphae become distorted and usually disintegrate while the conidia swell to become round, thick-walled adiaconidia (formerly called adiaspores). The adiaconidia of *E. crescens* are produced at 37°C and measure 20–140 μm in diameter. Adiaconidia *in vivo* are larger and have thicker walls.

Emmonsia crescens (continued)

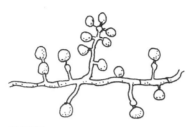

At 25°C.

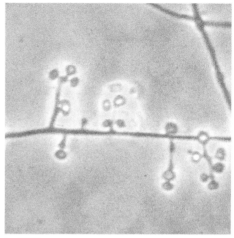

At 25°C.

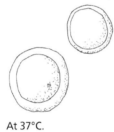

At 37°C.

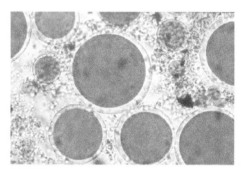

At 37°C.

For further information, see
Jiang et al., 2018
Schwartz et al., 2015

Thermally Monomorphic Moulds

Thermally monomorphic moulds are fungi that are filamentous at whatever temperatures they are able to grow (25–35°C). The growth of some are inhibited at 35–37°C.

Mucormycetes

PART II Identification of Fungi in Culture

THERMALLY MONOMORPHIC MOULDS • Mucormycetes

Introduction to Mucormycetes

The large majority of Mucormycetes that are encountered in the clinical laboratory belong to the order Mucorales. Infections caused by fungi in this order can correctly be described as mucormycosis; however, the misinterpretation that they are all caused by *Mucor* spp. must be avoided. *Rhizopus* spp. are the most common causes of mucormycosis. Among all causes of mucormycosis, the leading four genera are *Rhizopus* spp., *Mucor* spp., *Lichtheimia* spp., and *Cunninghamella* spp. The class Mucormycetes has now replaced the term "Zygomycetes." As the class of Zygomycetes was found to be polyphyletic (having more than one immediate common ancestor among the included species), the term was discarded and the two phyletically distinct orders of Mucorales and Entomophthorales were established.

Mucormycetes are a class of fungi that have broad hyphae (6–15 µm wide) and very rare septations (i.e., pauciseptate); in some preparations no septations may be seen. Septa are most often seen on sporangiophores just below the sporangia and elsewhere in older cultures. Asexual reproduction of the most commonly encountered species occurs in a saclike structure called a sporangium, in which the internal contents are cleaved into spores. Some species may rarely form zygospores in culture. Most genera are inhibited by cycloheximide.

The Mucorales are easily recognized by their grayish, floccose colonies that rapidly fill the tube or petri plate in a cotton candy-like fashion. The differentiation of the various genera is based on

- The presence and location (or absence) of rhizoids (rootlike structures along the vegetative hyphae)
- The branching or unbranched nature of the sporangiophores (the stalks bearing the saclike sporangia)

  Examining growth on a slant, angled to view the side, on a dissecting microscope can be very helpful in viewing the presence or absence of rhizoids and branching
- The shape of the columella (the small domelike area at the apex of the sporangiophore)
- The appearance of an apophysis (a broadening near the apex of the sporangiophore, just below the columella)
- The size and shape of the sporangia

See labeled diagram, p. 203.

A few genera (e.g., *Apophysomyces* and *Saksenaea*) require special media (p. 428) to enhance sporulation.

Patients who are predisposed by diabetes mellitus, neutropenia, corticosteroid therapy, hematological malignancies, transplantation, HIV/AIDS, severe burns, intravenous drug abuse, iron overload conditions, and malnutrition are at risk for severe disease by members of the order Mucorales. More recently, this group of fungi has been found to infect individuals suffering from COVID-19, likely exacerbated by the use of corticosteroids in treatment. The Mucorales also have caused devastating trauma-associated infections from military blast injuries, burns, and tornadoes. Infections have been reported from a wide range of anatomic sites but are most commonly sino-orbital, rhinocerebral, pulmonary, cutaneous, gastrointestinal, and disseminated. The organisms are angioinvasive, known for their disastrous ability to invade and clot blood vessels.

The Entomophthorales are considered to be an order of fungi that is phyletically distinct from the order of Mucorales. In comparison to mucormycosis, infections caused by members of the order of Entomophthorales occur in otherwise healthy individuals and are less commonly encountered. The two medically important genera of Entomophthorales (*Basidiobolus* and *Conidiobolus*) cause tropical subcutaneous mycoses and are discussed in the latter portion of this section (pp. 212–213). *Basidiobolus* has also been described to cause gastrointestinal infections.

For further information, see
Al-Tawfiq et al., 2021
Cornely et al., 2019
de Hoog et al., 2020
Garcia-Hermoso et al., 2023
Jeong et al., 2019
Kidd et al., 2023b
Ribes et al., 2000
Roden et al., 2005
Shaikh et al., 2016
Steinbrink and Miceli, 2021
St-Germain and Summerbell, 2011
Vilela and Mendoza, 2018
Walsh et al., 2019

TABLE 2.11 Differential characteristics of similar organisms in the class Mucormycetes[a]

Organism	Rhizoids	Sporangio-phores	Apophysis	Columellae	Sporangia	Maximum optimal growth temp (°C)
Rhizopus	Present, nodal	Single or in tufts; usually unbranched; mostly brownish	Mostly inconspicuous	Almost round or slightly elongated	Round, 50–275 µm	~40–50; species vary
Rhizomucor	Few, usually short, intranodal	Branched, dark brown	Absent (or very tiny)	Almost round	Round, 40–100 µm	~38–58; species vary
Mucor	Absent	Branched or unbranched; mostly hyaline	Absent	Various shapes	Round, 50–100 µm	≤37
Lichtheimia	Present, but often indistinct, intranodal	Finely branched; almost hyaline; form in groups of 2–5	Conspicuous, conical	Semicircle; may have projection at top	Pyriform (pear shaped), 20–90 µm	~45–50
Apophyso-myces	Present, variable location (nodal and intranodal)	Generally single and unbranched; grayish brown	Conspicuous, bell shaped	Semicircle; may be elongated	Pyriform, 20–60 µm	≥42

[a] Data from Scholer et al., 1983, with additions and updates.

TABLE 2.12 Differential characteristics of the clinically encountered *Rhizopus* spp.[a]

Organism	Patho-genic	Maximum growth temp (°C)	Rhizoid length (µm)	Sporan-giophore length (µm)	Sporan-gium diame-ter (µm)	Columellae	Sporangiospores
R. arrhizus (most common agent of mucormycosis)	+	40–46	150–300	500–2,000	50–250	Almost round	Variable size; average length, 6–8 µm; striated; elongate to lemon shaped
R. microsporus var. *rhizo-podiformis*[b] (second most common agent of mucormycosis)	+	50–52	100–120	200–500	40–120	Slightly elongated: distinct apophysis	Equal in size; average length, 4–6 µm; smooth to slightly striated; almost round to slightly elongated
R. stolonifer	0	30–32	300–350	1,500–4,000	150–350	Almost round	Variable in size; average length, 9–11 µm; very striated; elongate to polyhedric

[a] Abbreviations: +, positive; 0, negative.

[b] Other varieties of *R. microsporus* do not grow at 50°C.

Rhizopus spp.

TAXONOMY NOTES: The most common species of *Rhizopus, R. arrhizus,* was recently recognized by the species name *R. oryzae* but is now recognized as *R. arrhizus* again.

PATHOGENICITY: The most common etiologic agents of mucormycosis (see p. 44 for a description of the disease). They occasionally may be found as common contaminants, but should not be discarded without a clinical-pathologic-mycologic correlation given the severity of disease caused by these fungi.

RATE OF GROWTH: Rapid; mature within 5 days. The pathogenic species grow well at 37°C. Growth is inhibited by cycloheximide.

COLONY MORPHOLOGY: Quickly covers agar surface with dense growth that is cotton candy-like; colonies are white at first and then gray or yellowish brown. Reverse is white to pale shades of gray or brown.

MICROSCOPIC MORPHOLOGY: Broad hyphae (6–15 μm in diameter) have very rare septa. Numerous stolons run among the mycelia, connecting groups of long sporangiophores that usually are unbranched. At the point where the stolons and sporangiophores meet, root-like hyphae (rhizoids) are produced. The sporangiophores are long (up to 3 mm) and terminate with a dark, round sporangium (40–275 μm in diameter) containing a columella and many oval, colorless or brown sporangiospores (4–9 μm in diameter). No collarette remains when the sporangial wall dissolves. Large chlamydospores are sometimes seen. This genus is differentiated from *Mucor* spp. (p. 200) by the presence of stolons, rhizoids, and usually unbranched sporangiophores. It is differentiated from *Lichtheimia* (p. 202) by the location of the rhizoids in relation to the sporangiophores and by the size and shape of the sporangia.

See Tables 2.11 and 2.12 (p. 197) for identification of genus and species.

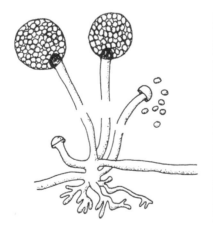
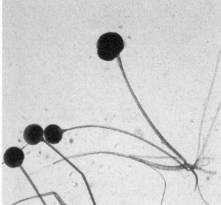

Rhizopus spp. *(continued)*

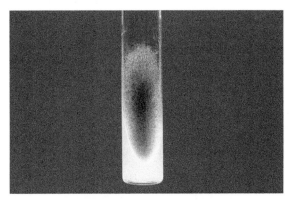

Rhizopus sp. slant. SDA, 30°C, 4 days. Note robust cotton candy-like growth.

Mucor spp.

PATHOGENICITY: Another important etiologic agent of mucormycosis (for a description of the disease, see p. 44). This fungus is also occasionally a contaminant, but should not be discounted until a clinical-pathologic-mycologic correlation is completed. The most common agent of human infection is *Mucor circinelloides*.

RATE OF GROWTH: Rapid; mature within 5 days. Growth is inhibited by cycloheximide. Some species do not grow well at 37°C.

COLONY MORPHOLOGY: Quickly covers agar surface with floccose colony resembling cotton candy; white, later turns gray or grayish brown. Reverse is white.

MICROSCOPIC MORPHOLOGY: Hyphae are wide (6–15 µm) and pauciseptate. Sporangiophores are long and often branched and bear terminal round, spore-filled sporangia (50–100 µm in diameter). The sporangial wall dissolves, scattering the round or slightly oblong spores (4–8 µm in diameter), revealing the columella and sometimes leaving a collarette at the base of the sporangium. There is no apophysis. No rhizoids are formed. Chlamydospores may form in some species.

See Table 2.11 (p. 197) for differentiation of similar organisms in the class Mucormycetes.

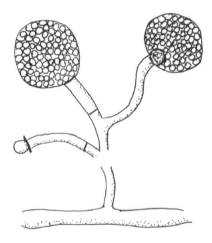
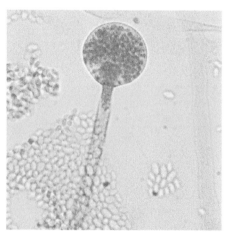

Rhizomucor spp.

PATHOGENICITY: An occasional etiologic agent of mucormycosis (for a description of the disease, see p. 44), primarily in leukemic patients. Incidence in the clinical laboratory is uncertain, as isolates may have been misidentified in the past.

RATE OF GROWTH: Rapid; mature within 5 days. Growth is inhibited by cycloheximide. Some members of the genus (*R. miehei* and *R. pusillus*) are thermophilic, with a maximum growth temperature of 54–58°C.

COLONY MORPHOLOGY: Very fluffy growth with texture of cotton candy; gray, becoming dark brownish with age. Reverse is white.

MICROSCOPIC MORPHOLOGY: Appears to be intermediate between *Rhizopus* (p. 198) and *Mucor* (p. 200) spp. Sporangiophores are long, and they branch in a sympodial manner, most often near the top of the sporangiophore. Sporangia are round and are usually 40–100 μm in diameter. A few primitive, short, irregularly branched rhizoids are formed, differentiating the organism from *Mucor* spp. It differs from *Rhizopus* spp. by having branched sporangiophores and by the poor development and location of the rhizoids (intranodal—at points between the sporangiophores).

See Table 2.11 (p. 197) for differentiation of similar organisms in the class Mucormycetes.

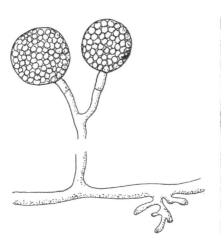
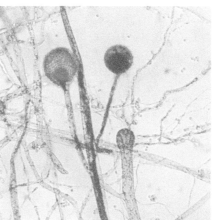

Lichtheimia corymbifera species complex

TAXONOMY NOTES: The species complex includes *Lichtheimia corymbifera sensu stricto*, *L. ornata*, and *L. ramosa*. These species are difficult to differentiate phenotypically. *Absidia corymbifera* and *Mycocladus corymbifer* are previous names.

PATHOGENICITY: An infrequent etiologic agent of mucormycosis (for a description of the disease, see p. 44). It has been particularly associated with wound infections involving burns, trauma, and surgical interventions. The organism is ubiquitous and may therefore be a contaminant in cultures, but should not be discounted until a clinical-pathologic-mycologic correlation is achieved.

RATE OF GROWTH: Rapid; mature within 5 days. Growth is inhibited by cycloheximide. Maximum growth temperature is 45–50°C.

COLONY MORPHOLOGY: Coarse woolly gray surface; rapidly covers agar slant with fluff resembling gray cotton candy. Reverse is white.

MICROSCOPIC MORPHOLOGY: Hyphae are wide (6–15 μm in diameter) and paucisepate. This mould is similar in structure to *Rhizopus* spp. (p. 198) except that the sporangiophores of *Lichtheimia* arise (often in small clusters) at points on the stolon that are between the rhizoids (i.e., intranodal), rather than at the base of the sporangiophore (i.e., nodal), as with *Rhizopus*. Also, the sporangiophores (up to 450 μm long) are branched and widen near the top, forming a conical apophysis just below the columella. The columella is typically shaped like a semicircle with a small, domelike projection on top. The sporangia are relatively small (20–90 μm in diameter) and slightly pear shaped instead of round. When the sporangial wall dissolves, a short collarette often remains where the wall met the sporangiophore. The sporangiospores are round to oval (3–5 μm in diameter).

Note: The rhizoids are often difficult to detect; they may be best observed by using a dissecting microscope to examine colonies on a slanted agar surface.

See p. 204 for differentiation from *Apophysomyces elegans*, which it closely resembles.

See Table 2.11 (p. 197) for differentiation of similar organisms in the class Mucormycetes.

Lichtheimia corymbifera species complex *(continued)*

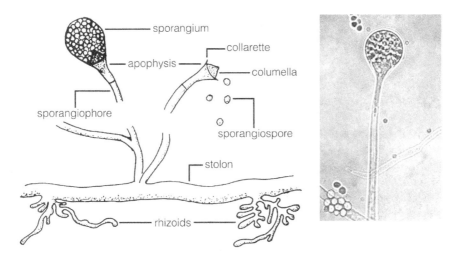

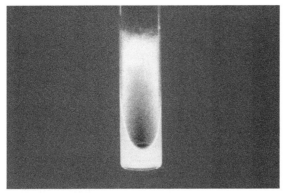

Lichtheimia corymbifera. SDA, 30°C, 4 days. Cotton candy-like growth.

For further information, see
Schwartze and Jacobsen, 2014

Apophysomyces elegans species complex

TAXONOMY NOTES: The species complex includes *Apophysomyces elegans sensu stricto*, *A. ossiformis*, *A. trapeziformis*, and *A. variabilis*. These species are difficult to differentiate phenotypically.

PATHOGENICITY: Occasional agent of mucormycosis (for a description of the disease, see p. 44). Infection is usually acquired by traumatic implantation, such as accidental injuries, surgery, insect bites, and contamination of burns. Systemic cases have also been reported. Some infected patients appear to be otherwise immunocompetent. The organism is found in soil. Mucormycosis following musculoskeletal injuries sustained in dry, arid, or desert soil has been particularly associated with this organism.

RATE OF GROWTH: Rapid; mature within 5 days (growth fills plate or tube); grows at temperatures up to 42°C. It grows on media containing cycloheximide, in contrast to other Mucormycetes.

COLONY MORPHOLOGY: Fluffy, cottony growth that fills tube or plate; surface is white when young, becoming cream to yellow or brownish gray with age. Reverse is white to pale yellow.

MICROSCOPIC MORPHOLOGY: Sporulation does not occur on routine media; only broad, pauciseptate hyphae form. A special culture method, such as water media, (p. 428) is required to induce sporulation. Hyphae are generally pauciseptate and branched (4–8 μm in diameter). Sporangiophores are long (up to 530 μm) and unbranched and arise singly from a hyphal segment that resembles the foot cells seen in *Aspergillus* spp. (p. 327); the apex of the sporangiophore widens to form a funnel-shaped or bell-shaped apophysis (11–40 μm in diameter at the widest part). The columella is a half circle. Sporangia are pear shaped, or pyriform (20–55 μm in diameter), and upon dissolution may leave a small collar at the base of the columella. The sporangiospores are smooth and mostly oblong (5–8 μm in length) and may appear pale brown in mass. Rhizoids may be between the points of origin of the sporangiophores or opposite the sporangiophore, depending on the medium.

Apophysomyces is similar to *Lichtheimia* but differs by having a more pronounced apophysis, which is bell shaped rather than conical, a "foot cell" at the base of the sporangiophore, and sporangiophores developing opposite rhizoids on plain agar. Darkening and thickening of the sporangiophore wall below the apophysis, failure to sporulate readily with routine culture methods, and resistance to cycloheximide also help distinguish the two genera.

Apophysomyces elegans **species complex** *(continued)*

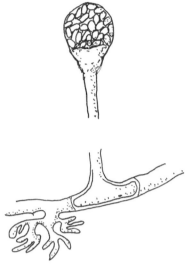 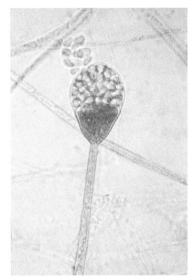

For further information, see
Kimura et al., 1999

Saksenaea vasiformis

PATHOGENICITY: Occasionally an agent of mucormycosis (for a description of the disease, see p. 44). Cases are usually preceded by traumatic implantation. Infections reported have been cutaneous, subcutaneous, osteomyelitic, rhinocerebral, and cranial; systemic infection is often fatal. Many of the patients appear to be otherwise immunocompetent.

RATE OF GROWTH: Rapid; mature within 5 days (growth fills plate or tube). Maximum growth temperature is 44°C.

COLONY MORPHOLOGY: Very cottony, fluffy white surface. Reverse is white.

MICROSCOPIC MORPHOLOGY: On routine media the organism does not sporulate; only broad, pauciseptate, branched, hyaline hyphae form. Water culture medium (p. 428) can be used for stimulation of sporulation. Sporulation can occasionally occur on Czapek agar after 7 days' incubation at 37°C. Sporangiophores (24–64 μm long) bear sporangia that are flask shaped (50–150 μm long), having a swollen portion near the base and a long neck that broadens at the apex. Sporangiospores are elongate (3–4 μm long) and smooth and are released through the top of the neck. Rhizoids form near the base of the sporangiophore, are dichotomously branched, and darken with age.

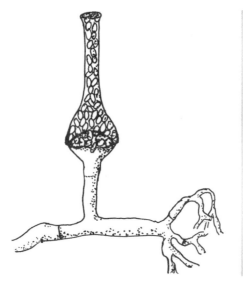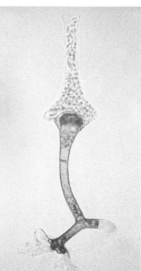

Cokeromyces recurvatus

PATHOGENICITY: Has been recovered several times from genitourinary sites (cervix, vagina, and bladder), but there was no tissue invasion demonstrated. It appears to have a predilection for colonization of those sites. It has very rarely been reported in infections at other sites; its possible role as an etiologic agent of disease is uncertain.

RATE OF GROWTH: Moderate; mature within 6–10 days. Growth more rapid at 37°C than at 30°C; growth also occurs at 42°C.

COLONY MORPHOLOGY: At 25–30°C, thermally dimorphic colonies are at first cream to tan, thin, feltlike or powdery, and radially folded; the central area later becomes heaped and dark; entire colony may become brown with age. Reverse is tan to brown.

At 35–37°C, preferably on enriched medium such as brain heart infusion agar, in 5–7% CO_2, tan to gray, slightly wrinkled yeastlike colonies develop in 2 days.

MICROSCOPIC MORPHOLOGY: At 25–30°C, broad, pauciseptate hyphae are seen. Sporangiophores (100–500 μm long) terminate in a round vesicle that produces recurving stalks, each bearing a round sporangiole (9–13 μm in diameter). The sporangiole contains 12–20 sporangiospores that are smooth walled and of variable size and shape, mostly oval (average, 2.5 × 4.5 μm). No rhizoids are formed. Zygospores are abundantly produced between pairs of hyphal segments, sporangiophores, or suspensors of mature zygospores. Mature zygospores are round (35–55 μm in diameter), brown, and rough walled.

At 35–37°C in 5–7% CO_2, thin-walled, round yeast cells (15–90 μm in diameter) develop, with single or multiple budding that may resemble the mariners's-wheel appearance of *Paracoccidioides brasiliensis* (p. 181).

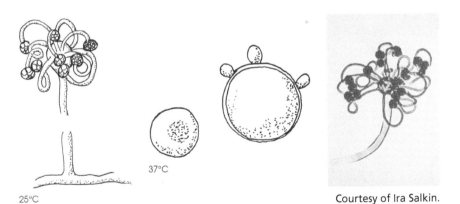

25°C

37°C

Courtesy of Ira Salkin.

Cokeromyces recurvatus *(continued)*

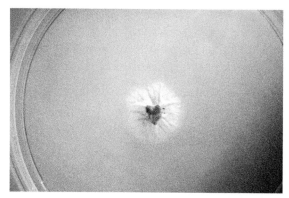

Cokeromyces recurvatus. PDA, 30°C, 5 days. Note lack of woolly growth.

For further information, see
Kemna et al., 1994
McGough et al., 1990
Ramani et al., 2000

Cunninghamella bertholletiae

PATHOGENICITY: Among the members of the order Mucorales, *Cunninghamella berthol-letiae* has been associated with the highest mortality, particularly in causing sinopulmonary and disseminated infections in patients with hematological malignancies. This property also is reflected by laboratory animal studies demonstrating increased virulence measured by mortality and degree of tissue injury in neutropenic hosts. It is an uncommon cause of cutaneous infections following traumatic inoculation. It also has been identified as a serious pathogen in patients with iron overload conditions.

RATE OF GROWTH: Rapid; mature within 5 days. Can grow at 40–45°C.

COLONY MORPHOLOGY: Floccose, like cotton candy; white, then gray. Reverse is white.

MICROSCOPIC MORPHOLOGY: Broad pauciseptate hyphae produce sporangiophores that are long, branched, and end in swollen vesicles (30–65 μm in diameter); vesicles on lateral branches are smaller (14–35 μm in diameter). The vesicles are covered with spinelike denticles, each supporting a round to oval sporangiolum (5–8 × 6–14 μm; each sporangiolum yields one spore). The walls of the sporangiola are often encrusted with needlelike crystals. Rhizoids may be seen. Zygospores and chlamydospores may also be formed.

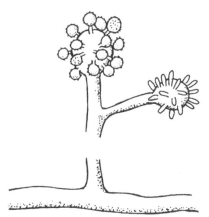 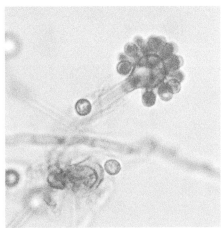

Cunninghamella bertholletiae (continued)

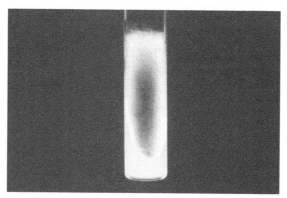

Cunninghamella bertholletiae slant. SDA, 30°C, 4 days. Cotton candy-like growth.

For further information, see
Hsieh et al., 2013
Petraitis et al., 2013

Syncephalastrum racemosum

PATHOGENICITY: Although seldom recovered in a health care setting, *Syncephalastrum racemosum* is occasionally involved in serious infections.

RATE OF GROWTH: Rapid; mature within 5 days. Maximum growth temperature is 40°C.

COLONY MORPHOLOGY: Quickly fills petri plate with white, cotton candy-like fluff, then turns dark gray to almost black. Reverse is white.

MICROSCOPIC MORPHOLOGY: Hyphae are broad and pauciseptate (irregular septa may form with age). Sporangiophores are rather short and branched and terminate in a large, round vesicle (30–80 µm). On the vesicle are fingerlike tubular merosporangia (4–6 × 12–40 µm) containing chains of round spores. Rhizoids are usually formed. This organism may at first resemble *Aspergillus niger* (p. 333), but careful examination reveals the merosporangia and the absence of phialides.

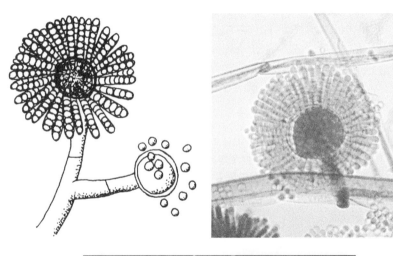

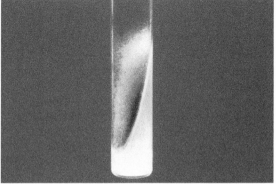

Syncephalastrum racemosum slant. SDA, 30°C, 3 days. Cotton candy-like growth.

For further information, see
Rodríguez-Gutiérrez et al., 2015

Basidiobolus spp.

PATHOGENICITY: Etiologic agent of entomophthoromycosis basidiobolae (subcutaneous mucormycosis), which is a chronic inflammatory or granulomatous disease generally restricted to the limbs, chest, back, or buttocks. The lesions are characteristically large, palpable, hard, nonulcerating subcutaneous masses. Gastrointestinal infections are also known to rarely occur, and disseminated disease may follow. Mainly seen in Asia and Africa, but is occasionally reported in other areas, including gastrointestinal infections in the United States. *Basidiobolus ranarum* is the species most often associated with human disease, and patients often have a history of exposure to lizards and other small reptiles.

RATE OF GROWTH: Rapid; mature within 5 days. Grows faster at 30°C than at 35–37°C. The organism does not survive well at 4°C.

COLONY MORPHOLOGY: Thin, flat, waxy; buff to gray. Becomes heaped up or radially folded, grayish brown, and covered with white aerial hyphae. Reverse is white. Although cultures are handled appropriately in a biological safety cabinet, some may appreciate an earthy odor similar to that of *Streptomyces* spp. The lid of the plate may become covered with ballistospores.

MICROSCOPIC MORPHOLOGY: Wide (8–20 μm) hyphae having occasional septa that become numerous with the production of spores. Short sporophores enlarge apically to form a swollen area from which a single-celled spore and a fragment of the sporophore are forcibly discharged (these are known as ballistospores). Other sporophores (not swollen) passively release club-shaped spores having a knoblike tip; these spores can function as sporangia, producing more sporangiospores. The organism also produces many round intercalary zygospores (20–50 μm in diameter) with smooth (occasionally rough), thick walls and a prominent beaklike appendage (remnant of a copulatory tube) on one side.

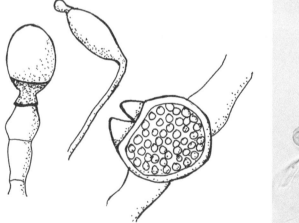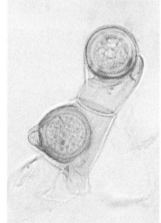

For further information, see
Lyon et al., 2001

Conidiobolus coronatus

PATHOGENICITY: Etiologic agent of entomophthoromycosis conidiobolae, which is a tropical chronic inflammatory or granulomatous disease usually restricted to the nasal mucosa; it can spread to adjacent subcutaneous tissue and cause disfigurement of the face. The disease is characterized by polyps or palpable subcutaneous masses. On rare occasions, this and other species of the genus have caused deeply invasive, life-threatening infections.

RATE OF GROWTH: Rapid; mature within 5 days.

COLONY MORPHOLOGY: Flat, waxy; buff or gray, becoming sparsely covered with short, white aerial hyphae. With age, colony becomes tan to brown. Reverse is white. Satellite colonies form, and sides of culture tube or lid of plate become covered with spores forcibly discharged by the sporophores.

MICROSCOPIC MORPHOLOGY: Hyphae have few septa; unbranched sporophores bear single-celled, round spores (20–40 μm in diameter). At maturity, the spores (ballistospores) are forcibly ejected and bear a broad, tapering projection at the site of former attachment. The spores may germinate and produce long hyphal tubes that become sporophores, each bearing another spore. A spore may also develop a number of short extensions that give rise to a corona of secondary spores. Some spores may produce short, hairlike, villous appendages.

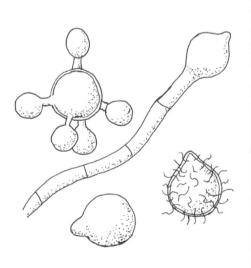
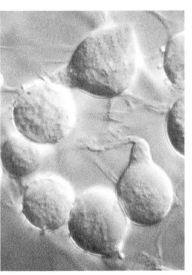

Dematiaceous Fungi

THERMALLY MONOMORPHIC MOULDS • Dematiaceous Fungi

PART II Identification of Fungi in Culture

Introduction to Dematiaceous Fungi

Dematiaceous fungi include a large group of organisms that produce dark (olive, brown, gray, or black) colonies due to a melanin pigment in their cell walls.

The diseases produced by some of the dematiaceous fungi are classified according to the clinical presentation and the appearance of the organism in tissue.

- **Chromoblastomycosis:** The fungi are seen in tissue as sclerotic bodies (also known as medlar bodies, or copper pennies). These structures are round (5–12 μm in diameter), brownish, usually with a single septum or two intersecting septa. The infection is chronic and causes the development of warty nodules, tumorlike masses, or raised, rough, cauliflowerlike lesions containing the sclerotic bodies that involve the subcutaneous soft tissues but spare muscle, tendon, and bone. The lesions usually develop in the subcutaneous tissue of the lower extremities but are sometimes on other exposed areas, such as the hands, head, or trunk. On rare occasions, the etiologic agents have been known to spread to the central nervous system, lungs, or muscular tissues.

- **Phaeohyphomycosis:** The etiologic agents occur in tissue as darkly pigmented septate hyphae, yeastlike cells, pseudohyphaelike elements, variously shaped hyphae, or any combination of these forms. The most common infections are cutaneous, subcutaneous, brain abscesses, or sinusitis. Disseminated infection can occur in immunocompromised individuals.

- **Mycetoma:** The infection is a chronic subcutaneous infection involving muscle, tendon, and bone and characterized by swollen tumorlike lesions that yield granular pus through draining sinuses. The granules of eumycotic mycetoma may be dark or light (many of the etiologic agents are not dematiaceous) and contain variously shaped fungal elements. The infection occurs most often in the feet or hands but may occur on any exposed parts of the body.

For more detailed clinical descriptions of these infections, see pp. 41, 52, and 53. For tinea nigra clinical features, see p. 51.

Tinea nigra and black piedra are also caused by dematiaceous fungi. Each disease is caused by one specific fungus; *Hortaea werneckii* causes tinea nigra and *Piedraia hortae* causes black piedra. The infections are described on the individual page for each organism.

Many of the infections caused by the dematiaceous fungi are due to traumatic implantation of the organism from the environment into cutaneous or subcutaneous tissue, but pulmonary or disseminated infections have been initiated by inhalation of conidia.

Although the dematiaceous fungi are not highly virulent, some are regularly seen as etiologic agents of disease while others usually are encountered as saprophytes or contaminants and only occasionally act as opportunistic pathogens.

Sporothrix schenckii grows as a dematiaceous fungus when incubated at 25–30°C, but it has a yeast phase and is relatively nonpigmented at 35–37°C and is therefore placed with the thermally dimorphic fungi (p. 186).

For further information, see

Anaissie et al., (ed.), 2009

de Hoog et al., 2020

Kidd et al., 2023b

Queiroz-Telles et al., 2017

Revankar and Sutton, 2010

St-Germain and Summerbell, 2011

Fonsecaea spp.

TAXONOMY NOTES: Medically important species include *F. monophora*, *F. pedrosoi*, *F. pugnacious*, and *F. nubica*. These species are difficult to differentiate based on morphology. The previously named species *F. compacta* is rarely encountered and is considered a mutant form of *F. pedrosoi*.

PATHOGENICITY: *F. monophora*, *F. pedrosoi*, *F. pugnacious*, and *F. nubica* are recognized as the most common worldwide cause of human chromoblastomycosis (for a description of the disease, see p. 53). *F. monophora* and *F. pugnacious* may also be involved in disseminated infection and have been recovered from brain, bile, and cervical lymph nodes.

RATE OF GROWTH: Slow; mature after 10 days.

COLONY MORPHOLOGY: Surface is dark green, gray, or black, covered with silvery, velvety mycelium; colonies are usually flat and then develop a convex, cone-shaped protrusion in the center. The colony becomes slightly embedded in the medium. Reverse is black.

MICROSCOPIC MORPHOLOGY: Hyphae are septate, branched, and brown; conidiophores and conidia are dark. Conidia are smooth and thin-walled.

Conidiation is enhanced on cornmeal agar or potato dextrose agar. Four types of conidial formation may be seen. Most colonies display two or three types of conidiation.

1. *Fonsecaea* type: Conidiophores are septate, erect, and compactly sympodial. The tip of the conidiophore develops swollen denticles that bear primary single-celled, ovoid conidia. Denticles on the primary conidia support secondary single-celled conidia that may produce a third row of conidia, but long chains are not formed. Elongate conidia often form in verticils at fertile sites along the conidiophore, producing an asterisk-like appearance.
2. *Rhinocladiella* type: Conidiophores are septate, erect, and sympodial; swollen denticles bear one-celled ovoid conidia at the tip and along the side of the conidiophore. Usually only primary conidia develop per conidiation site; secondary conidia are rare.
3. *Cladosporium* type: Conidiophores are erect and give rise to large, primary, shield-shaped cells that in turn produce short, branching chains of oval conidia having small, dark hila (scars of attachment).
4. *Phialophora* type: Phialides are vase shaped with terminal cuplike collarettes. Round to oval conidia accumulate at the apex of the phialide. This type of conidiation is often scant or lacking.

In tissues, *Fonsecaea*, as well as the other etiologic agents of chromoblastomycosis, appear as large (5–12 μm in diameter), round, brownish, thick-walled cells (sclerotic bodies) with horizontal and vertical septa. When cultured at 25, 30, or 37°C, the organisms are filamentous.

Fonsecaea spp. *(continued)*

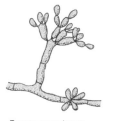

Fonsecaea-type
conidiation.

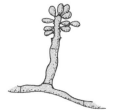

Rhinocladiella-type
conidiation.

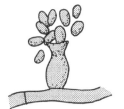

Phialophora-type
conidiation.

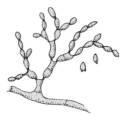

Cladosporium-type
conidiation.

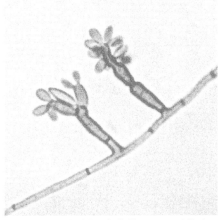

Fonsecaea- and *Rhinocladiella*-type conidiation.

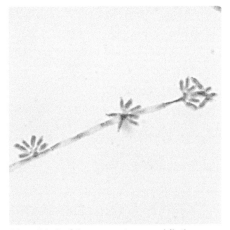

"Asterisks" of *Fonsecaea*-type conidiation.

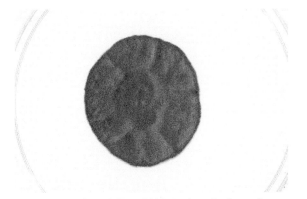

Fonsecaea pedrosoi. SDA, 30°C, 14 days. Surface of colony.

Fonsecaea spp. *(continued)*

Fonsecaea pedrosoi. SDA, 30°C, 14 days. Reverse of colony, typical of completely dark, dematiaceous fungi.

For further information, see de Azevedo et al., 2015

Myrmecridium schulzeri

TAXONOMY NOTES: This species was formerly known as *Ramichloridium schulzeri* and *Rhinocladiella schulzeri*.

PATHOGENICITY: An uncommon soil saprophyte that has been implicated as the cause of "Golden Tongue" after isolation from golden-yellow erosive lesions on the tongue of a neutropenic patient in the United States. It has also been isolated from bronchoscopy specimens from a man in the Netherlands.

RATE OF GROWTH: Moderate (mature within 6–10 days) to slow (mature after 10 days).

COLONY MORPHOLOGY: Surface is velvety, pale orange to orange, and becomes powdery due to sporulation. Reverse is pink to orange.

MICROSCOPIC MORPHOLOGY: Hyphae are septate. Conidiophores are unbranched, reddish-brown, erect, long (up to 250 µm in length), thin-walled, and become paler at the tip. Conidiophores bear scattered pimple-shaped denticles that produce conidia. Conidia (3–4 × 6.5–10 µm) proliferate sympodially and are solitary, subhyaline (not colorless, but not distinctly pigmented), thin-walled, smooth or slightly rough-walled, ellipsoid, obovoid or fusiform, tapering to a narrowly truncate base with an unpigmented hilum.

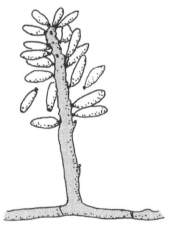 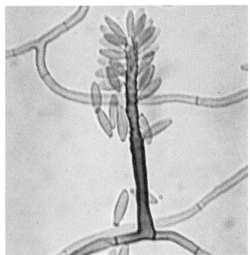

Courtesy of Deanna A. Sutton, doctorfungus.org.

For further information, see Arzanlou et al., 2007

Rhinocladiella mackenziei

TAXONOMY NOTES: *Rhinocladiella mackenziei* was formerly known as *Ramichloridium mackenziei*.

PATHOGENICITY: *R. mackenziei* is a recognized cause of fatal intracerebral infections in the Middle East, India, Afghanistan, and Pakistan. Several species have very occasionally been involved in chromoblastomycosis and mycetoma.

RATE OF GROWTH: Moderate (mature within 6–10 days) to slow (mature after 10 days).

COLONY MORPHOLOGY: Surface may be smooth, velvety, or woolly; dark gray, olivaceous brown to greenish black. Center may be slightly mucoid. Reverse is dark.

MICROSCOPIC MORPHOLOGY: Hyphae are septate. Conidiophores arise at right angles; are relatively short, thick-walled, brown; and usually not well-differentiated from vegetative hyphae. Conidia (4–5 × 8.5–12 µm) are attached to conidiophores with short-cylindrical denticles and are produced sympodially. They are scant, ellipsoidal, brown and thick walled, with a prominent basal scar. *Rhinocladiella* species are superficially similar and sequencing is recommended for accurate identification to species level.

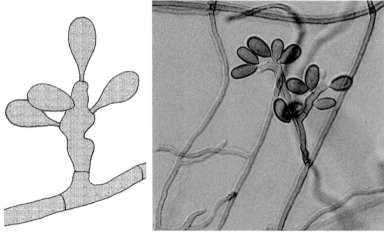

Reprinted from Badali H et al. *J Clin Microbiol* 48:646–649.

For further information, see
Arzanlou et al., 2007
Chowdhary et al., 2014b
Taj-Aldeen et al., 2010

Phialophora verrucosa

PATHOGENICITY: Causes chromoblastomycosis, of which it is the second most common etiologic agent worldwide (members of the genus *Fonsecaea* are the most common) and the most common cause in North America. It is also an etiologic agent of phaeohyphomycosis and, on rare occasions, mycetoma. For descriptions of these diseases, see pp. 53, 52, and 41, respectively.

RATE OF GROWTH: Moderate (mature within 6–10 days) to slow (mature after 10 days).

COLONY MORPHOLOGY: Surface is dark greenish brown to black with a close, matlike, olive to gray woolly mycelium. Some strains are heaped and granular; others are flat. Colonies often become embedded in the agar medium. Reverse is olive-black.

MICROSCOPIC MORPHOLOGY: Hyphae are brown, branched, and septate. Phialides are vase-shaped with a dark, flared, cuplike collarette; they usually have a distinct septum at the base. Round to oval conidia (1–3 × 2–4 µm) accumulate at the apex of the phialide, giving the appearance of a vase of flowers.

To differentiate *Phialophora* from other similar genera, see Table 2.13 (p. 224). They must be distinguished from *Phaeoacremonium* spp. and from *Fonsecaea* spp., which can also display *Phialophora*-type conidiation.

Note: In tissue with chromoblastomycosis, the organism appears as dark, round cells, 5–12 µm in diameter, with horizontal and vertical septa.

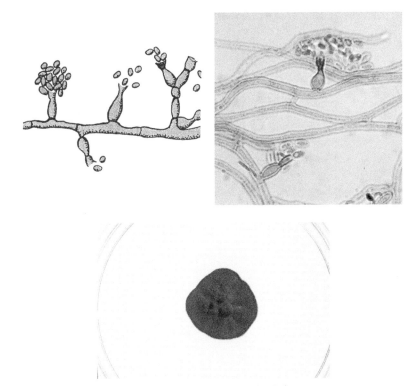

Phialophora verrucosa. SDA, 30°C, 12 days.

PART II Identification of Fungi in Culture

TABLE 2.13 Characteristics of *Phialophora*, *Pleurostoma* (formerly *Pleurostomophora*), *Phaeoacremonium*, *Acremonium and Sarocladium*, *Phialemonium*, and *Coniochaeta* (formerly *Lecythophora*)

| Organism | Colony | Phialide | | | Conidia | Illustration |
		Basal septum	Shape	Collarette		
Phialophora (p. 223)	Dark greenish brown to black	Yes, usually	Flask or vase shaped	Flared, distinct	Oval or round; clusters	
Pleurostoma (formerly *Pleurostomophora*) (p. 225)	Olive brown to brownish gray	Yes, usually	Flask or vase shaped	Flared, distinct (*Pleurostoma repens* is an exception)	Oval or round; clusters	
Phaeoacremonium (p. 226)	Dark olive gray to brown	Yes, usually	Cylindrical; rough at base; tapered toward tip	Almost inconspicuous; tubular or slightly funnel shaped	Oblong; some curved; clusters	
Acremonium and Sarocladium (p. 365)	White, gray, or rose; cottony	Yes, usually	Erect, cylindrical; elongated, unbranched, tapered	Inconspicuous	Oblong; clusters	
Phialemonium (p. 228)	White, then yellow, gray, light brown, or greenish; may become dark	No, usually not	Short, peglike or long, cylindrical	Inconspicuous	Tear shaped or oblong; curved or straight; clusters	
Coniochaeta (formerly *Lecythophora*) (p. 369)	Pink or salmon; moist to slimy	No, usually not	Short; volcano shaped along hyphae	Parallel sided	Oval to oblong; straight or slight curve; no clusters	

Pleurostoma richardsiae

TAXONOMY NOTES: This species was formerly known as *Pleurostomophora richardsiae* and prior to that as *Phialophora richardsiae*. Other medically important species in this genus include *Pleurostoma ochraceum* (formerly *Pleurostomophora ochracea*) and *Pleurostoma repens* (formerly *Pleurostomophora repens*).

PATHOGENICITY: An uncommon agent of cystic subcutaneous phaeohyphomycosis (see p. 52 for a description of the disease). Most reported cases have been in debilitated or immunocompromised patients. *P. ochraceum* is an agent of human mycetoma with yellow grains.

RATE OF GROWTH: Moderate; mature within 6–10 days.

COLONY MORPHOLOGY: Surface is olive brown to brownish gray, woolly to velvety or powdery; brown diffusing pigment may develop with age. Reverse is dark.

MICROSCOPIC MORPHOLOGY: Septate hyphae are at first colorless and become brown. The distinguishing phialides usually (but not always) have a distinct septum at the base and are slightly flask shaped with a characteristic flared, saucer-shaped collarette; they produce conidia that are brown and almost round (2–3.5 µm in diameter). Simple, short, unflared phialides may also form along the hyphae and produce conidia that are hyaline and cylindrical or slightly curved (2–3 × 3–6 µm).

To differentiate *Phialophora* and *Pleurostoma* from other similar genera, see Table 2.13 (p. 224).

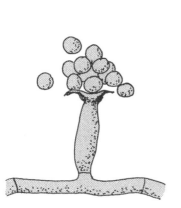 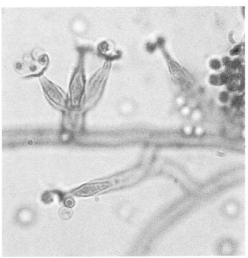

For further information, see
Levenstadt et al., 2012
Mhmoud et al., 2012

Phaeoacremonium parasiticum

TAXONOMY NOTES: This species was formerly known as *Phialophora parasitica*.

PATHOGENICITY: Has been reported in cases of subcutaneous phaeohyphomycoses, mycetoma, arthritis, endocarditis, and infection of various sites including disseminated infection, particularly in immunocompromised patients.

RATE OF GROWTH: Moderate; mature within 6–10 days.

COLONY MORPHOLOGY: Surface initially cream colored and velvety, then becomes grayish beige to olive-brown with radial furrows and a lighter edge and develops clusters of aerial hyphae. Reverse tan to brown.

MICROSCOPIC MORPHOLOGY: Young hyphae appear hyaline, later brown and rough or warty; they may accumulate side by side to form thick bundles (fascicles). Phialides form along the hyphae or on branched or unbranched conidiophores that may be rough walled near the base; phialides are brown, cylindrical (2–3×15–35 µm), slightly tapering toward the apex; they usually have a basal septum and a collarette that is small and tubular or vaguely funnel shaped. Conidia are hyaline, oblong (1–2×3–6 µm), some curved, gathering in clusters at end of phialide.

To differentiate *Phaeoacremonium* from other similar genera, see Table 2.13 (p. 224).

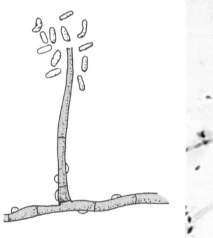
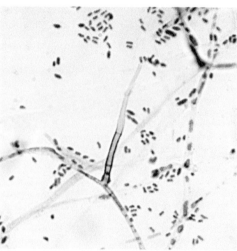

Phaeoacremonium parasiticum (continued)

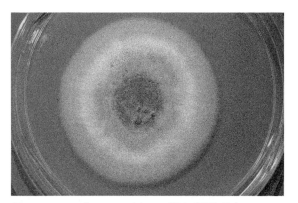

Phaeoacremonium parasiticum. PDA, 30°C, 7 days.

For further information, see
El-Herte et al., 2014

Phialemonium spp.

TAXONOMY NOTES: *Phialemonium curvatum* is currently recognized as *Thyridium curvatum*.

PATHOGENICITY: Occasionally isolated from clinical specimens. Has been reported in a subcutaneous phaeohyphomycotic cyst; an endocarditis mixed infection; peritonitis; osteomyelitis; brain abscesses; fungemia due to contaminated venous catheters; and infection of cutaneous, subcutaneous, and spleen tissue in a burn patient. Infections tend to be invasive and all of the involved patients were immunocompromised. Cutaneous phaeohyphomycosis has also been reported in immunocompetent individuals.

RATE OF GROWTH: Rapid (mature within 5 days) to moderate (mature within 6–10 days).

COLONY MORPHOLOGY: Broadly spreading. Surface is at first white or cream, becoming yellow, grayish, or slightly greenish (the pale yellow or green pigment may diffuse into the agar); with age, light brown or gray areas may develop; some colonies produce chlamydoconidia and develop dark centers. Texture may be smooth or slightly fuzzy or may have superficial radiating hyphal strands. Reverse is light with pale wine-buff or brown areas sometimes developing. Although the colonies are pale in culture, melanin pigmentation of the cell walls of *Phialemonium* in tissue can be demonstrated with Fontana-Masson stain and therefore *Phialemonium* is considered a dematiaceous fungus.

MICROSCOPIC MORPHOLOGY: Hyphae are septate and hyaline or very pale yellow-brown; they may accumulate side by side to form thick bundles (fascicles). Phialides form singly along the hyphae, usually with no septum at the base to delimit it from the hypha; they may be short and peglike (0.5–1.5×1.0–9.0 μm) or longer and cylindrical (up to 30 μm long, 1–2 μm wide), usually lacking a visible collarette when grown on routine mycology media (rarely forms a very inconspicuous cylindrical, parallel-walled collarette). Conidia are single celled (1.0–2.5×3.0–6.0 μm), hyaline, and smooth walled and form clusters. Chlamydoconidia sometimes form in older cultures and result in brown spots or a black center on the colony.

Phialemonium obovatum can be differentiated from *Phialemonium dimorphosporum* and *T. curvatum* as follows.

- *P. obovatum* produces conidia that are oval to tear shaped, may appear slightly cut off at the base, are consistently straight; old colonies become greenish; pale brown chlamydoconidia may develop in old cultures and result in brown spots or a black center on the colony.
- *Phialemonium dimorphosporum* and *T. curvatum* produce conidia that are oval, elongate, and curved (some may remain straight). Chlamydoconidia are not formed. Colonies may develop pale wine-buff zones on reverse side.

Phenotypic characteristics of this genus show significant variation depending on culture medium and temperature. Therefore, it is recommended to standardize conditions, e.g., use potato dextrose agar and incubate at 24–25°C.

To differentiate *Phialemonium* from other similar genera, see Table 2.13 (p. 224).

Phialemonium spp. *(continued)*

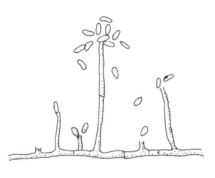 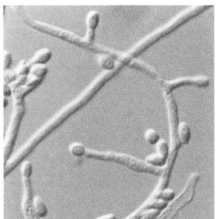

Courtesy of Wiley Schell.

For further information, see
Harrington et al., 2018
Proia et al., 2004
Singh et al., 2021

Cladosporium spp.

TAXONOMY NOTES: There are three prominent species complexes in the genus: *Cladosporium cladosporioides* species complex, *C. herbarum* species complex, and *C. sphaerospermum* species complex. Members of the genus are difficult to differentiate except by molecular methods but differentiation beyond genus level is unnecessary.

PATHOGENICITY: Commonly considered saprophytic contaminants; however, several species have been implicated as plant pathogens and some are also able to rarely infect animals and humans. Allergic rhinitis, keratitis, pulmonary infection, central nervous system infections, and cutaneous phaeohyphomycosis have been reported, mostly in immunocompromised individuals.

RATE OF GROWTH: Moderate; mature within 6–10 days at 25°C. Most strains do not grow at 37°C, but some do.

COLONY MORPHOLOGY: Surface is greenish brown or black with grayish velvety nap, becoming heaped and slightly folded. Reverse is black.

MICROSCOPIC MORPHOLOGY: Hyphae are septate and dark; conidiophores are dark and may be branched in the apical region, vary in length, and usually produce two or more conidial chains. Conidia are brown, round to oval (3–6 × 4–12 μm), and usually smooth; they form branching tree-like chains and are easily dislodged, showing dark spots (hila) at the point where they were attached to the conidiophore or other conidia. The cells bearing the conidial chains are large, sometimes septate, resemble shields (therefore called "shield cells"), and may be mistaken for macroconidia when seen alone.

See Table 2.14 (p. 232) for differentiation from *Cladophialophora* spp.

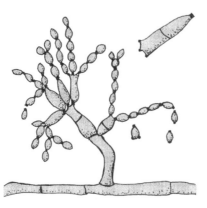
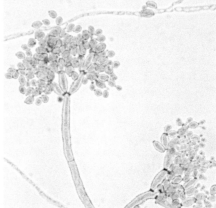

Cladosporium spp. *(continued)*

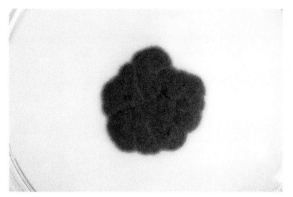

Cladosporium sp. SDA, 30°C, 7 days.

For further information, see
Bensch et al., 2012
Grava et al., 2016
Kantarcioğlu et al., 2002
Polack et al., 1976
Sandoval-Denis et al., 2015
Tamsikara et al., 2006
Vieira et al., 2001

TABLE 2.14 Characteristics of *Cladosporium* spp. and *Cladophialophora* spp.[a]

Organism	Distinct conidio-phores	"Shield cells"	Shape of conidia	Distinct hila on conidia	Conidial chain length	Conidial chain branching	Maximum growth temp (°C)[c]	MDG[b] assimilation	Growth with 15% NaCl	Pathogenicity
Cladosporium spp.	+	+	Oval	+	Short	Frequent	<37 (V)[c]		+	Occasionally pathogenic
Cladophialophora carrionii	±	±	Oval	±	Medium	Moderate	35–37	+	0	Causes chromoblastomycosis
Cladophialophora bantiana	0	0	Oval	0	Long	Sparse	42–43	+	0	Causes cerebral phaeohyphomycosis
Cladophialophora boppii	0	0	Round	0	Long	Sparse	<37	0		Causes skin infection, chromoblastomycosis, and lung infection

[a] Reprinted (updated) by permission of the publisher from Larone, 1989. Copyright by Elsevier Science Inc. Abbreviations: +, positive; 0, negative; ±, sometimes difficult to distinguish; V, variable.

[b] Methyl-α-D-glucoside (MDG) assimilation test is commonly used in the identification of yeasts. The substrate is included in the API 20C AUX (bioMérieux, Inc., Durham, NC) and perhaps other commercial systems; extended period of incubation is required.

[c] 29% grow at 40°C.

Cladophialophora carrionii

TAXONOMY NOTES: This species was formerly known as *Cladosporium carrionii*.

PATHOGENICITY: Causes chromoblastomycosis, most commonly in Australia, Venezuela, and South Africa (for a description of the disease, see p. 53).

RATE OF GROWTH: Slow; mature after 10 days.

COLONY MORPHOLOGY: Dark surface; flat with slightly raised center; covered with velvety dull gray, gray-green, or purplish brown, short-napped mycelium. Reverse is black.

MICROSCOPIC MORPHOLOGY: Hyphae are septate and dark with lateral and terminal conidiophores of various sizes. Conidiophores often poorly differentiated from hyphae. Conidiophores produce long, heavily branched chains of brown, smooth-walled, oval, lemon-shaped, conidia (~2.5 × 4.5–7 μm) that easily break apart during preparation for microscopy. The youngest conidium is at the tip of the chain. The conidia typically have relatively pale scars of attachment (i.e., hila that are not as dark and prominent as those of *Cladosporium* spp.). Phialides with wide collarettes occasionally form on nutritionally deficient media.

For differentiation from *Cladosporium* spp. and other species of *Cladophialophora*, see Table 2.14 (p. 232).

In tissue, the organism appears as large (5–12 μm in diameter), dark, round, septate cells.

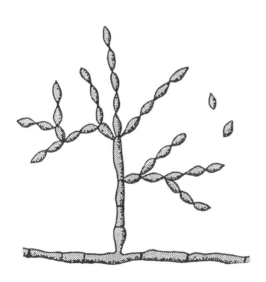 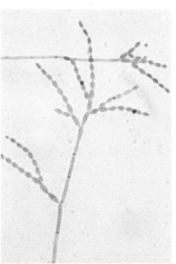

Cladophialophora carrionii (continued)

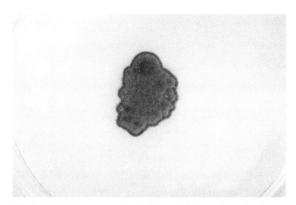

Cladophialophora carrionii. SDA, 30°C, 14 days. Surface of colony.

Cladophialophora boppii

TAXONOMY NOTES: This species was formerly known as *Taeniolella boppii*.

PATHOGENICITY: Has been involved in superficial human skin and nail lesions and in cases of phaeohyphomycosis and chromoblastomycosis-like infections (but typical sclerotic bodies were not always seen in tissue). Pulmonary infection in a lung transplant recipient has been reported but the method of identification was not specified in this report.

RATE OF GROWTH: Slow; mature after 10 days.

COLONY MORPHOLOGY: Surface is olive-gray to black and velvety. Reverse is black.

MICROSCOPIC MORPHOLOGY: Brown, septate hyphae. Conidia are fairly round (3–4 µm in diameter) and form long, mostly unbranched chains directly from the sides of the hyphae; the conidia do not display conspicuous scars of attachment.

For differentiation from *Cladosporium* spp. and other species of *Cladophialophora*, see Table 2.14 (p. 232).

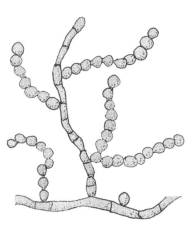
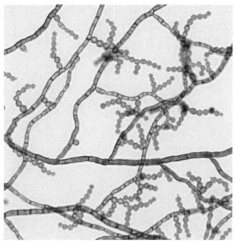

For further information, see
Jang et al., 2018
Saito et al., 2020

Cladophialophora bantiana

TAXONOMY NOTES: This species was formerly known as *Cladosporium bantianum* and *Xylohypha bantiana*.

PATHOGENICITY: Has a predilection for the central nervous system and consequently causes cerebral phaeohyphomycosis. The infection may present initially as a brain tumor. Cerebral lesions that are solitary and encapsulated carry a more favorable prognosis, while lesions with satellite abscesses, or ones that are poorly encapsulated, carry a worse prognosis. Optimal outcome has been best achieved with combined medical and surgical interventions. Infection might be contracted through inhalation; extreme care and a biological safety cabinet should be used when handling this organism. Slide cultures should NOT be made. This organism is only rarely involved in cutaneous and subcutaneous infections.

RATE OF GROWTH: Slow; mature after 10 days.

COLONY MORPHOLOGY: Surface is olive-gray to brown or black and velvety to hairy, sometimes powdery. Reverse is black.

MICROSCOPIC MORPHOLOGY: Brown, septate hyphae with conidiophores that are similar to the vegetative hyphae; long, sparsely branched, wavy chains of smooth, oval lemon-shaped conidia ($2.5–5 \times 6–11$ µm); the conidia do not display conspicuous scars of attachment. The youngest conidium is at the tip of the chain and chains do not fall apart when prepared for microscopy.

For differentiation from similar organisms, see Table 2.14 (p. 232).

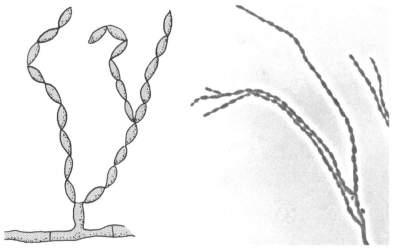

From Michael McGinnis, *Manual of Clinical Microbiology*, 4th ed.

For further information, see
Ajantha and Kulkarni, 2011
McCarthy et al., 2014

Scedosporium apiospermum species complex

TAXONOMY NOTES: The species complex includes *Scedosporium apiospermum sensu stricto* (teleomorph, *Pseudallescheria apiospermum*), *S. boydii*, *P. ellipsoidea*, *P. fusoidium*, and *P. angusta*. Other medically important species in this genus that are not part of the *S. apiospermum* species complex include *S. aurantiacum*, *S. dehoogii*, and *S. minutisporum*. All of these species are morphologically very similar and are difficult to identify to species level without molecular means.

The term "graphium" is descriptive and represents a morphologically distinct phase of growth, not an independent genus. If observed, the culture report should indicate *S. apiospermum* species complex or genus and species name, if determined.

PATHOGENICITY: Found in soil and polluted or stagnant waters. Although commonly considered an agent of phaeohyphomycosis, the hyphae are hyaline. Infection occurs most often in the upper and lower extremities but may occur on any exposed parts of the body. The most common cause of white grain eumycetoma in North America. They can infect subcutaneous tissues, muscle, tendon, and bones, as well as lungs, sinuses, eyes, central nervous system, and other body sites. They are the most common cause of fatal lung and central nervous system infections complicating near-drowning accidents in immunocompetent victims. Disseminated infection is most commonly seen in immunocompromised patients. Invasive *Scedosporium* lung disease in immunocompromised patients may clinically resemble invasive pulmonary aspergillosis. Patients with cystic fibrosis have a high frequency of colonization by *Scedosporium* spp. or chronic infection in the form of fungus balls in the lower respiratory tract, but seldom with progression to locally invasive disease or dissemination. Clinical differences between the member of the genus are not known. Among the different antifungal agents, members of the *S. apiospermum* species complex have the lowest MICs to voriconazole. They tend to have high MICs to amphotericin B.

RATE OF GROWTH: Moderate; mature within 6–10 days. The asexual state grows on media containing cycloheximide, but the cleistothecia of the sexual state are often inhibited.

COLONY MORPHOLOGY: Surface has a spreading, white, cottony aerial mycelium that later turns gray or brown. Reverse is at first white but usually becomes gray or black over time. *Scedosporium aurantiacum* colonies have a concentric growth pattern with a yellow-gray to brown surface and white margin, yellow-orange reverse, and a pale yellow, diffusible pigment.

MICROSCOPIC MORPHOLOGY: Produce septate hyphae (2–4 μm in diameter), with simple, long or short conidiophores bearing conidia singly or in small groups (may resemble mould phase of *Blastomyces* [p. 177]). Conidia (4–7 × 5–12 μm) are unicellular and fairly oval or clavate, with the larger end toward the apex, and appear cut off at the base (i.e., truncate); they become dark with age. In the sexual state (teleomorph), large, brown, thick-walled cleistothecia (50–200 μm in diameter) are formed and release elliptical ascospores when ruptured. They seldom develop in routine clinical cultures, but may sometimes be

Scedosporium apiospermum species complex *(continued)*

induced by culturing on cornmeal agar or potato dextrose agar; the cleistothecia are most likely to form in the center of the colony.

The graphium form of asexual synanamorph conidiation is seen occasionally; it is characterized by septate hyphae with simple, long, dark conidiophores that are cemented together forming synnemata. At the apex of each synnema is a cluster of oval, colorless, single-celled conidia (2–3 × 5–7 μm), some exhibiting a narrowed, truncate base. Delicate, rhizoid-like structures appear at the base of the synnema. See Table 2.2 (p. 124) for differentiation of species.

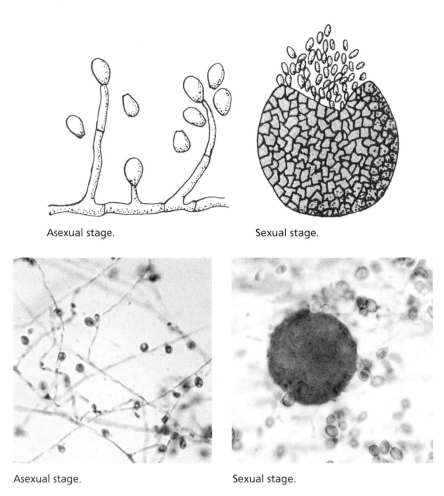

Asexual stage.

Sexual stage.

Asexual stage.

Sexual stage.

Scedosporium apiospermum species complex *(continued)*

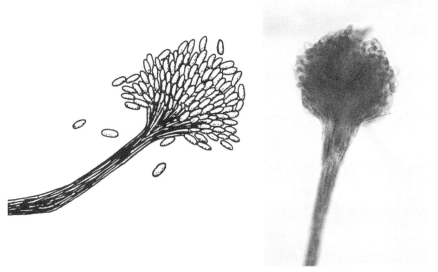

Scedosporium, graphium phase.

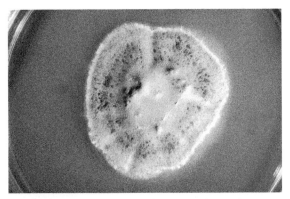

S. apiospermum species complex. SDA, 30°C, 7 days.
Surface of colony.

Scedosporium apiospermum species complex *(continued)*

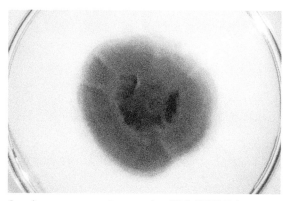

S. apiospermum species complex. SDA, 30°C, 7 days.
Reverse of colony.

For further information, see

Choi et al., 2019

Cortez et al., 2008

Kantarcioglu et al., 2012

Kravitz et al., 2011

Lackner et al., 2012

Lackner et al., 2014

Leek et al., 2016

McCarthy et al., 2014

Ramirez-Garcia et al., 2018

Taj-Aldeen et al., 2015

TABLE 2.15 Differentiating phenotypic characteristics of the clinically encountered members of *Scedosporium* spp. and *Lomentospora prolificans*[a]

Species	Conidiogenous cells	Colony reverse orangish[b]	Yellow diffusible pigment[b]	Growth at 40°C	Growth at 45°C	Growth in presence of cyclo-heximide
Scedosporium apiospermum/ boydii	Cylindrical	0	V	+	0	+
Scedosporium aurantiacum	Cylindrical or slightly flask shaped	+	+	+	+	+
Scedosporium dehoogii	Cylindrical or slightly flask shaped	0	0	0	0	+
Scedosporium minutisporum	Cylindrical	0	0	+	0	+
Lomentospora prolificans	Flask shaped with basal swelling	0	0	+	V	0

[a] Source: Chen *et al.*, 2021a, Gilgado *et al.*, 2008, Ramirez-Garcia *et al.*, 2018. Abbreviations: +, positive; 0, negative; V, variable.

[b] On potato dextrose agar at 25°C.

Lomentospora prolificans

TAXONOMY NOTES: This species was formerly known as *Scedosporium prolificans* and *Scedosporium inflatum.*

PATHOGENICITY: Causes invasive infection that is often characterized by arthritis or osteomyelitis, often occurring by traumatic inoculation, in immunocompetent patients, while disseminated and hematogenous infections occur in immunocompromised hosts. Localized and disseminated infections occur in a variety of sites, especially lung, brain, and bone. The isolates are usually resistant to virtually all available antifungal agents, and disseminated infections are often fatal.

RATE OF GROWTH: Rapid; mature within 5 days. Growth is inhibited by cycloheximide.

COLONY MORPHOLOGY: Young colony is cottony or moist (yeasty) and light gray to black. Mature colony becomes dark gray to black and may develop white mycelial tufts with age. Reverse is gray to black.

MICROSCOPIC MORPHOLOGY: Hyphae are septate, with conidiogenous cells (annellides) having a swollen base and elongated "neck"; conidia form small clusters at the apex. Conidia (2–5 × 3–12 μm) are olive to brown, one celled, smooth, and ovoid with a slightly narrowed, truncated (cut-off) base. As the colony matures, the inflated bases of the conidiophores become less prominent.

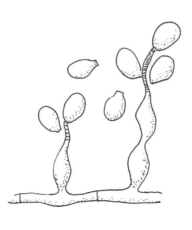 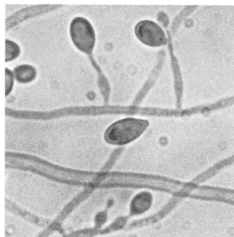

Lomentospora prolificans (continued)

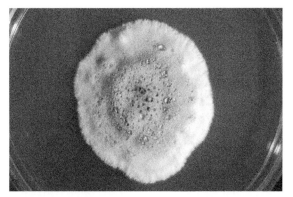

Lomentospora prolificans. SDA, 30°C, 7 days. Surface of colony.

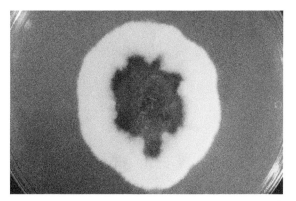

Lomentospora prolificans. SDA, 30°C, 7 days. Reverse of colony.

For further information, see
Clinical and Laboratory Standards Institute M38M51S, 2022
Lackner et al., 2014
Ramirez-Garcia et al., 2018

Verruconis gallopava

TAXONOMY NOTES: This species was formerly known as *Ochroconis gallopava* and *Dactylaria constricta* var. *gallopava*.

PATHOGENICITY: Has caused subcutaneous and disseminated infections in immunocompromised patients, especially those with solid organ transplantation and hematological malignancies. The organism is thermophilic (grows at 40°C) and is known to have a predilection for the central nervous system. It is a recognized agent of brain infection in humans and is a relatively common cause of encephalitis in turkeys, chickens, and other birds. Pulmonary infections in immunocompetent humans have also been reported.

RATE OF GROWTH: Rapid; mature within 5 days. Growth is inhibited by cycloheximide.

COLONY MORPHOLOGY: Surface is feltlike and dark olive-gray, reddish brown, or brownish black. Reverse is dark; a red to brown pigment usually diffuses into the medium.

MICROSCOPIC MORPHOLOGY: Hyphae are hyaline to pale brown, thick-walled and septate with conidiophores that are hyaline, erect, and sometimes knobby or bent at the point of conidial formation. Conidia (2.5–4.5 × 11–18 μm) form on threadlike denticles; the conidia are brownish, two celled, oval to tear shaped, and typically have a marked constriction at the central septum. A frill of the denticle often remains on the base of the conidium after detachment from the conidiophore. Young conidia may be round and single celled.

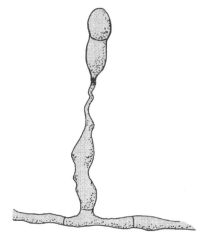 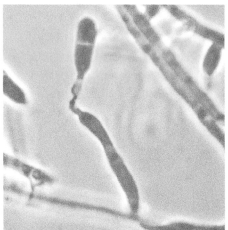

Courtesy of Dennis Dixon.

Verruconis gallopava *(continued)*

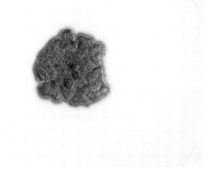

Verruconis gallopava. SDA, 30°C, 7 days.

For further information, see
Giraldo et al., 2014

TABLE 2.16 Characteristics of some of the "black yeasts"[a]

Organism	Decomposition of:		Growth in 15% NaCl	KNO$_3$ assimilation	Maximum growth temp (°C)
	Casein (% positive)	Tyrosine (% positive)			
Exophiala jeanselmei species complex	0	+ (78)	0	+	≤37
Exophiala dermatitidis	0	+ (83)	0	0	42
Hortaea werneckii	+ (78)	0 (22)	+	+	<37

[a] Reprinted by permission of the publisher from Larone, 1989. Copyright by Elsevier Science Inc. Abbreviations: +, positive; 0, negative. (Updated 2011.)

Exophiala jeanselmei species complex

TAXONOMY NOTES: The species complex includes *E. heteromorpha*, *E. lecanii-corni*, and *E. jeanselmei sensu stricto*. These species are difficult to differentiate phenotypically.

PATHOGENICITY: Causes black grain mycetoma and phaeohyphomycosis. Chromoblastomycosis-like infections have only rarely been reported. For descriptions of diseases, see pp. 41, 52, and 53, respectively.

RATE OF GROWTH: Slow; mature after 10 days when incubated at 25–30°C. Grows more slowly or not at all at 37°C.

COLONY MORPHOLOGY: Surface is at first brownish black or greenish black and skin-like; it then becomes covered with short, velvety, grayish hyphae. Reverse is black.

MICROSCOPIC MORPHOLOGY: Young culture consists of many yeastlike budding cells. Eventually, septate hyphae form with numerous conidiogenous cells (annellides) that are slender, tubular, sometimes branched, and characteristically tapered to a narrow, elongated tip. The conidia (1–3 × 2–6 μm) are oval and gather in clusters at the end and sides of the conidiophore and at points along the hyphae. Conidium formation is often best exhibited on cornmeal agar or potato dextrose agar. Chlamydospores may be present.

See Table 2.16 (p. 246) for differentiation from similar organisms.

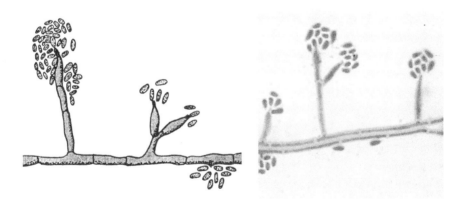

Exophiala jeanselmei species complex *(continued)*

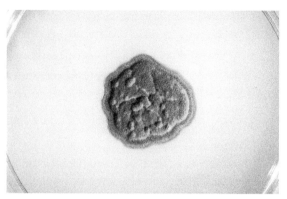

Exophiala jeanselmei species complex. SDA, 30°C,
14 days. Surface of colony.

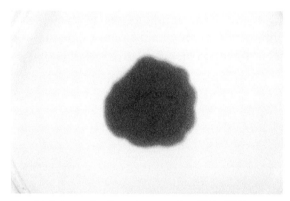

Exophiala jeanselmei species complex. SDA, 30°C,
14 days. Reverse of colony.

For further information, see
Badali et al., 2010

Exophiala dermatitidis

TAXONOMY NOTES: This species was formerly known as *Wangiella dermatitidis*.

PATHOGENICITY: Causes phaeohyphomycosis (for a description of the disease, see p. 52). The organism has a predilection for the central nervous system; it has been involved in infections of various sites, including the brain, lung (especially in cystic fibrosis patients), and eye, as well as cutaneous and subcutaneous tissue.

RATE OF GROWTH: Slow; mature and filamentous after 10 days (typically within 25 days) (yeastlike within 10 days).

COLONY MORPHOLOGY: At first the colony is black, moist, shiny, and yeastlike. After 3 or 4 weeks or upon repeated subculture, olive-gray aerial hyphae develop at the periphery and sometimes near the center of the colony. Reverse is dark.

MICROSCOPIC MORPHOLOGY: Young cultures are composed of dark (may originally be hyaline), oval to round, budding, yeastlike cells. These cells eventually produce dark, septate hyphae and cylindrical to flask-shaped conidiogenous cells that usually have a somewhat truncate apex without collarette or conspicuous extension. Round to oval, single-celled, pale brown conidia (2–3 × 3–6 µm) accumulate at the apex of the conidiogenous cell and down the sides of the conidiophore. Conidia may also be produced at projections along the hyphae. Production of conidia is sometimes sparse. See Table 2.16 (p. 246) for differentiation from similar organisms.

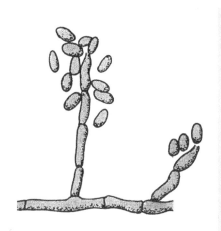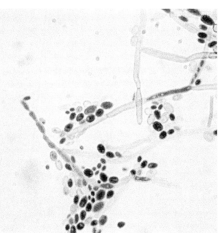

Exophiala dermatitidis (continued)

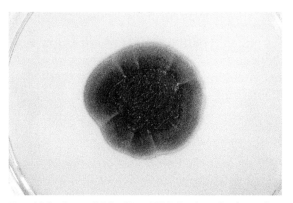

Exophiala dermatitidis. SDA, 30°C, 21 days. Surface of colony.

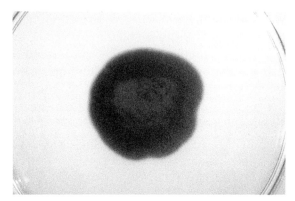

Exophiala dermatitidis. SDA, 30°C, 21 days. Reverse of colony.

For further information, see
Kirchhoff et al., 2019
Mills et al., 2021
Yu et al., 2021

Hortaea werneckii

TAXONOMY NOTES: This species was formerly known as *Phaeoannellomyces werneckii*.

PATHOGENICITY: Etiologic agent of most cases of tinea nigra, a superficial, asymptomatic fungal infection of the skin, usually on the palms of the hands and occasionally on other parts of the body. The lesions are flat, smooth, and not scaly and appear as irregularly shaped brown to black spots resembling silver nitrate stains. The palmar and plantar lesions may also resemble melanoma. Tinea nigra is more common in tropical regions of Central America, South America, Africa, and Asia. Although rare, it has been reported in individuals in the United States who live along southeast or southern coastal areas (e.g., Alabama, Florida, Louisiana, North Carolina, Texas, and Virginia) or who have acquired the infection on travel to areas where it is more common. Other dematiaceous fungi, such as *Stenella araguata* and *Cladophialophora saturnica* have been reported to cause similar lesions.

RATE OF GROWTH: Slow; mature after 10 days (typically within 21 days).

COLONY MORPHOLOGY: Surface is at first light colored, moist, shiny, and yeastlike but soon becomes olive-black. Later, grayish green hyphae may form at the periphery, and the center may lose its shine and become olive colored due to thin layer of mycelium. Reverse is black.

MICROSCOPIC MORPHOLOGY: The very early phase consists mainly of pale or dark brown, yeastlike cells. Mature forms are one or two celled (3–5 × 7–10 µm); they are actually annellides, round at one end while tapered and elongated with striations at the other end where conidia are formed. With age, dark, closely septated, thick-walled hyphae develop. Annelloconidia may form and accumulate at annellidic points along the hyphae. Each conidium can function as an annellide and produce new conidia. Chlamydoconidia may develop with age.

See Table 2.16 (p. 246) for differentiation from similar organisms.

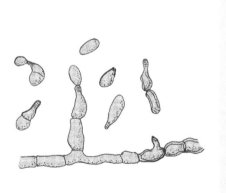
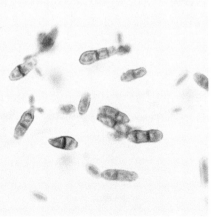

For further information, see
Rezusta et al., 2010

Madurella mycetomatis

PATHOGENICITY: Causes black grain mycetoma (for a description of the disease, see p. 41) that may result in chronic debilitating deformity and osteoarticular destruction usually of the lower extremities. Most common in South America, India, and East Africa. Rare cases of cerebral abscess have also been reported.

RATE OF GROWTH: Moderate; mature within 6-10 days. Best growth at 37°C; much slower at 25–30°C.

COLONY MORPHOLOGY: Varies greatly; may be smooth or folded and glabrous or powdery and ranges in color from white to yellowish brown. There is usually a brown, diffusible pigment in the agar. Reverse is dark brown.

MICROSCOPIC MORPHOLOGY: On Sabouraud dextrose agar, forms only septate hyphae (1–6 μm in diameter) with numerous chlamydoconidia-like, enlarged cells. On cornmeal agar, some strains produce phialides that bear round or oval conidia at their tips. May form large, black masses of modified hyphae (sclerotia) in old cultures.

M. mycetomatis can be distinguished from *Trematosphaeria grisea* by growth at 37°C and production of brown diffusible pigment.

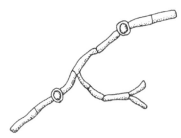

On Sabouraud dextrose agar.

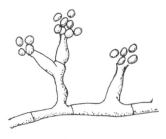

On cornmeal agar.

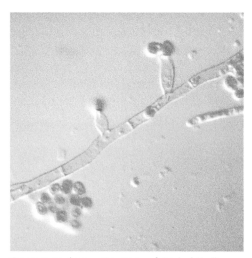

On cornmeal agar. Courtesy of Arvind Padhye.

For further information, see

Mir et al., 2013

Verma and Jha, 2019

Zaid et al., 2021

Trematosphaeria grisea

TAXONOMY NOTES: This species was formerly known as *Madurella grisea*.

PATHOGENICITY: Causes black grain mycetoma (for a description of the disease, see p. 41). Occurs in India, Africa, Central and South America, and occasionally in the United States.

RATE OF GROWTH: Slow; mature after 10 days. Best growth at 25–30°C; does not grow well, if at all, at 37°C.

COLONY MORPHOLOGY: Surface is somewhat folded in the center with radial grooves toward the periphery. Very short, tan or gray aerial hyphae cover a dark gray or olive-brown mycelial mat. Reverse is dark. May form diffusible pigment, but not as commonly as does *Madurella mycetomatis*.

MICROSCOPIC MORPHOLOGY: Hyphae are septate, mostly wide (3–5 µm), branched, and dark. The hyphae sometimes appear to be made up of chains of rounded cells, suggesting a budding process. Thinner (1–3 µm in diameter), cylindrical, branched hyphae are also present. Conidia are not commonly formed. Some strains may produce pycnidia; chlamydoconidia are occasionally produced.

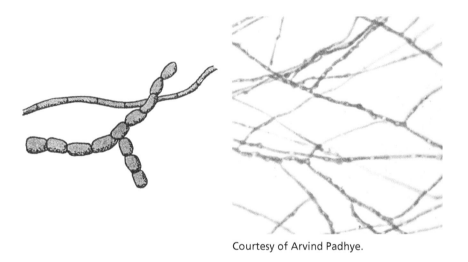

Courtesy of Arvind Padhye.

*For further information, see
Verma and Jha, 2019*

Piedraia hortae

PATHOGENICITY: Causes black piedra, a fungal infection of the hairs of the scalp seen most commonly in the tropics. It is characterized by the formation of small, stony hard, dark nodules along the hair shafts. White piedra is caused by *Trichosporon ovoides* and *Trichosporon inkin* (p. 163).

RATE OF GROWTH: Slow; mature after 10 days (typically within 21 days).

COLONY MORPHOLOGY: Colonies are small, adherent, compact, somewhat raised, and dark greenish brown to black and may be glabrous or covered with very short aerial hyphae. Reddish brown, diffusible pigment may form. Reverse is black.

MICROSCOPIC MORPHOLOGY: Hyphae are closely septate, dark, and thick walled and vary in diameter, with many intercalary chlamydoconidia-like cells. Asci may be produced in culture. The walls of the asci readily dissolve, releasing single-celled, curved ascospores (5–10 × 30–35 μm) that taper at the ends to form whiplike extensions. The ascospores are more likely to be seen on direct microscopic examination of the specimen than on culture.

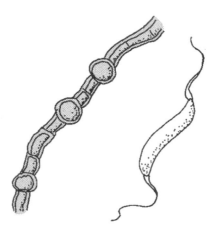

For further information, see Schwartz, 2004

Aureobasidium pullulans

PATHOGENICITY: Relatively rare agent of phaeohyphomycosis; reported cases include corneal, peritoneal, cutaneous, pulmonary, and systemic infections, particularly as a result of traumatic implantation. May also be encountered as a contaminant in clinical specimens.

RATE OF GROWTH: Rapid; growth appears within 5 days, but pigment production and characteristic morphology may require extended incubation.

COLONY MORPHOLOGY: Colony is at first white, very occasionally pale pink; appears moist and creamy. Eventually develops areas of brown or black (when chlamydoconidia develop) and becomes shiny, with a white to grayish fringe. Reverse is dark when colony is mature.

MICROSCOPIC MORPHOLOGY: Young colonies consist of unicellular, budding, yeastlike cells. Two types of hyphae (3–12 μm in diameter) develop: (i) hyaline, delicate, and thin walled, producing blastoconidia directly from the walls at certain fertile points, and (ii) thick-walled, dark, and closely septated segments that become chlamydoconidia that may also produce blastoconidia. The blastoconidia are hyaline and oval, vary in size (average, 3–6 × 6–12 μm), and may continue to multiply by budding; they form synchronously (i.e., simultaneously, each from a separate fertile point), mostly on the hyaline hyphae. The early yeastlike form may be similar to *Candida* spp. or young cultures of *Exophiala dermatitidis* (p. 249) and *Hortaea werneckii* (p. 251), but it can be distinguished by careful examination of growth rate and mature microscopic morphology.

A. pullulans is most likely to be confused with *Hormonema dematioides* (p. 258); for differentiation of these two fungi, see Table 2.17 (p. 257).

THERMALLY MONOMORPHIC MOULDS • Dematiaceous Fungi

Aureobasidium pullulans (continued)

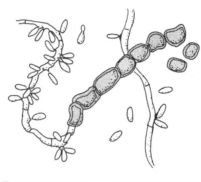

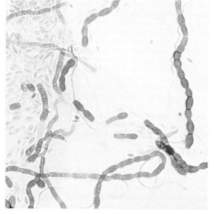

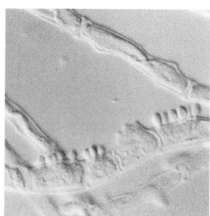

Synchronous production of blastoconidia.

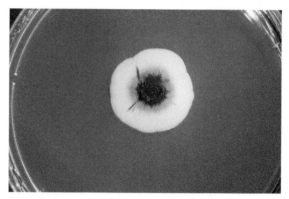

Aureobasidium pullulans. SDA, 30°C, 7 days.

*For further information, see
Mittal et al., 2018*

TABLE 2.17 Differential characteristics of *Aureobasidium pullulans* versus *Hormonema dematioides*

Organism	Assimilation of MDG[a]	Formation of hyaline blastic conidia[b]	
Aureobasidium pullulans (p. 255)	Positive	Form mostly on hyaline hyphae Develop in a synchronous fashion (i.e., conidia are formed simultaneously, each **from a separate fertile point**; these points are often very close together, producing clusters of conidia)	
Hormonema dematioides (p. 258)	Negative	Form on both hyaline and dematiaceous hyphae Develop in an asynchronous fashion (i.e., conidia are produced in succession **from the same single fertile point**; the conidia may form short chains or gather in loose clusters)	

[a] Methyl-α-D-glucoside (MDG) assimilation can be tested with the API 20C AUX panel (bioMérieux, Inc., Durham, NC); extended incubation is required. This one substrate appears to give credible results with these organisms, but the overall identification profile number cannot be accepted.

[b] The microscopic morphology of these organisms is best demonstrated by utilizing the Dalmau method (p. 454) on cornmeal-Tween 80 medium incubated at 25°C for an extended period of time (until dematiaceous hyphae develop).

Hormonema dematioides

PATHOGENICITY: Has been reported to cause peritonitis, fungemia, and cutaneous phaeohyphomycosis. Exposure to birds has been related to deep infection by *H. dematioides*. It may also be encountered as a contaminant.

RATE OF GROWTH: Rapid; growth appears within 5 days, but pigment production and characteristic morphology may require extended incubation.

COLONY MORPHOLOGY: Colony is initially white to cream, sometimes pinkish; appears smooth and becomes moister as conidia develop; poorly conidiating strains may have a woolly mycelial mat; color eventually becomes brownish black as chlamydoconidia develop. Reverse is dark when colony is mature.

MICROSCOPIC MORPHOLOGY: Young colonies consist of unicellular, budding, yeast-like cells. Two types of hyphae (3–12 μm in diameter) develop: (i) hyaline, delicate, and thin walled, producing blastoconidia directly from the walls at certain fertile points, and (ii) thick-walled, dark, and closely septated segments that become chlamydoconidia. The blastoconidia are hyaline and oval, vary in size (average, 3–6 × 6–12 μm), and may continue to multiply by budding; they are produced asynchronously (i.e., in succession, from the same single fertile point) on both the hyaline and dematiaceous hyphae.

H. dematioides can easily be mistaken for *Aureobasidium pullulans* (p. 255); for differentiation of these two fungi, see Table 2.17 (p. 257).

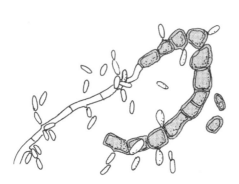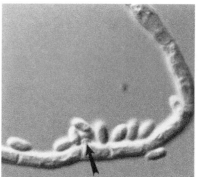

Asynchronous production of blastoconidia.
Courtesy of Wiley Schell.

For further information, see
Kent et al., 1998
Shin et al., 1998

Neoscytalidium dimidiatum

TAXONOMY NOTES: This species was formerly known as *Fusicoccum dimidiatum*, *Neoscytalidium hyalinum*, *Scytalidium dimidiatum*, and *Scytalidium hyalinum*.

PATHOGENICITY: Known to commonly cause nail and skin infections, as well as keratitis; there are also rare reports of more deep-seated infections, such as subcutaneous abscess, sinusitis, endophthalmitis, lymphadenitis, brain infection, empyema, and fungemia predominantly in immunocompromised patients. Infection is principally in individuals who live in or have visited tropical or subtropical areas, while several cases have been reported in individuals who have never left temperate zones.

RATE OF GROWTH: Rapid; mature within 5 days. Growth is inhibited by cycloheximide; therefore, the organism will not grow on most media specifically designed for dermatophytes.

COLONY MORPHOLOGY: Colonies are usually woolly, and growth quickly fills the agar plate or covers the agar slant; some isolates do not spread across the agar as robustly. The surface is gray to brown or black with a dark reverse or may be white to cream or gray with a buff to yellowish reverse in melanin-deficient mutants.

MICROSCOPIC MORPHOLOGY: Hyphae are hyaline, septate and branched, but no conidiophores are formed. Arthroconidia (3–6 × 5–13 µm) develop that have one or two cells, are flattened on the ends, and may be rectangular, square, oval, or roundish and become barrel shaped; they are consecutive; i.e., there are no empty cells between the arthroconidia. The wider hyphae (6–10 µm) and arthroconidia of *N. dimidiatum* are brown, while the narrower side branches of hyphae tend to produce pale arthroconidia. Melanin-free mutants occur (previously known as *Scytalidium hyalinum*); they produce hyphae and arthroconidia that are invariably colorless but are identical to those of *N. dimidiatum* in every other way.

A pycnidial form very occasionally develops in old cultures. The pycnidia are large (100–300 µm in diameter); pycnidial conidia are hyaline when young and with age develop one to five septa and a dark brown central area.

See Table 2.21 (p. 320) for differential characteristics of fungi in which arthroconidia predominate.

Neoscytalidium dimidiatum (continued)

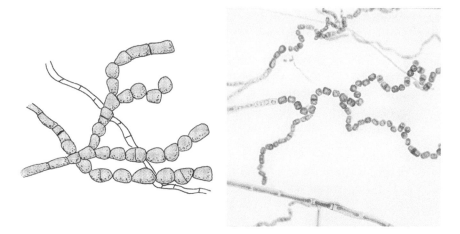

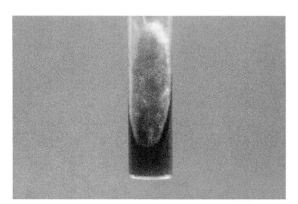

Neoscytalidium dimidiatum slant. SDA, 30°C, 3 days.

For further information, see
Jo et al., 2021

Botrytis cinerea

PATHOGENICITY: Considered a contaminant when encountered in the mycology laboratory. Its normal habitat is plants. It spoils strawberries and most other fruits, vegetables, and flowers by forming "gray mould," but when on grapes under the proper conditions, it is a valuable contributor to the development of the sweetness of some dessert wines.

RATE OF GROWTH: Rapid; mature within 5 days.

COLONY MORPHOLOGY: Surface is at first white and then gray or brown, sometimes with blackish spots; woolly. Reverse is usually dark.

MICROSCOPIC MORPHOLOGY: The term *Botrytis* derives from the ancient Greek word *botrys*, meaning "grapes." Wide, septate hyphae with dark, septate, long conidiophores that branch only at the apex. The branches have swollen tips that bear round to oval, colorless to pale brown conidia on short denticles. Conidia also form at points along the conidiophore. The swollen apices bearing conidia on short denticles may be suggestive of *Cunninghamella* (p. 209), but close examination of macroscopic and microscopic morphology and the presence of melanin will provide differentiation of the two.

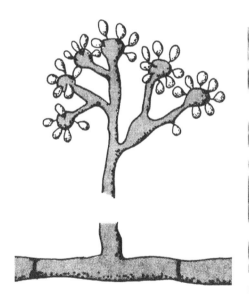

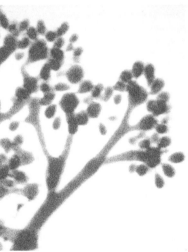

From Rippon, 1988.

Stachybotrys chartarum

TAXONOMY NOTES: This species was formerly known as *S. alternans* and *S. atra*.

PATHOGENICITY: Produces several mycotoxins that appear to have the ability to adversely affect humans and animals after ingestion, inhalation, or percutaneous absorption. The fungus has been associated with pulmonary hemorrhage and hemosiderosis in animals. It has also been implicated in illnesses (with a variety of symptoms), including hypersensitivity pneumonitis, in occupants (of all ages) of water-damaged homes and other buildings. Additional studies are needed to establish a firm causal relationship.

RATE OF GROWTH: Moderate; mature within 6–10 days but can be rather fastidious on routine laboratory media; prefers medium with high cellulose content, e.g., cellulose Czapek agar.

COLONY MORPHOLOGY: Surface is at first white, becoming dark gray to black with age; powdery to cottony, spreading. Reverse is at first light and then dark.

MICROSCOPIC MORPHOLOGY: Hyphae are septate and colorless to dark. Conidiophores are simple or branched, may become pigmented and rough with age, and bear clusters of 3–10 phialides. The phialides are colorless or pigmented, nonseptate, and cylindrical, with a swollen upper portion. Conidia are dark, oval (average, 4.5 × 9 μm), single celled, and smooth or rough walled and usually form in clusters on the phialides.

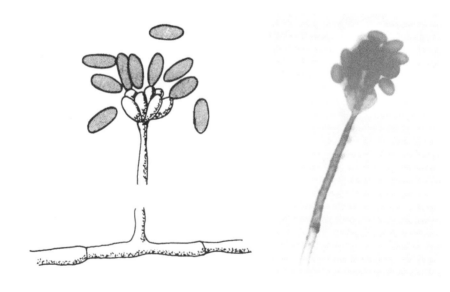

Stachybotrys chartarum (continued)

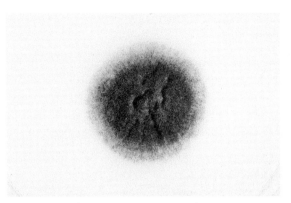

Stachybotrys chartarum. SDA, 30°C, 7 days.

For further information, see
Kuhn and Ghannoum, 2003
Vance and Weissfeld, 2007

Thermothelomyces thermophilus

TAXONOMY NOTES: This species was formerly known as *Thermothelomyces thermophila* and *Myceliophthora thermophila*.

PATHOGENICITY: A rarely encountered agent of phaeohyphomycosis. Pulmonary and disseminated infections have been observed in immunocompromised patients, while post-traumatic and post-surgical focal non-pulmonary infections have been reported in immunocompetent individuals. The organism appears to have a vascular tropism. Cross-reactivity with the *Aspergillus* galactomannan assay has been described.

RATE OF GROWTH: Rapid; mature within 5 days. Best growth at elevated temperatures of 35°C and 42°C (growth up to 55°C).

COLONY MORPHOLOGY: Initially white and cottony, then turn cinnamon brown and powdery-to-cottony with an ill-defined margin.

MICROSCOPIC MORPHOLOGY: Contains melanin within its cell wall; however, septate hyphae appear hyaline. Conidiophores are hyaline and smooth-walled. Ovoid-to-pyriform conidia are produced from flask-shaped swellings, and begin smooth and hyaline but with maturation become dark and rough. Conidia are 3.0–4.5 × 4.5–11 μm, arise terminally or laterally, and may occur singly or cluster.

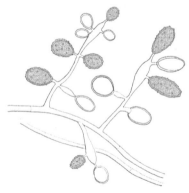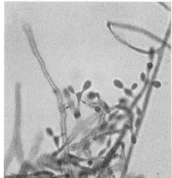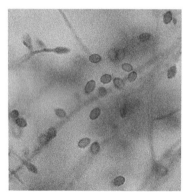

Reprinted from Morio F et al. 2011. *Med Mycol* 49:883–886.

For further information, see
Bourbeau et al., 1992
Destino et al., 2006
Marin-Felix et al., 2015
Nourrisson et al., 2017

Curvularia spp.

TAXONOMY NOTES: The genus *Curvularia* has undergone extensive taxonomic revision. Human pathogenic *Bipolaris* spp. have been moved to the genus *Curvularia*. This includes the former species *B. australiensis*, *B. hawaiiensis*, and *B. spicifera*. Other medically important species in the genus *Curvularia* include *C. geniculata* and *C. lunata*. There are many other species of *Curvularia* that may be capable of causing infections in immunocompromised hosts.

PATHOGENICITY: Etiologic agents of opportunistic infections, most commonly causing keratitis and allergic/chronic sinusitis. May also cause onychomycosis as well as dark grain mycetoma and phaeohyphomycosis at various sites, including subcutaneous tissue and deep tissues. Keratitis, sinusitis, cutaneous and subcutaneous infections, peritonitis, onychomycosis, endocarditis, endophthalmitis, and pneumonia as well as disseminated disease have also been reported. Dissemination to the brain is known to occur occasionally in immunocompetent and immunocompromised individuals, often following sinusitis or lung infection. There is also an apparent association between heavy marijuana use and *Curvularia* infection, presumably from inhalation of the organism on contaminated marijuana leaves.

RATE OF GROWTH: Rapid; mature within 5 days.

COLONY MORPHOLOGY: Surface of *Curvularia* spp. (*C. geniculata*, *C. lunata*, and other species) is dark olive-green to brown or black with a pinkish gray, woolly surface. Reverse is dark.

Surface of former *Bipolaris* spp. (*B. australiensis*, *B. hawaiiensis*, and *B. spicifera*) that are now recognized as *Curvularia* is at first grayish brown, becoming black with a matted center and raised grayish periphery. Reverse is dark brown to black.

MICROSCOPIC MORPHOLOGY: *Curvularia* spp. (*C. geniculata*, *C. lunata*, and other species) have dark, septate hyphae. Conidiophores are simple or branched and bent or knobby at points of conidium formation (sympodial geniculate growth). Conidia are large (8–14 × 21–35 μm), usually contain four cells and eventually appear curved due to swelling of a central cell (the curving may take 5 or more days to develop).

The former *Bipolaris* spp. (*B. australiensis*, *B. hawaiiensis*, and *B. spicifera*) that are now recognized as *Curvularia* have dark, septate hyphae. Conidiophores elongate and bend at the point where each conidium is formed (sympodial geniculate growth); this produces a knobby, zigzag appearance. Conidia are hyaline when immature, brown when mature, oblong to cylindrical (6–13 × 14–39 μm), appear thick walled, rounded at both ends, have three to five transverse septations, and a slightly protruding hilum.

See Table 2.18 for differentiation from similar organisms.

Curvularia spp. *(continued)*

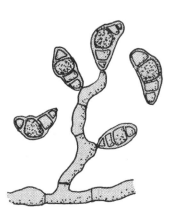 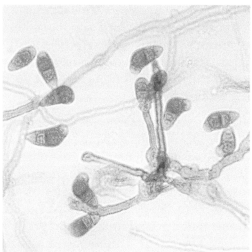

Curvularia sp.

Curvularia sp. SDA, 30°C, 5 days.

Curvularia spp. *(continued)*

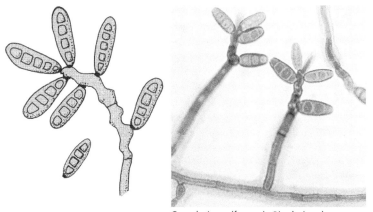

Curvularia sp. (formerly *Bipolaris* sp.).

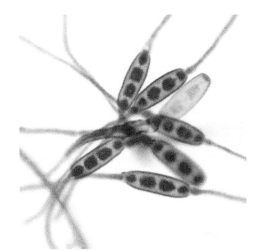

Curvularia sp. (formerly *Bipolaris* sp.), bipolar germ tubes. When tested for, germ tubes develop at both poles of the conidium (hence the former genus name).

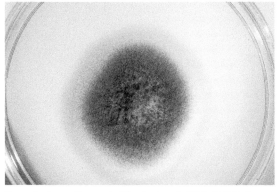

Curvularia sp. (formerly *Bipolaris* sp.). SDA, 30°, 5 days. Surface of colony.

THERMALLY MONOMORPHIC MOULDS   **267**

Curvularia **spp.** *(continued)*

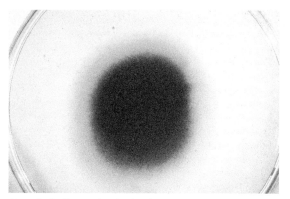

Curvularia (formerly *Bipolaris*). SDA, 30°, 5 days. Reverse of colony.

For further information, see
da Cunha et al., 2012
Gonzales Zamora and Varadarajalu, 2019
Manamgoda et al., 2012
Skovrlj et al., 2014
Vachharajani et al., 2005
Wilhelmus and Jones, 2001

TABLE 2.18 Characteristics of *Curvularia* spp. and *Exserohilum rostratum*.

Genus	Conidiation	Conidia			Illustration
		Avg. size (μm)	No. of septa	Hilum	
Curvularia	Profuse, dark, curved due to swelling of central cell	8–14 × 21–35	Usually 3	Does not protrude	
Curvularia (former *Bipolaris* species)	Profuse, dark, straight or slightly curved, oblong to cylindrical	6–13 × 14–39	3–5	Protrudes slightly	
Exserohilum rostratum	Profuse; ellipsoidal to fusoid	14 × 90 or greater	5–12	Protrudes slightly	

Exserohilum rostratum

PATHOGENICITY: In 2012, caused an epidemic outbreak of iatrogenic meningoencephalitis, meningoradiculitis, epidural abscesses, and vertebral osteomyelitis following intrathecal or lumbosacral injection of contaminated methylprednisolone solution. Before this outbreak, *E. rostratum* was known to cause other infections, including phaeohyphomycosis (see p. 52 for a description of the disease), sinusitis, subcutaneous infection, and keratitis. Fatal disseminated infections also have been reported to occur in immunocompromised hosts.

RATE OF GROWTH: Rapid; mature within 5 days.

COLONY MORPHOLOGY: Surface is dark gray to black, cottony. Reverse is black.

MICROSCOPIC MORPHOLOGY: Dark, septate hyphae. Conidiophores elongate and bend (sympodial geniculate growth) at the point where each conidium is formed; this produces a knobby, zigzag appearance. The conidia are brown, long (average, 14 × 90 μm or greater), fusiform, appear thick walled, and usually have 7–11 septa. The hilum (scar of attachment) on each conidium is seen as a dark, conspicuous, square protrusion. Displays a distinctive dark septum at each end cell of the mature conidium.

See Table 2.18 (p. 269) for differentiation from similar organisms.

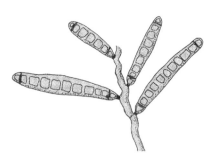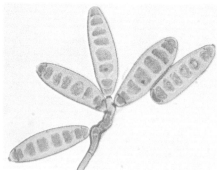

Exserohilum rostratum (continued)

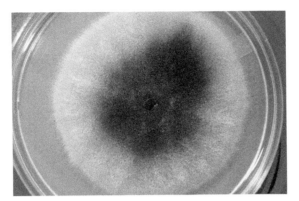

Exserohilum sp. SDA, 30°C, 7 days.

For further information, see
Katragkou et al., 2014
Larone and Walsh, 2013
Lyons et al., 2012

Helminthosporium spp.

PATHOGENICITY: Commonly considered a contaminant. Natural habitat is soil and grass; plant pathogen but not known to cause human infection.

RATE OF GROWTH: Rapid; mature within 5 days.

COLONY MORPHOLOGY: Surface is dark gray to black, cottony. Reverse is black.

MICROSCOPIC MORPHOLOGY: Hyphae are septate. Conidiophores are brown, determinate (i.e., not elongating at the point of conidium formation), erect, slightly curved, unbranched, smooth, and often in clusters. Conidia form along the sides of the conidiophores, frequently in whorls. Conidia are large (~9 × 40 μm), pale to dark brown, thick-walled, club-shaped with the broader end toward the conidiophore, and usually contain six or more cells. Isolates identified as *Helminthosporium* are often confirmed to be either *Curvularia* or *Exserohilum*. *Helminthosporium* differs from *Curvularia* and *Exserohilum* by forming parallel-walled, erect conidiophores (i.e., no sympodial geniculate growth).

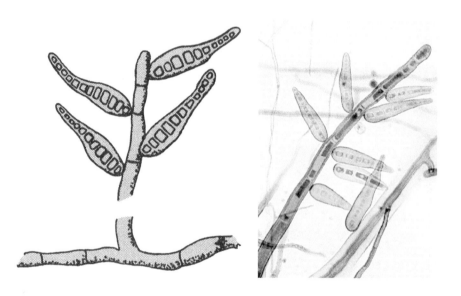

*For further information, see
Weber, 2005*

Alternaria spp.

TAXONOMY NOTES: The genus *Ulocladium* is currently recognized as *Alternaria*. *Alternaria chartarum* (formerly *Ulocladium chartarum*) and *A. botrytis* (formerly *U. botrytis*) are the species most commonly reported in published cases.

PATHOGENICITY: *Alternaria* spp. are commonly considered saprobic contaminants but are also known to cause phaeohyphomycosis, most commonly in subcutaneous tissue of immunocompromised patients. There have also been reports of onychomycosis, keratitis, and noninvasive rhinosinusitis. Locally invasive sinusitis may occur in hematopoietic stem cell transplant recipients. *Alternaria* spp. also may play an important role in asthma and hypersensitivity pneumonitis.

RATE OF GROWTH: Rapid; mature within 5 days.

COLONY MORPHOLOGY: Surface of *Alternaria* spp. is at first grayish white and woolly and later becomes greenish black or brown with a light border. May eventually become covered by short, grayish aerial hyphae. Reverse is black.

Surface of former *Ulocladium* spp. that are now recognized as *Alternaria* is dark brown to black, cottony. Reverse is black.

MICROSCOPIC MORPHOLOGY: *Alternaria* hyphae are septate and dark. Conidiophores are septate, of variable length, and are geniculate (have a zigzag appearance). Conidia are large (usually 8–16 × 23–50 μm) and brown, have both transverse and longitudinal septations (i.e., muriform) and typically form chains; they are usually club-shaped with the broader end nearest the conidiophore while narrowing at the apex to form a long or short beak. Conidia with long beaks often do not form chains.

The former *Ulocladium* spp. that are now recognized as *Alternaria* have light to dark brown septate hyphae. Conidiophores are simple or branched and bent at points of conidial production, giving a zigzag appearance. Conidia are brown to black, smooth or rough, and round to oval or slightly egg shaped (7–12 × 18–24 μm) with the narrowest end at the base, with transverse and longitudinal septations.

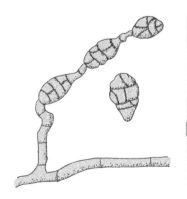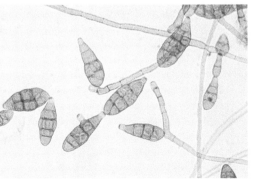

Alternaria sp.

Alternaria **spp.** *(continued)*

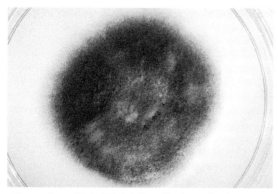

Alternaria sp. SDA, 30°C, 5 days. Surface of colony.

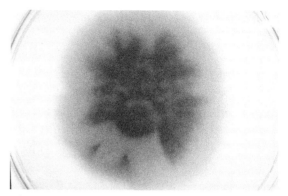

Alternaria sp. SDA, 30°C, 5 days. Reverse of colony.

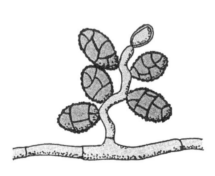

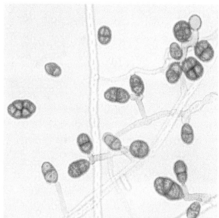

Alternaria sp. (formerly *Ulocladium* sp.).

For further information, see
de Hoog and Horré, 2002
Hernandez-Ramirez et al., 2021
Kaur et al., 2010
Pastor and Guarro, 2008

Stemphylium spp.

PATHOGENICITY: Commonly considered a contaminant.

RATE OF GROWTH: Rapid; mature within 5 days.

COLONY MORPHOLOGY: Surface is brown to black, cottony.

MICROSCOPIC MORPHOLOGY: Septate hyphae, light to dark brown. Conidiophores are septate and are simple or occasionally branched, with a dark, swollen terminus bearing individual conidia; the conidiophore develops a nodular or knobby appearance as it ages and produces more conidia. Conidia (12–20 × 15–30 μm) are dark, smooth or rough, and round or oval and have transverse and longitudinal septations, often with marked constriction at the central septum.

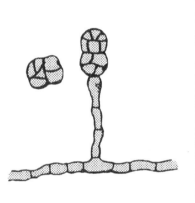
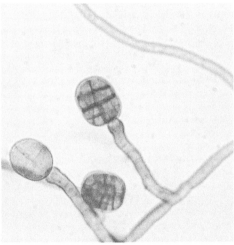

Pseudopithomyces spp.

TAXONOMY NOTES: *Pseudopithomyces chartarum* and *Pseudopithomyces sacchari* were formerly known as *Pithomyces chartarum* and *Pithomyces sacchari*, respectively.

PATHOGENICITY: Commonly considered a contaminant. *Pseudopithomyces chartarum* causes facial eczema in a variety of animals, but sheep are especially susceptible. *P. chartarum* and *P. sacchari* are the species most commonly recovered from clinical specimens (cutaneous, respiratory, and nasal specimens) but their role in human disease has not been conclusively proven.

RATE OF GROWTH: Rapid; mature within 5 days.

COLONY MORPHOLOGY: Surface is light to dark brownish black, cottony. Reverse is dark.

MICROSCOPIC MORPHOLOGY: Septate hyphae, hyaline or light brown. Conidiophores are short, simple, and peglike and are poorly differentiated from vegetative hyphae. Conidia are single, oval (10–20 × 20–30 µm), yellow to dark brown, and usually rough, with transverse and longitudinal septations.

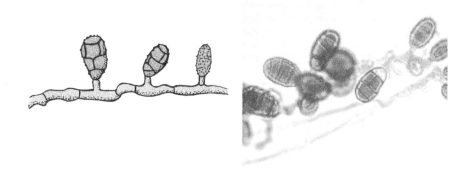

For further information, see
Ariyawansa et al., 2015
da Cunha et al., 2014

Epicoccum spp.

PATHOGENICITY: Commonly known as a contaminant; not known to cause disease.

RATE OF GROWTH: Moderately rapid; mature within 6–10 days.

COLONY MORPHOLOGY: Colonies are irregularly cottony and usually yellow to orange at first (due to the color of the hyphae), becoming brown to black where the dark mature conidia eventually form. Reverse is sometimes red or may be dark brown or grayish. A diffusible pigment may color the medium yellow, orange, red, or brown.

MICROSCOPIC MORPHOLOGY: Hyphae are septate and hyaline to dark brown. Clusters of short conidiophores form on hyphae by repeated branching to form a dense mass (sporodochium) from which conidia arise. Young conidia are round to pear shaped, pale, smooth, and nonseptate. Mature conidia (15–30 μm in diameter) are almost round, multiseptate both longitudinally and transversely, dark brown or black, and often rough walled and warty. Characteristically, all stages of conidia will be present simultaneously in the clusters.

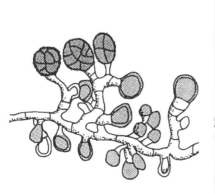 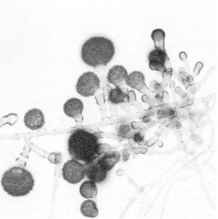

Epicoccum spp. *(continued)*

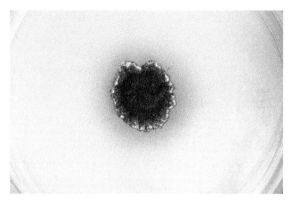

Epicoccum sp. PDA, 30°C, 7 days. Surface of colony. Note yellow-orange diffusing pigment.

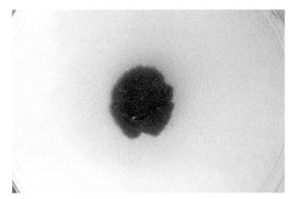

Epicoccum sp. PDA, 30°C, 7 days. Reverse of colony. Note yellow-orange diffusing pigment.

Nigrospora spp.

PATHOGENICITY: Commonly considered a contaminant; possible involvement in disease has very rarely been reported.

RATE OF GROWTH: Rapid; mature within 5 days.

COLONY MORPHOLOGY: Compact, woolly; at first white, then gray. With age, black areas of conidiation appear. Reverse is black.

MICROSCOPIC MORPHOLOGY: Hyphae are septate and become darkly pigmented with age. Short translucent conidiophores rise from the hyphae at right angles. Conidiophores are swollen at the base and then taper at the point of conidium formation. The conidia are large, single-celled, smooth, densely black, and almost round, slightly flattened (~14–20 μm in diameter).

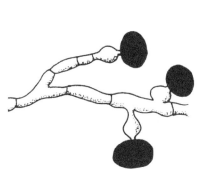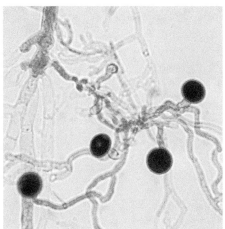

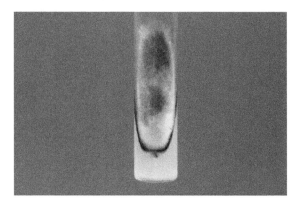

Nigrospora sp. slant. SDA, 30°C, 4 days.

Chaetomium spp.

PATHOGENICITY: Occasionally implicated in infections of the nails and skin and in subcutaneous and systemic phaeohyphomycosis. Peritonitis and sinusitis have been reported in immunocompetent individuals and cases of empyema, otitis externa, and pneumonia in immunocompromised individuals. Several species that grow at 42°C are neurotropic and have caused cerebral phaeohyphomycosis in immunocompromised individuals and intravenous drug abusers. They more commonly occur as contaminants.

RATE OF GROWTH: Rapid; mature within 5 days.

COLONY MORPHOLOGY: Surface is cottony, spreading, and usually white, becoming tannish gray, grayish olive, or brown with age. Reverse is usually orange-tan tinted with red but may be brown to black.

MICROSCOPIC MORPHOLOGY: Hyphae are hyaline and septate with large (90–170 × 110–280 μm), round, oval, or flask-shaped perithecia (best seen on potato dextrose agar) that are olive to brown, fragile, and have wavy and/or straight brownish filamentous appendages called setae. Asci are stalked and cylindrical, ovoid, or club-shaped; contain four to eight ascospores; and usually dissolve soon after release from the ostiole (opening) of the perithecium. Ascospores, readily observed, are oval or lemon-shaped, single-celled, and usually olive-brown but may occur in a variety of sizes, shapes, and colors.

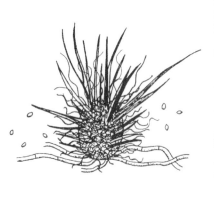 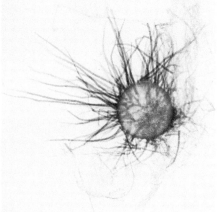

Chaetomium spp. *(continued)*

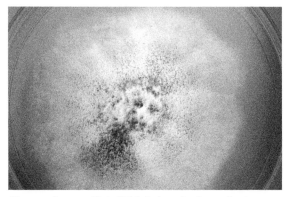

Chaetomium sp. PDA, 30°C, 5 days. Surface of colony.

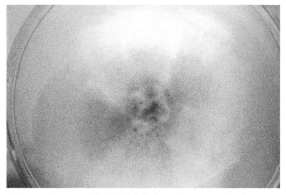

Chaetomium sp. PDA, 30°C, 5 days. Reverse of colony.

For further information, see
Cárdenas Del Castillo et al., 2021
Hubka et al., 2011

Phoma spp.

PATHOGENICITY: Commonly considered contaminants. Occasional agents of phaeohyphomycosis occurring primarily on exposed areas of the skin on the hands, feet, and face. Most cases of *Phoma* infection occurred in immunocompromised individuals although several cases have been described in healthy people following trauma. *Phoma* spp. have also been reported as the cause of eye infections including corneal ulcers due to trauma or use of contact lenses and endophthalmitis following trauma, lung infections, onychomycosis, and invasive rhinosinusitis.

RATE OF GROWTH: Rapid; mature within 5 days (may take longer for pycnidia to form).

COLONY MORPHOLOGY: Colony is powdery or velvety, spreading, and grayish brown or greenish; some species may develop pink or reddish areas. Reverse is brown to black. A reddish to brown, diffusible pigment is produced by some species.

MICROSCOPIC MORPHOLOGY: Septate hyphae; large (~60–400 μm in diameter), asexual fruiting bodies (pycnidia). The pycnidia are dark and round or flask shaped and have openings (ostioles) through which conidia are dispersed. The conidia, formed on phialidic cells inside the pycnidia, are mostly one celled, hyaline to pale brown, and may be round, oval, or cylindrical. Chlamydoconidia resembling the conidia of *Alternaria* spp. (p. 273) are produced in some species.

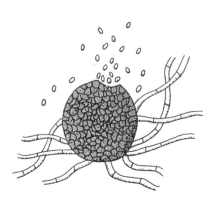
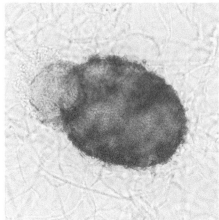

Phoma spp. *(continued)*

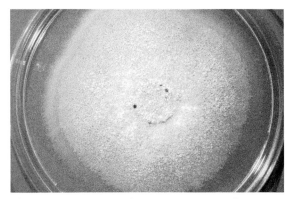

Phoma sp. SDA, 30°C, 5 days.

For further information, see
Bennett et al., 2018

Dermatophytes

Introduction to Dermatophytes

Dermatophytes are filamentous fungi that are able to digest and obtain nutrients from keratin (a relatively insoluble protein; the primary component of skin, hair, and nails). Infection usually involves only the keratinized layer of the skin, as well as hair follicles, hair shafts, and nails. The "disease" known as tinea or ringworm is the result of the host reaction to the cell wall of the fungus and to the enzymes released by the fungus during its digestive process. Dermatophytes are among the few fungi that have evolved a dependency on human or animal infection for the survival of the species. It is therefore not surprising that these fungi are among the most common infectious agents of humans.

The group has three longstanding genera that can generally be differentiated by their conidium formation.

Microsporum: —Macroconidia numerous, thick walled, rough.

—Microconidia usually present.

(*M. audouinii* is an exception; it seldom forms conidia.)

Trichophyton: —Macroconidia rare, thin walled, smooth.

—Microconidia numerous.

(Some species do not produce any conidia.)

Epidermophyton: —Macroconidia numerous, thin and thick walled, smooth.

—Microconidia are not formed.

Molecular taxonomic studies have led to the recognition of additional dermatophyte genera and resulted in the reclassification of many organisms. Most anthropophilic (infecting humans) species and several zoophilic (infecting animals and humans) species that frequently infect humans have been retained in the genera *Trichophyton* and *Epidermophyton*. The majority of geophilic (recovered from soil) species and those zoophilic species that rarely cause human infection are divided between *Arthoderma*, *Lophophyton*, *Nannizzia*, and *Paraphyton*. *Microsporum* has been reduced to three species.

Molecular and proteomic diagnostics tools are being used increasingly in reference laboratories for rapid identification of dermatophytes to complement existing morphological studies and biochemical profiles.

Latin Terms for Dermatophyte Infections

The clinical dermatophyte diseases are designated in many references by their Latin names. These are constructed by adding to "tinea" the Latin word for the specific body part affected:

Tinea barbae = infection of the bearded areas of the face and neck

Tinea capitis = infection of the scalp and hair shaft

Tinea corporis = infection of the glabrous skin on body parts not otherwise specified (usually the trunk of the body)

Tinea cruris = infection of the groin, perineum, and perianal region

Tinea manuum = infection of the hand

Tinea pedis = infection of the feet

Tinea unguium = infection of the nails (onychomycosis is infection of the nail caused by any fungus, not necessarily caused by a dermatophyte)

For further information, see
Aly, 1994
Borman and Summerbell, 2023
Degreef, 2008
de Hoog et al., 2017
de Hoog et al., 2020
Havlickova et al., 2008
Kane et al., 1997
Kidd et al., 2023b
Lipner and Scher, 2019
Rebell and Taplin, 1970
Segal and Elad, 2021
St-Germain and Summerbell, 2011
White et al., 2014

Microsporum audouinii

PATHOGENICITY: This anthropophilic dermatophyte formerly caused widespread epidemics of tinea capitis in children. The relatively few cases seen now usually have a connection with sub-Saharan Africa. Also known to infect skin on other parts of the body. Very rarely infects adults.

RATE OF GROWTH: Moderate; mature within 6–10 days.

COLONY MORPHOLOGY: Surface is flat, downy to silky, with a radiating edge; it is grayish or tannish white. Reverse is light salmon with reddish brown center (pigment is best seen on potato dextrose agar).

MICROSCOPIC MORPHOLOGY: Hyphae are septate with terminal chlamydoconidia that are often pointed on the end. Pectinate (comblike) hyphae are commonly seen. This species is usually almost devoid of conidia but sometimes forms poorly shaped, abortive macroconidia suggestive of *Microsporum canis* (p. 290). The occasional microconidia that form are identical to those occurring in other species of the genus *Microsporum*.

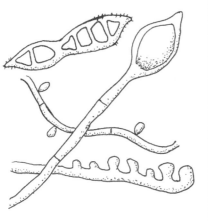 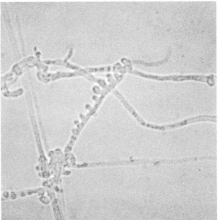

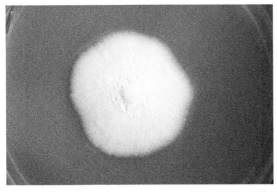

Microsporum audouinii. PDA, 30°C, 7 days. Surface of colony.

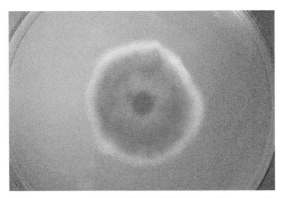

Microsporum audouinii. PDA, 30°C, 7 days. Reverse of colony.

Microsporum canis

PATHOGENICITY: This zoophilic dermatophyte causes infections of scalp (tinea capitis) and skin (tinea corporis); it is most prevalent in children. This organism is one of the most commonly recognized causes worldwide of tinea capitis and other dermatophytoses. Most infections in humans are acquired from infected dogs or cats or from other animals in an agricultural environment. *M. canis* is a common cause of dermatophytosis in patients who may have lived and worked in a rural or farm setting. This organism is a classical ectothrix pathogen, which destroys the hair shaft from the cuticle inward.

RATE OF GROWTH: Rapid (mature within 5 days) to moderate (mature within 6–10 days).

COLONY MORPHOLOGY: Surface is whitish, coarsely fluffy, hairy to silky or furlike, with yellow pigment at periphery and closely spaced radial grooves. Reverse is deep yellow and turns brownish yellow with age.

MICROSCOPIC MORPHOLOGY: Hyphae are septate with numerous macroconidia, which are long (10–25 × 35–110 μm), spindle shaped, rough, and thick walled and characteristically taper to beaklike ends. The rough surface of the macroconidia is seen especially at the beak. Usually more than six cells are seen in the macroconidia. A few microconidia are sometimes observed; they are club shaped and smooth walled and form along the hyphae.

Microsporum canis var. *distortum* is a variant of *M. canis* with distinctive distorted and very bent macroconidia. The macroconidia have fewer cells than *M. canis* and are produced best on potato dextrose agar, and club-shaped microconidia are often abundant (an uncommon finding in *M. canis*). The patterns of infections are indistinguishable from those of *M. canis*.

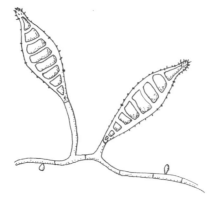 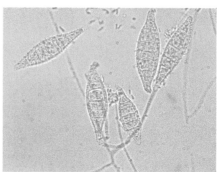

Microsporum canis

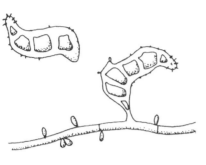

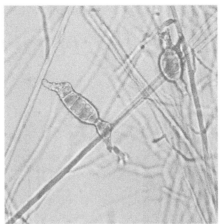

Microsporum canis var. *distortum*

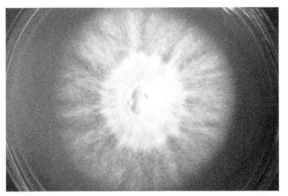

Microsporum canis. PDA, 30°C, 7 days. Surface of colony.

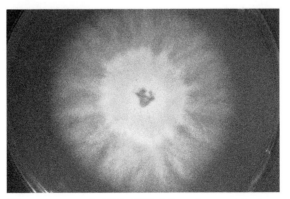

Microsporum canis. PDA, 30°C, 7 days. Reverse of colony.

PART II Identification of Fungi in Culture

THERMALLY MONOMORPHIC MOULDS • Dermatophytes

Paraphyton cookei species complex

TAXONOMY NOTES: This species complex was formerly known as *Microsporum cookei* species complex. The species complex includes *Paraphyton cookei sensu stricto* and *P. mirabile*. These species are difficult to differentiate phenotypically.

PATHOGENICITY: This geophilic fungus is occasionally involved in infections in humans; it is not known to infect hair *in vivo*.

RATE OF GROWTH: Moderate; mature within 6–10 days.

COLONY MORPHOLOGY: Surface is coarse, powdery; yellowish or dark tannish central area surrounded by thin, downy, white peripheral zone. Under the aerial mycelium is a characteristic deep grape-red pigment. Reverse is deep purplish red.

MICROSCOPIC MORPHOLOGY: Hyphae are septate and branched. Macroconidia are oval (10–15 × 30–50 μm), thick walled, and rough, with approximately five to eight cells. Thick walls serve to distinguish this species from reddish isolates of *Nannizzia gypsea*. Club-shaped microconidia are usually abundant.

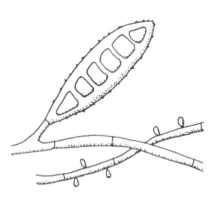
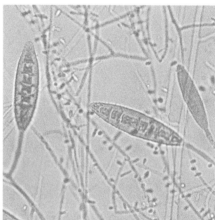

Nannizzia gypsea species complex

TAXONOMY NOTES: This species complex was formerly known as *Microsporum gypseum* species complex. The species complex includes *Nannizzia duboisii*, *N. fulva*, *N. gypsea sensu stricto*, and *N. incurvata*. These species are difficult to differentiate phenotypically.

PATHOGENICITY: This geophilic dermatophyte occasionally infects the scalp and skin on various parts of the body; infections are more common in lower animals than in humans.

RATE OF GROWTH: Moderate; mature within 6–10 days.

COLONY MORPHOLOGY: Surface is flat and spreading and powdery to granular, developing an irregularly fringed border; it is buff at first, then tan to cinnamon brown. Colony often develops a sterile white hyphal border or cottony white center. Reverse may be yellow, orange-tan, brownish red, or purplish red in spots.

MICROSCOPIC MORPHOLOGY: Septate hyphae. Macroconidia (8–16 × 22–60 μm) appear in enormous numbers and are symmetric, rough, and relatively thin walled, with no more than six cells. The ends are rounded, not pointed as in *M. canis*. Microconidia, club shaped, are usually present along the hyphae.

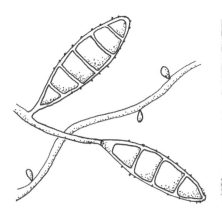 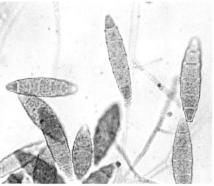

Nannizzia gypsea species complex *(continued)*

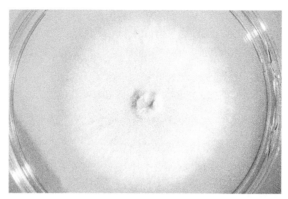

Nannizzia gypsea species complex. PDA, 30°C, 6 days.
Surface of colony.

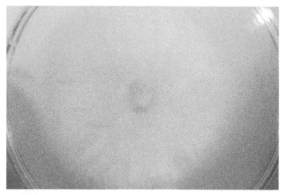

Nannizzia gypsea species complex. SDA, 30°C, 6 days.
Reverse of colony.

Lophophyton gallinae

TAXONOMY NOTES: *Microsporum gallinae*, a zoophilic species associated with poultry, is currently recognized as *Lophophyton gallinae*. *Microsporum vanbreuseghemii*, a soil-dwelling organism (i.e., geophilic), is also currently recognized as *L. gallinae* but is morphologically distinct from the zoophilic form.

PATHOGENICITY: The zoophilic form (formerly *M. gallinae*) is a rare cause of tinea capitis and tinea corporis that may be seen as a cause of dermatophytosis in chickens or other fowl. The geophilic form (formerly *M. vanbreuseghemii*) is a rare cause of ringworm in humans and lower animals.

RATE OF GROWTH: Moderate; mature within 6–10 days.

COLONY MORPHOLOGY: Surface of the zoophilic form (formerly *M. gallinae*) is slightly fluffy or satiny and white, becoming pinkish with age. Reverse is yellow at first and later has a red pigment that diffuses into the medium.

Surface of the geophilic form (formerly *M. vanbreuseghemii*) is powdery or fluffy; cream, pink, or tan in color. Reverse is colorless or yellow to orange-tan.

MICROSCOPIC MORPHOLOGY: Hyphae are septate. Macroconidia (6–8 × 15–50 μm) of the zoophilic form (formerly *M. gallinae*) have walls that are relatively thin and usually smooth but sometimes slightly rough at the tip; they contain 4–10 cells, are blunt tipped, and are often distinctively curved with a tapering base. Microconidia are usually abundant.

Macroconidia of the geophilic form (formerly *M. vanbreuseghemii*) are long (10–12 × 58–62 μm), tapered, thick walled, and usually rough and spiny surfaced, with seven or more cells. The macroconidia are in abundance singly, laterally, or terminally. Microconidia are also present. Care must be taken not to confuse the geophilic form (formerly *M. vanbreuseghemii*) with *Arthroderma uncinatum* (formerly *Trichophyton ajelloi*) (p. 314).

The zoophilic form (formerly *M. gallinae*) is negative for urease (urea broth) and *in vitro* hair perforation tests, while the geophilic form (formerly *M. vanbreuseghemii*) is positive for both.

Lophophyton gallinae (continued)

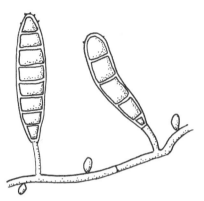
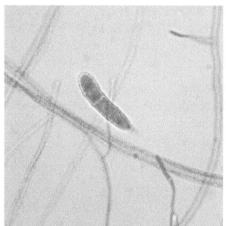

Zoophilic form *Lophophyton gallinae*
(formerly *Microsporum gallinae*).

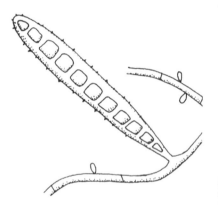
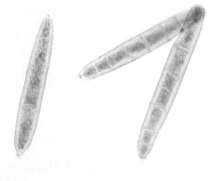

Geophilic form *Lophophyton gallinae*
(formerly *Microsporum vanbreuseghemii*).

Nannizzia nana

TAXONOMY NOTES: This species was formerly known as *Microsporum nanum*.

PATHOGENICITY: This zoophilic organism is a rare cause of dermatophytosis in humans; more common in pigs.

RATE OF GROWTH: Moderate; mature within 6–10 days.

COLONY MORPHOLOGY: Surface is at first white and then yellowish, peachy, or beige; spread thin, downy or powdery, with fringed edges. Reverse is initially orange and later reddish brown.

MICROSCOPIC MORPHOLOGY: Septate hyphae; macroconidia (4–8 × 12–18 µm) are rough, fairly thin walled (as in *Nannizzia gypsea*), and egg shaped with truncate base, having one to three cells (usually two). Microconidia, club shaped and smooth walled, may also be present.

The short conidiophores, singly formed macroconidia with rough walls and no footlike attachment points, and presence of microconidia serve to distinguish this organism from *Trichothecium roseum* (p. 370).

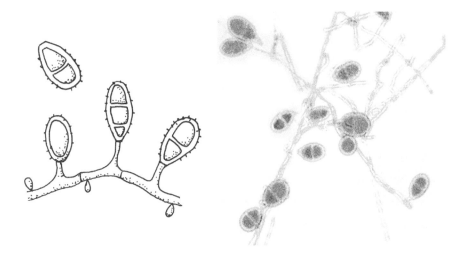

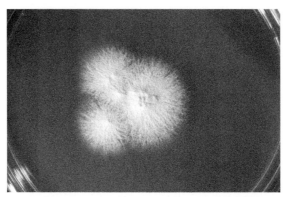

Nannizzia nana. SDA, 30°C, 7 days. Surface of colony.

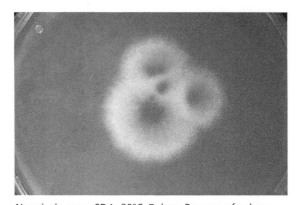

Nannizzia nana. SDA, 30°C, 7 days. Reverse of colony.

Microsporum ferrugineum

PATHOGENICITY: This anthropophilic species primarily causes tinea capitis in children. It occasionally causes tinea corporis and onychomycosis.

RATE OF GROWTH: Slow; mature after 10 days.

COLONY MORPHOLOGY: Isolates from the Far East have a surface that is usually yellow to rusty orange, smooth, waxy, and heaped; on repeated subculture, the pigment is often lost. Another colony type (typical in the Balkans) is also waxy, but white to pale yellow and flatter. Either form may develop a fine velvety overgrowth. Reverse is cream to brownish.

MICROSCOPIC MORPHOLOGY: Hyphae are septate; some are characteristically long and straight with prominent cross walls; these are called "bamboo" hyphae. Other hyphae are irregularly branched, clubbed, and fragmented and may have intercalary chlamydoconidia-like cells. Macroconidia, rarely produced, resemble those of *Microsporum canis* (p. 290) and *Paraphyton cookei* (p. 292).

Note: The orange form of this organism may be differentiated from *Trichophyton soudanense* (p. 309), which it somewhat resembles, by the formation of light yellowish colonies on Lowenstein-Jensen medium; *T. soudanense* will form dark reddish-brown-to-blackish colonies.

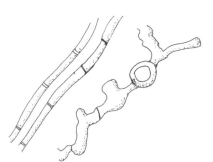 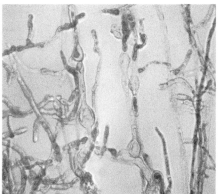

Courtesy of Michael Rinaldi.

Trichophyton mentagrophytes species complex

TAXONOMY NOTES: The species complex includes *Trichophyton africanum*, *T. benhamiae* var. *benhamiae*, *T. benhamiae* var. *luteum*, *T. europaeum*, *T. eriotrephon*, *T. japonicum*, *T. mentagrophytes sensu stricto*, *T. indotineae*, *T. interdigitale*, and *T. quinckeanum*. These species are difficult to differentiate phenotypically.

PATHOGENICITY: Members of the complex are zoophilic, with the exception that *T. indotinae* and *T. interdigitale* behave as anthropophilic species. Commonly invades all parts of the body surface, including hair and nails. A common cause of tinea pedis and onychomycosis. It also infects a wide range of domestic and agricultural animals. *T. indotineae* is associated with severe infections and allylamine and azole resistance.

RATE OF GROWTH: Moderate; mature within 6–10 days.

COLONY MORPHOLOGY: Varies greatly; surface may be buff and powdery or white and downy. May become pinkish or yellowish. Powdery form exhibits concentric and radial folds. Colonies rapidly develop a dense fluff with little or no conidiation. Reverse is usually brownish tan but may be colorless, yellow, or red.

MICROSCOPIC MORPHOLOGY: Septate hyphae. Microconidia in powdery cultures are very round (4–6 μm in diameter) and clustered on branched conidiophores or, in fluffy strains, are smaller, fewer in number, tear shaped, and more easily confused with those of *Trichophyton rubrum* (p. 303). Macroconidia (4–8 × 20–50 μm) are sometimes, but not always, present; they are cigar shaped and thin walled, have narrow attachments to hyphae, contain one to six cells, and are more readily found in young primary cultures 5–10 days old. Coiled spiral hyphae are often seen. Nodular bodies are seen in some strains.

See Table 2.19 (p. 302) to differentiate *T. mentagrophytes* from similar species of *Trichophyton* and *Arthroderma*.

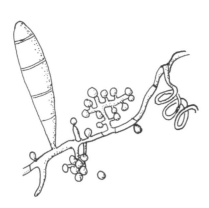 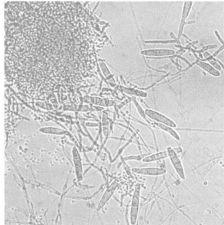

Trichophyton mentagrophytes species complex *(continued)*

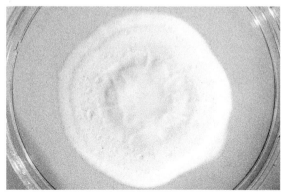

Trichophyton mentagrophytes. PDA, 30°C, 7 days.
Surface of colony.

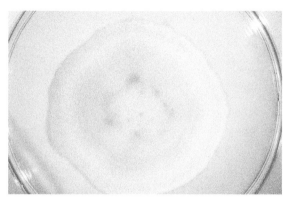

Trichophyton mentagrophytes. PDA, 30°C, 7 days.
Reverse of colony.

For further information, see
Gupta et al., 2022
Kano et al., 2020
Tang et al., 2021

TABLE 2.19 Differentiation of similar conidia-producing *Trichophyton* spp. and *Arthroderma* spp.[a]

Organism	Growth on *Trichophyton* agars		Urease (7 days)	*In vitro* hair perforation	Red pigment on cornmeal with 1% dextrose	Growth at 37°C	Growth on *Trichophyton* agars[b]	
	No. 1 (casein base)	No. 4 (casein + thiamine)					No. 6 (NH_4NO_3 base)	No. 7 (NH_4NO_3 + histidine)
T. mentagrophytes	4+	4+	+	+	0	+	4+	2+
T. rubrum	4+	4+	0 or W	0	+	+	3+	4+
T. tonsurans	± or +	4+	+	0[v]	0	+	±	±
A. terrestre (formerly *T. terrestre*)	4+	4+	+	+	V	0	2+	2+
T. megninii	4+	2+	+[V, c]	0		+	0	4+

[a] Abbreviations: +, positive; 0, negative; W, weak; ±, trace; 4+, maximum growth; V, variable.

[b] As *T. megninii* is the only dermatophyte that requires histidine, *Trichophyton* agar no. 6 and 7 are used only when it is suspected.

[c] Use urea broth, not agar, to ensure positive result in 7 days with *T. megninii*.

Trichophyton rubrum

PATHOGENICITY: Infects the skin and nails and only rarely the beard, hair, or scalp. *T. rubrum* is one of the most commonly recognized causes of dermatophytosis and onychomycosis in humans (i.e., anthropophilic) worldwide. The most common sites of infection are the feet (tinea pedis) and the nails.

RATE OF GROWTH: Slow; mature after 10 days.

COLONY MORPHOLOGY: Surface is granular or fluffy, white to buff. Reverse is deep red or purplish; occasionally it is brown, yellow-orange, or even colorless. The pigment production is best seen on potato dextrose agar (p. 460) or cornmeal dextrose agar (p. 454).

MICROSCOPIC MORPHOLOGY: Septate hyphae. Tear-shaped microconidia (2–3.5 × 3–5.5 μm) usually form singly all along the sides of the hyphae resembling birds on a wire (not clustered like *T. mentagrophytes* [p. 300]). Macroconidia (4–8 × 40–60 μm) may be abundant, rare, or absent; when present, they are long, narrow, and thin walled, with parallel sides (pencil-like), and have 4–10 cells. Macroconidia may form directly on ends of thick hyphae singly or in groups. Microconidia characteristically form directly on hyphae. Arthroconidia tend to form from both hyphae and macroconidia. Granular cultures have more macroconidial formation and larger, rounder microconidia than the fluffy form.

See Table 2.19 (p. 302) for differentiation from similar species of *Trichophyton* and *Arthroderma*.

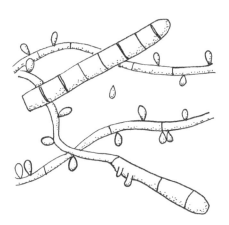 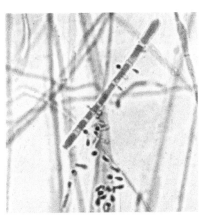

Trichophyton rubrum (continued)

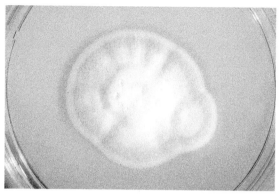

Trichophyton rubrum. PDA, 30°C, 7 days. Surface of colony.

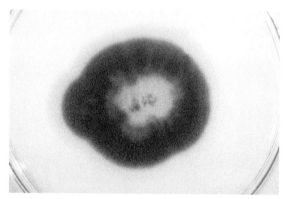

Trichophyton rubrum. PDA, 30°C, 7 days. Reverse of colony.

Trichophyton tonsurans

PATHOGENICITY: This anthropophilic species is the principal etiologic agent of tinea capitis in the United States; it also infects the skin and nails. *T. tonsurans* causes tinea capitis principally in children who live in large urban areas.

RATE OF GROWTH: Slow; mature after 10 days.

COLONY MORPHOLOGY: Highly variable. Surface may be white, grayish, yellow, rose, or brownish. Surface is usually suedelike, with many radial or concentric folds. Reverse is usually reddish brown (pigment may diffuse into the medium); sometimes it is yellow or colorless.

MICROSCOPIC MORPHOLOGY: Hyphae are septate, with many variably shaped microconidia along the hyphae or on short stalks that are perpendicular to the parent hyphae. Microconidia are usually teardrop or club shaped but may be elongate or enlarge to round "balloon" forms. Intercalary and terminal chlamydoconidia are common in older cultures. Macroconidia are rare, irregular in form, and a bit thick walled. The organism may have spiral coils and arthroconidia. This species has a partial requirement for thiamine.

See Table 2.19 (p. 302) for differentiation from similar species of *Trichophyton* and *Arthroderma*.

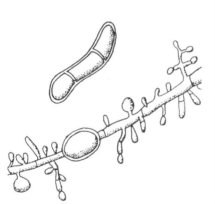 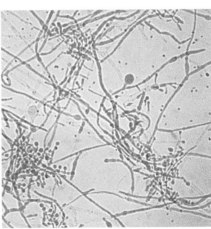

Trichophyton tonsurans (continued)

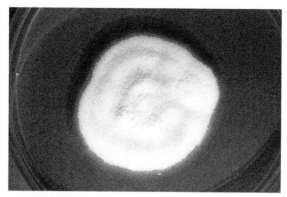

Trichophyton tonsurans. SDA, 30°C, 7 days. Surface of colony, yellowish rose strain.

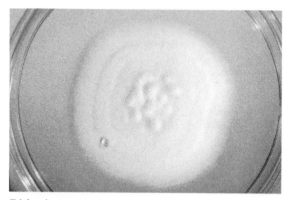

Trichophyton tonsurans. SDA, 30°C, 7 days. Surface of colony, white and yellow strain.

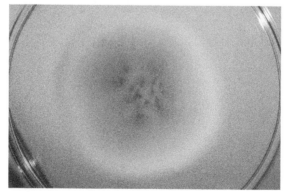

Trichophyton tonsurans. SDA, 30°C, 7 days. Reverse of colony.

Arthroderma terrestre species complex

TAXONOMY NOTES: Formerly known as *Trichophyton terrestre* species complex. The species complex includes *Arthroderma crocatum*, *A. eboreum*, *A. insingulare*, *A. lenticulare*, *A. melbournense*, *A. melis*, *A. thuringiense*, and *A. quadrifidum*. These species are difficult to differentiate phenotypically.

PATHOGENICITY: This soil-associated organism is not known to cause infection in humans but may be confused with *Trichophyton* spp.

RATE OF GROWTH: Moderate; mature within 6–10 days. It does not grow at 35–37°C.

COLONY MORPHOLOGY: Surface is white to yellow and velvety or granular. Reverse is colorless, yellow, reddish, or brown.

MICROSCOPIC MORPHOLOGY: Hyphae are septate, with club-shaped microconidia (often on short stalks) or characteristic larger, peg-shaped microconidia that usually exhibit transition forms to rather numerous smooth, thin-walled macroconidia (4–5 × 8–50 μm). The conidia often stain more intensely with lactophenol cotton blue than do the hyphae and are cut off on a relatively broad base.

See Table 2.19 (p. 302) for differentiation from similar species of *Trichophyton* and *Arthroderma*.

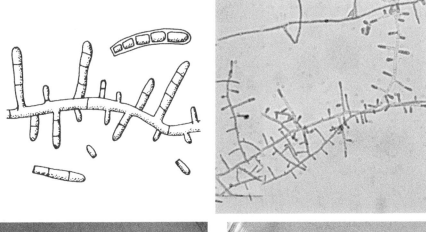

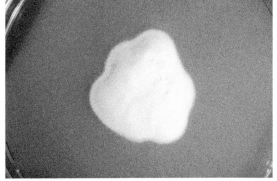

Arthroderma terrestre. SDA, 30°C, 7 days. Surface of colony.

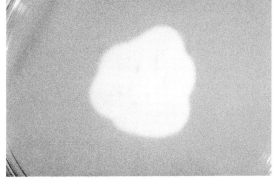

Arthroderma terrestre. SDA, 30°C, 7 days. Reverse of colony.

Trichophyton megninii

TAXONOMY NOTES: This species has been suggested as a synonym of *Trichophyton rubrum* but there are notable differences in physiology and infection symptomatology that have prevented widespread acceptance.

PATHOGENICITY: This anthropophilic organism primarily infects the beard, but it also infects the scalp and the skin on various parts of the body. Very rarely encountered in the Americas; it is endemic in parts of southern Europe and in north and east central Africa.

RATE OF GROWTH: Moderate; mature within 6–10 days.

COLONY MORPHOLOGY: Surface is suedelike, at first white and then pink to violet with widely spaced radial grooves. Reverse is red.

MICROSCOPIC MORPHOLOGY: Hyphae are septate, with teardrop-shaped microconidia along the sides. Macroconidia, infrequently produced, are long, narrow, thin walled, and pencil shaped. There is a close resemblance to *Trichophyton rubrum* (p. 303), but *T. megninii* differs by requiring histidine (in *Trichophyton* agar no. 7) and often giving a positive test for urease within 7 days.

See Table 2.19 (p. 302) for differentiation from similar species of *Trichophyton* and *Arthroderma*.

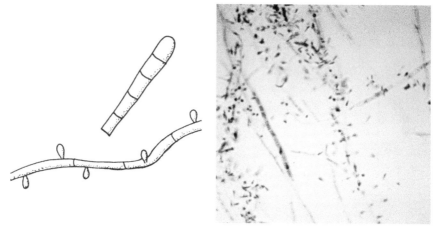

Courtesy of Michael Rinaldi.

Trichophyton soudanense

PATHOGENICITY: This anthropophilic dermatophyte primarily infects the scalp and hair and may spread to other parts of the body. It is endemic in Central and West Africa and has occasionally been reported in Europe, the United States, and South America.

RATE OF GROWTH: Slow; mature after 10 days. Growth factor requirements are variable.

COLONY MORPHOLOGY: Surface is yellow to orange, suedelike, and flat to folded, with a radiating fringe. Purplish red variants exist. Reverse is similar in color to the surface.

MICROSCOPIC MORPHOLOGY: Septate hyphae that often break up to form arthroconidia. Characteristically, branches form at both forward and backward angles to the parent hypha (i.e., in directions that are both the same as and opposite to that of the elongating hypha). This is known as "reflexive" branching; when adjacent branches point in opposite directions, they often give the appearance of barbed wire. The unique characteristic microscopic formations are most likely to be found in the radiating fringe of the colony. Teardrop-shaped microconidia may also form along the hyphae; no macroconidia are seen. Chlamydoconidia may develop in older cultures.

Note: The orange form of this organism may be differentiated from *M. ferrugineum* (p. 299), which it somewhat resembles, by the formation of dark reddish-brown-to-blackish colonies on Lowenstein-Jensen medium; *M. ferrugineum* forms pale yellow colonies on this medium.

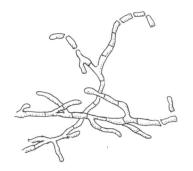

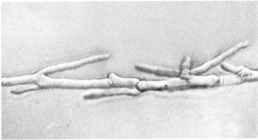

Courtesy of Stanley Rosenthal.

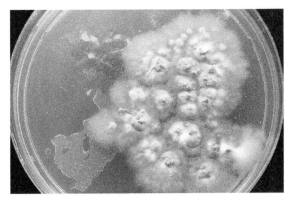

Trichophyton soudanense. (Courtesy of Joel Mortensen.)

TABLE 2.20 Growth patterns of *Trichophyton* spp. and *Arthroderma* spp. on nutritional test media[a] (p. 465)

Organism	Percent	Growth on *Trichophyton* agar no.						
		1	2	3	4	5	6	7
USUALLY NO CONIDIA ON ROUTINE MEDIA; INCUBATE *TRICHOPHYTON* AGARS AT 37°C								
T. verrucosum	84	0	±	4+	0			
	16	0	0	4+	4+			
T. schoenleinii		4+	4+	4+	4+			
T. concentricum[b]	50	4+	4+	4+	4+			
	50	2+	2+	4+	4+			
T. violaceum[c]		± or 1+			4+ (in 3 weeks)			
USUALLY PRODUCES MICROCONIDIA AND SOMETIMES MACROCONIDIA ON ROUTINE MEDIA; INCUBATE *TRICHOPHYTON* AGARS AT ROOM TEMPERATURE								
T. tonsurans		± or 1+			4+			
T. rubrum[d]		4+			4+			
T. mentagrophytes[d]		4+			4+	4+		
T. equinum[e]		0				4+		
T. megninii[f]		4+			2+		0	4+
A. terrestre (formerly *T. terrestre*)[g]		4+			4+			

[a] Abbreviations: 1, casein agar base (vitamin free);

2, casein + inositol;

3, casein × inositol and thiamine;

4, casein + thiamine;

5, casein + nicotinic acid;

6, ammonium nitrate agar base;

7, ammonium nitrate + histidine;

0, no growth;

+, growth;

1+, ¼ as much growth as 4+;

2+, ½ as much growth as 4+;

3+, ¾ as much growth as 4+;

4+, maximum growth.

[b] For more information, see Kane et al., 1997 (pp. 135–136), or Rebell and Taplin, 1970 (p. 61).

[c] Usually has distinct pigment on primary isolation.

[d] Differentiation of *T. rubrum* and *T. mentagrophytes* is by morphology, urease test, *in vitro* hair perforation test, and pigment production on cornmeal dextrose agar. See Table 2.19 (p. 302).

[e] Commonly found in horses; has been confused with *T. mentagrophytes*, but *T. equinum* usually requires nicotinic acid. For more information, see Kane et al., 1997 (pp. 136–138), or Rebell and Taplin, 1970 (p. 45).

[f] No other dermatophyte shows this regular requirement for histidine.

[g] Not known to cause infections, but may be confused with some pathogenic species. See Table 2.19 (p. 302).

Trichophyton schoenleinii

PATHOGENICITY: This anthropophilic species is the agent of favus, a severe, chronic, scarring scalp infection that results in permanent hair loss; sometimes infects the nails and skin.

RATE OF GROWTH: Slow; mature after 10 days.

COLONY MORPHOLOGY: Colony is whitish, waxy, or slightly downy; heaped or folded; primary isolates are sometimes yeastlike. Growth is often submerged and splits the agar medium. Reverse is colorless or pale yellowish orange to tan.

MICROSCOPIC MORPHOLOGY: Hyphae are septate, highly irregular, and knobby. The subsurface hyphae usually form characteristic antlerlike branching structures commonly called favic chandeliers; they have swollen tips that resemble nail heads. Chlamydoconidia are numerous. Microconidia and macroconidia are absent. Initial growth from clinical specimen may resemble yeast both macroscopically and microscopically.

See Table 2.20 (p. 310) for growth pattern on *Trichophyton* agars.

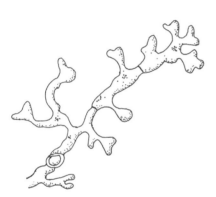
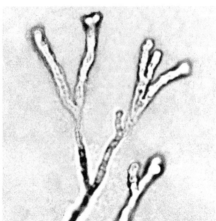

Trichophyton verrucosum

PATHOGENICITY: This zoophilic pathogen, which is usually contracted from cattle, infects the scalp, beard, nails, and skin on various parts of the body.

RATE OF GROWTH: Slow; mature after 10 days. Unlike other dermatophytes, this fungus grows best at 37°C.

COLONY MORPHOLOGY: Usually small, heaped, and buttonlike but sometimes flat. Texture skinlike, waxy, or slightly downy. Usually white, but can be gray or yellow. Reverse varies from nonpigmented to yellow.

MICROSCOPIC MORPHOLOGY: On routine mycology media at 37°C, forms hyphae with many intercalary chlamydoconidia (typically in chains) and some antlerlike branches. On enriched media with thiamine, produces many small, delicate, single microconidia and occasional long, thin, irregular macroconidia shaped like string beans or rats' tails.

See Table 2.20 (p. 310) for growth patterns on *Trichophyton* agars. This species requires thiamine and usually inositol as well.

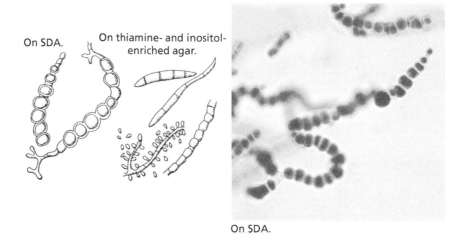

On SDA.

On thiamine- and inositol-enriched agar.

On SDA.

Trichophyton violaceum

PATHOGENICITY: This endothrix anthropophilic organism most commonly infects the scalp and hair but also causes infection in skin and nails. It is one of the most common causes of tinea capitis in West Asia and North Africa.

RATE OF GROWTH: Slow; mature after 10 days.

COLONY MORPHOLOGY: Original cultures are waxy, wrinkled, heaped, and deep purplish red. Subcultures are more downy, and they decrease in color. Reverse is lavender to purple.

MICROSCOPIC MORPHOLOGY: Hyphae are tangled, branched, irregular, and granular, with intercalary chlamydoconidia. Microconidia and macroconidia are not usually seen on routine media, but a few may form on thiamine-enriched media.

See Table 2.20 (p. 310) for growth pattern on *Trichophyton* agars. This species has a partial requirement for thiamine.

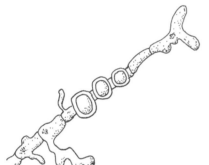
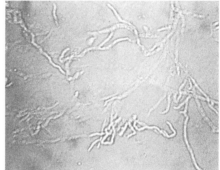

Courtesy of Michael Rinaldi.

Arthroderma uncinatum

TAXONOMY NOTES: This species was formerly known as *Trichophyton ajelloi*.

PATHOGENICITY: Has only rarely been reported as a possible cause of infections in humans.

RATE OF GROWTH: Moderate; mature within 6–10 days.

COLONY MORPHOLOGY: Surface is cream to orange-tan, rather powdery, and flat or folded. Reverse may be colorless or have a reddish purple or bluish black pigment that diffuses into the medium.

MICROSCOPIC MORPHOLOGY: Hyphae are septate with many macroconidia that are long (5–10 × 20–65 µm) and cigar shaped or cylindrical with tapering ends. They are smooth surfaced and moderately thick walled and contain 5–12 cells. Microconidia are sparse in most isolates but may be absent in others. Care must be taken not to confuse this organism with the geophilic form of *Lophophyton gallinae* (formerly *Microsporum vanbreuseghemii*) (p. 295) or *Epidermophyton floccosum* (p. 315).

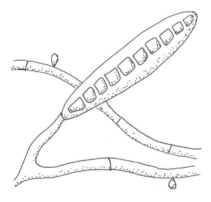 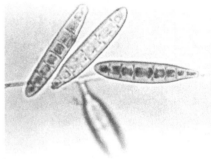

From Murray et al. (ed.), 1999, Manual of Clinical Microbiology, 7th ed., chapter 100.

Epidermophyton floccosum

PATHOGENICITY: This anthropophilic dermatophyte causes tinea corporis, tinea cruris, and onychomycosis. It does not infect hair.

RATE OF GROWTH: Moderate; mature within 6–10 days.

COLONY MORPHOLOGY: Surface is brownish yellow to olive-gray or khaki; it is at first lumpy and sparse and then folded in the center and grooved radially, becoming velvety. After several weeks, fluffy white sterile mycelium covers the colony. Reverse is orange to brownish, sometimes with a thin yellow border.

MICROSCOPIC MORPHOLOGY: Septate hyphae; no microconidia. Macroconidia (7–12 × 20–40 µm), seen best in young cultures, are smooth, both thin and slightly thick walled, and club shaped with rounded ends (often referred to as paddles or beaver tails); they contain two to six cells and are found singly or in characteristic clusters. With age, macroconidia often transform into chlamydoconidia; it is therefore imperative to observe the microscopic morphology before the culture passes its prime. Arthroconidia are also commonly formed with age. Older cultures commonly develop white sterile hyphae. Stock cultures may be best maintained on Sabouraud dextrose agar containing 3–5% sodium chloride.

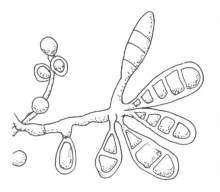 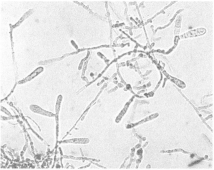

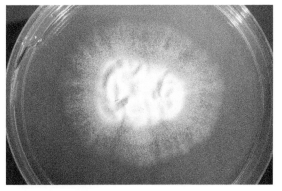

Epidermophyton floccosum. PDA, 30°C, 12 days. Surface of colony.

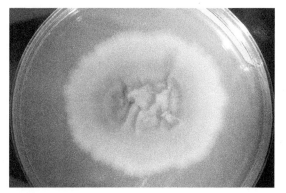

Epidermophyton floccosum. PDA, 30°C, 12 days. Reverse of colony.

Hyaline Hyphomycetes

Introduction to Hyaline Hyphomycetes

This section contains the fungi that have not been discussed earlier in this guide. These moulds have colorless, septate hyphae and produce conidia that may be colorless or pigmented. Their colony surfaces can be many different colors including white, gray, tan, yellow, pink, or green; the reverse is white or lightly pigmented. Most of these organisms are opportunistic and cause disease only in immunocompromised patients.

Fungi were previously categorized as pathogens or saprophytes; however, organisms that were once considered to be saprobic have been identified as important pathogens in immunocompromised patients. Almost any fungus isolated from a clinical specimen might be an etiologic agent of infection in a predisposed individual. All fungal isolates should be identified; most of those commonly considered as saprobic are identified in many laboratories only to genus level, as it often requires additional expertise or molecular methods to differentiate the species and further identification often does not provide additional guidance for clinical management.

In the medical laboratory, the saprophytic fungi are frequently encountered as contaminants. The source of the organism may be the transport container, the medium, or the laboratory environment, but may also be the result of specimen handling. Every effort should be made to instruct clinicians on proper techniques for specimen collection.

For further information, see
Anaissie et al. (ed.), 2009
de Hoog et al., 2020
Kidd et al., 2023b
St-Germain and Summerbell, 2011

THERMALLY MONOMORPHIC MOULDS • Hyaline Hyphomycetes

PART II Identification of Fungi in Culture

TABLE 2.21 Differential characteristics of fungi in which arthroconidia predominate[a]

Genus	Dark pigment	Pseudohyphae	Conidiophores	Alternating arthroconidia[b]	Arthroconidia barrel shaped	Blastoconidia	Illustration of microscopic morphology
Geotrichum (p. 167)	0	0	0	0	0	0	
Trichosporon and Cutaneotrichosporon (p. 163)	0	+	0	0	0	+	
Arthrographis (p. 324)	0	0	+	0	0	+[v]	
Hormographiella (p. 326)	0	0	+	0	0	0	
Pseudogymnoascus (formerly Geomyces) (p. 323)	0	0	+	+	+	0	
Coccidioides (p. 179)	0	0	0	+	+	0	
Malbranchea (p. 321)	0	0	0	+	0	0	
Neoscytalidium (p. 259)	+[v]	0	0	0	+[v]	0	

[a] Abbreviations: +, positive; 0, negative; V, variable.
[b] Empty cells appear between the arthroconidia.

Malbranchea spp.

PATHOGENICITY: Commonly considered a contaminant. At least one case of sinusitis has been reported.

RATE OF GROWTH: Moderate; mature within 6–10 days.

COLONY MORPHOLOGY: Surface may be white, yellow, beige, orange, pinkish, or brownish; texture is granular, powdery, or woolly. Reverse is light.

MICROSCOPIC MORPHOLOGY: Hyphae are septate, hyaline; no conidiophores are formed. Straight or curved arthroconidia alternating with empty cells develop in the hyphae. The arthroconidia may be of various lengths but are the same width as the fairly narrow hypha (usually <3 μm). Arthroconidia are released by breakage of the empty cells, and a portion of the adjacent empty cell often remains attached to separated arthroconidia. The arthroconidia are not swollen and not thick walled, differentiating them from those of *Coccidioides* spp. (p. 179). In its sexual state (which is rarely seen in routine culture), large, round, asci-producing fruiting bodies (gymnothecia) are formed; they have no opening and are surrounded by loosely organized hyphae. One species of *Malbranchea* forms large, round, dark masses of cells (sclerotia).

If the identification is questionable, and there is suspicion that the isolate could be *Coccidioides*, safety precautions must be diligently observed; wet preps should be made rather than slide cultures.

See Table 2.21 (p. 320) for differential characteristics of fungi in which arthroconidia predominate.

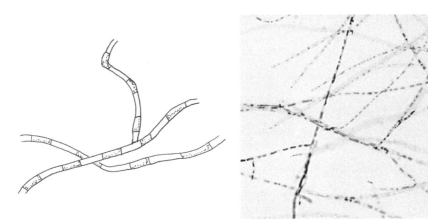

Malbranchea spp. *(continued)*

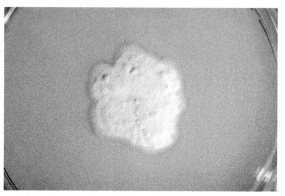

Malbranchea sp. PDA, 30°C, 7 days. Surface of colony.

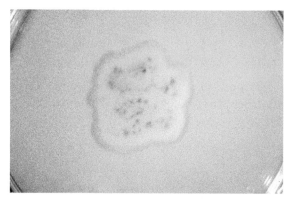

Malbranchea sp. PDA, 30°C, 7 days. Reverse of colony.

Pseudogymnoascus pannorum

TAXONOMY NOTES: This species was formerly known as *Geomyces pannorum*. Another significant species is *Pseudogymnoascus destructans*.

PATHOGENICITY: Commonly considered a contaminant; encountered in specimens of skin and nails; only rarely reported as an etiologic agent of infection in humans. There are rare reports of it causing cutaneous infection in dogs. *P. destructans* is the causative agent of bat white-nose syndrome, and has caused widespread decimation of bat populations in the eastern United States.

RATE OF GROWTH: Moderate (mature within 6–10 days) to slow (mature after 10 days). Grows well at 5–25°C; no growth at 37°C. Grows on media with cycloheximide.

COLONY MORPHOLOGY: Surface is white, pale yellow, gray, or tan; usually cottony or powdery. May be flat or elevated in the center; radial grooves sometimes form. Reverse can be colorless, but yellow is more typical, and a yellow or tan pigment may diffuse into the agar.

MICROSCOPIC MORPHOLOGY: Hyphae are septate. Conidiophores are erect, narrow, and measure 10–100 μm long; branches form in whorls around the central structure. Conidia (2–4 × 2–6 μm) are smooth or rough and form at the tips of the branches and also in intercalary positions separated by short empty spaces to create chains of two to four alternating, barrel-shaped arthroconidia. Conidia may also form along the sides of the conidiophore. Terminal and lateral conidia are somewhat clavate, having a rounded apex and truncate (cut-off, flattened) base.

See Table 2.21 (p. 320) for differential characteristics of fungi in which arthroconidia predominate.

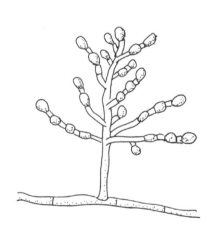 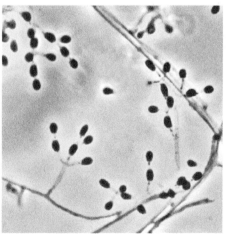

Courtesy of Lynne Sigler.

For further information, see
Gianni et al., 2003

Arthrographis kalrae

PATHOGENICITY: Reported rarely as a cause of mycetoma, septic arthritis, pulmonary infection, fungemia, and keratitis, as well as onychomycosis. It also has been isolated from various sites with questionable etiologic significance. It is commonly considered a contaminant in skin and nails. *Scytalidium cuboideum* (formerly *Arthrographis cuboidea*) is not known to cause infection.

RATE OF GROWTH: Moderate (mature within 6–10 days) to slow (mature after 10 days) at 25–30°C. Growth is enhanced at 37°C; also grows at 45°C. Grows on media containing cycloheximide. *S. cuboideum* is a rapid grower, reaching maturity within 5 days at 25–30°C but does not grow at 45°C and produces a pink-to-lavender pigment at 35–37°C that may form slowly and diffuse into the medium.

COLONY MORPHOLOGY: Surface at first smooth and yeastlike, later velvety; cream to pale yellow or tan. Reverse pale yellow, may become tan.

MICROSCOPIC MORPHOLOGY: Yeastlike cells seen on early growth; later hyphae are septate and colorless. Conidiophores, sometimes in bundles, are simple or branched in a treelike fashion; they produce chains of consecutive arthroconidia that are mostly rectangular, some oval (2–3.5 × 3–7 μm). Intercalary arthroconidia also form. Round blastoconidia (3.5–5.5 μm in diameter) may develop directly on the hyphae (most commonly on submerged hyphae).

See Table 2.21 (p. 320) for differential characteristics of fungi in which arthroconidia predominate.

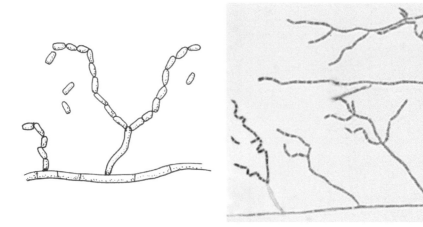

Arthrographis kalrae (continued)

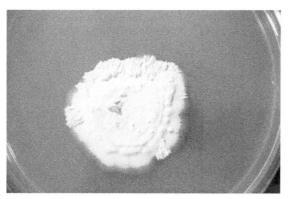

Arthrographis kalrae. PDA, 30°C, 8 days.

Hormographiella aspergillata

TAXONOMY NOTES: This species is a basidiomycete mushroom (gray shag mushroom) better known by the teleomorph name *Coprinopsis cinerea*, which was formerly known as *Coprinus cinereus*.

PATHOGENICITY: Has only occasionally been reported in immunocompromised patients to cause fatal pulmonary infections, cases of endocarditis following valve replacement, and skin and eye infections.

RATE OF GROWTH: Rapid; mature within 5 days. Growth is inhibited by cycloheximide.

COLONY MORPHOLOGY: Surface is white to cream colored, may become tan. Texture is dense, suedelike with cottony tufts; the edges are irregular. Reverse is pale.

MICROSCOPIC MORPHOLOGY: Hyphae septate, 2–5 µm wide. Conidiophores are broad based, septate, and may be branched or unbranched; at the apex or along the sides are fertile points from which are produced short hyphae that break at their septa, forming clusters of thin-walled, rectangular arthroconidia (1.5–3.0 × 2.5–6.5 µm). The arthroconidia are much narrower than the conidiophores; they are cylindrical, most with flat ends, but the terminal cells are usually rounded at their distal end. Rapid growth and susceptibility to cycloheximide further differentiate this organism from *Arthrographis kalrae*.

See Table 2.21 (p. 320) for differential characteristics of fungi in which arthroconidia predominate.

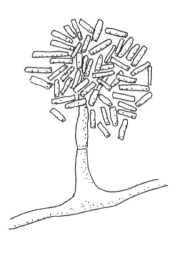 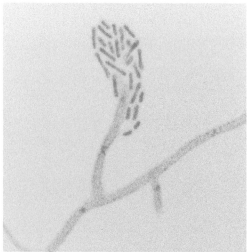

For further information, see
Conen et al., 2011
Moniot et al., 2020

The genus *Aspergillus*

TAXONOMY NOTES: *Aspergillus* spp. are divided into sections. A section is a taxonomic rank between genus and species. Many *Aspergillus* spp. have also been divided into species complexes because they are phylogenetically distinct but morphologically indistinguishable. While members of sections and species complexes largely overlap for the aspergilli, they do not always. In this text, we use species complex rather than section.

PATHOGENICITY: Members of the genus *Aspergillus* cause a group of diseases known as aspergillosis; the diseases may be in the forms of invasive infection, colonization, toxicoses, or allergy. The organisms are opportunistic invaders, the most common moulds to infect various sites in patients with lowered resistance due to neutropenia and/or treatment with high-dose corticosteroids or immunomodulatory drugs. *Aspergillus* spp. are the most common causes of acute fungal pneumonia and sinus infection in immunocompromised patients with neutropenia, iatrogenic immunosuppression, or following transplantation. Acute pulmonary aspergillosis may be complicated by dissemination to multiple sites including brain, liver, and bone. Chronic pulmonary aspergillosis may develop in less immunocompromised patients as a progressive necrotizing cavitary process or as an aspergilloma in a preexisting lung cavity. *Aspergillus* spp. may also cause allergic bronchopulmonary aspergillosis, particularly in patients with cystic fibrosis. *Aspergillus* keratitis is an important worldwide cause of mycotic corneal infection. *Aspergillus flavus* in agriculture produces aflatoxin, which is a potent environmental carcinogen and hepatotoxic agent. *Aspergillus* spp. are widespread in the environment and are commonly found as contaminants in cultures. Approximately 180 species of *Aspergillus* are known, but less than a quarter of them have been found to cause human disease. The species included on the following pages are the most commonly encountered in clinical specimens.

RATE OF GROWTH: Usually rapid; mature within 5 days; some species are slower growing.

COLONY MORPHOLOGY: Surface is at first white and then any shade of green, yellow, orange, brown, or black, depending on species. Texture is velvety or cottony. Reverse is usually white, golden, or brown.

MICROSCOPIC MORPHOLOGY: Hyphae are septate (2.5–8.0 µm in diameter); an unbranched conidiophore arises from a specialized foot cell. The conidiophore is enlarged at the tip, forming a swollen vesicle. Vesicles are completely or partially covered with flask-shaped phialides (formerly referred to as sterigmata), which may develop directly on the vesicle (uniseriate form) or be supported by a cell known as a metula (biseriate form). The phialides produce chains of mostly round, sometimes rough conidia (2–8 µm in diameter).

See Table 2.22 (p. 329) for differentiation of species most commonly encountered in the clinical laboratory.

The genus *Aspergillus* (continued)

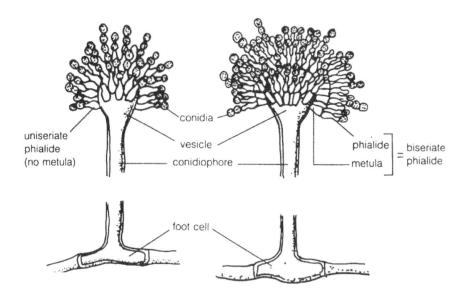

For further information, see
Anaissie et al. (ed.), 2009
de Hoog et al., 2020
Kidd et al., 2023b
Kousha et al., 2011
Patterson et al., 2016
Segal, 2009
St-Germain and Summerbell, 2011
Thompson and Young, 2021

TABLE 2.22 Differentiating characteristics of the most common *Aspergillus* spp.[a, b]

Species	Pathogenicity	Macroscopic morphology[b]	Microscopic morphology of conidiophores	Microscopic morphology of phialides	Illustration of microscopic morphology
A. fumigatus[c] (p. 331)	Most common cause of invasive disseminated aspergillosis; frequent agent of sinusitis	Velvety or powdery; at first white, then turning dark greenish to gray. Reverse white to tan	Short (<300 μm) Smooth	Uniseriate; usually only on upper two-thirds of vesicle, parallel to axis of conidiophore	
A. niger (p. 333)	Most common in ear infections; frequently in aspergilloma; rarely disseminated	Deep cottony; at first white to yellow, then turning black. Reverse white to yellow	Long (400–3,000 μm) Smooth	Biseriate; cover entire vesicle; form "radiate" head	
A. flavus (p. 334)	Involved in pulmonary, systemic, sinus, ear, and other infections; produces aflatoxins	Velvety; yellow to green or brown. Reverse goldish to red-brown	Medium (400–800 μm) Rough; pitted; spiny	Uniseriate and biseriate; cover entire vesicle; point out in all directions	
A. versicolor (p. 336)	Only occasionally involved in pulmonary or other infections	Velvety; at first white, then yellow, orangey, tan, green, or occasionally pinkish. Reverse white; may be yellow, orange, or red	Medium (200–500 μm) Smooth	Biseriate; loosely radiate; cover most of vesicle (Hülle cells may be present)	
A. ustus (p. 338)	Occasional cause of infection in various body sites	Velvety; brownish or olive-gray. Reverse yellowish brown	Short (130–300 μm) Smooth; brown when mature	Biseriate; loosely cover upper half to three-quarters of vesicle (can form irregular, elongate Hülle cells)	

Table continues on next page.

TABLE 2.22 Differentiating characteristics of the most common *Aspergillus* spp.[a, b] *(continued)*

Species	Pathogenicity	Macroscopic morphology[b]	Microscopic morphology of conidiophores	Microscopic morphology of phialides	Illustration of microscopic morphology
A. nidulans (p. 342)	Can cause infection at various sites; seen in patients with chronic granulomatous disease	Velvety; usually green, but buff to yellow where cleistothecia form. Reverse tan or purplish red	Short (<250 μm) Smooth; brown	Biseriate; short; columnar; cleistothecia usually present with reddish ascospores; Hülle cells often abundant	
A. glaucus (p. 344)	Rarely involved in nail, ear, and systemic disease	Feltlike; green with yellow areas. Reverse yellow (osmophilic, growth enhanced by 20% sucrose in medium)	Medium (300–700 μm) Smooth	Uniseriate; radiate to very loosely columnar; cover entire vesicle (cleistothecia generally present)	
A. terreus (p. 345)	Involved in infections in wide variety of body sites	Usually velvety; cinnamon-brown. Reverse yellow to brown	Short (<300 μm) Smooth	Biseriate; compactly columnar (round hyaline cells produced on mycelium submerged in agar)	
A. clavatus (p. 347)	An agent of allergic aspergillosis; rarely involved in infections in various body sites	Dense; green. Reverse white or tan	Long (500–2,000 μm) Smooth	Uniseriate; closely crowded on huge clavate vesicle (~200 × 40 μm)	

[a] In most cases the description applies to all members of the species complex (see detailed description of genus and species on pp. 327–347).

[b] *A. tanneri* is not included in Table 2.22 because conidial structures develop only when grown on Czapek agar or malt extract agar. See p. 340.

[c] Classically studied on Czapek-Dox agar; color of colonies may be somewhat different on various media.

[d] *A. fumigatus* grows well at 45°C or higher.

Aspergillus fumigatus species complex

For general information about the genus *Aspergillus*, see p. 327.

TAXONOMY NOTES: The species complex includes *Aspergillus felis*, *A. fischeri* (teleomorph, *Neosartorya fischeri*), *A. fumigatiaffinis*, *A. fumigatus sensu stricto*, *A. fumisynnematus*, *A hiratsukae*, *A. lentulus*, *A. novofumigatus*, *A. pseudoviridinutans*, *A. thermomutatus* (teleomorph, *N. pseudofischeri*), *A. udagawae* (teleomorph, *N. udagawae*), *A. viridinutans*, and *A. wyomingensis*. These species are difficult to differentiate phenotypically and most are rare in clinical specimens. These species are also grouped within *Aspergillus* section Fumigati.

PATHOGENICITY: It is the most common species of *Aspergillus* to cause invasive pulmonary aspergillosis, disseminated aspergillosis, allergic bronchopulmonary aspergillosis, fungal sinusitis, and mycotic keratitis. The organism is usually susceptible to antifungal triazoles and amphotericin B, which are considered first-line therapies for treatment of aspergillosis. However, studies indicate the emergence of resistance of *A. fumigatus* to triazoles.

RATE OF GROWTH: Rapid; mature within 5 days. Differs from the other common *Aspergillus* species by its ability to grow at 45°C.

COLONY MORPHOLOGY: Surface is velvety or powdery, various shades of green at prime with a narrow white border; colony turns dark gray with age. Reverse is white to tan.

MICROSCOPIC MORPHOLOGY: Septate hyphae; conidiophores smooth, relatively short (usually <300 μm long), and 5–10 μm in diameter. The phialides are uniseriate, close together (compact), forming only on the upper two-thirds of the vesicle, parallel to the axis of the conidiophore (known as columnar formation). Conidia are round, smooth, or slightly rough and 2–3.5 μm in diameter. *A. lentulus*, which also causes pulmonary aspergillosis, phenotypically resembles *A. fumigatus sensu stricto*; however, it is slower sporulating, tends to be more resistant, does not grow well at 48°C (*A. fumigatus* does so), and occurs uncommonly among clinical isolates. *A. lentulus* is best distinguished from *A. fumigatus* by molecular methods.

See Table 2.22 (p. 329) for differential characteristics of the most commonly encountered *Aspergillus* species.

Aspergillus fumigatus species complex *(continued)*

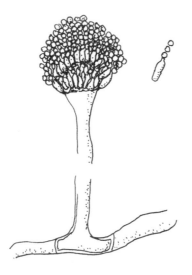
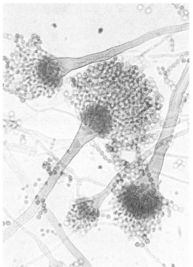

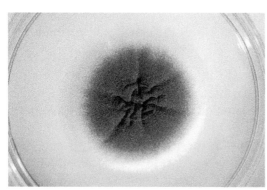

Aspergillus fumigatus. SDA, 30°C, 4 days. Surface of colony.

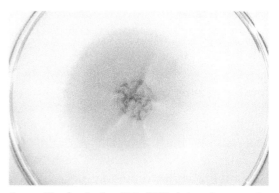

Aspergillus fumigatus. SDA, 30°C, 4 days. Reverse of colony.

For further information, see
Arastehfar et al., 2021
Latgé and Chamilos, 2019
Verweij et al., 2016
Wiederhold and Verweij, 2020

Aspergillus niger species complex

For general information about the genus *Aspergillus*, see p. 327.

TAXONOMY NOTES: The species complex includes *Aspergillus awamori*, *A. brasiliensis*, *A. japonicus*, *A. neoniger*, *Aspergillus niger sensu stricto*, *A. tubingensis*, and *A. welwitschiae*. These species are difficult to differentiate phenotypically and most are rare in clinical specimens. These species are also grouped within *Aspergillus* section Nigri.

PATHOGENICITY: Ubiquitous in nature. Most commonly isolated from the external ear, causing otomycosis; also a frequent agent of aspergilloma (fungus balls) in preexisting pulmonary cavities, in nasal sinuses, and in bronchiectatic airways. It occasionally causes acute and chronic invasive pulmonary and disseminated disease. *Aspergillus tubingensis* is more common in clinical specimens than *A. niger sensu stricto*.

RATE OF GROWTH: Rapid; mature within 5 days.

COLONY MORPHOLOGY: Surface is black with white border; thallus is deep, visibly composed of long, white to cream, erect hyphae with clusters of black conidia at the apices. Reverse white to cream.

MICROSCOPIC MORPHOLOGY: Septate hyphae. Conidiophores long (400–3,000 × 12–17 μm), smooth, may be brownish near top. Vesicles 30–75 μm in diameter. Phialides radiate around entire vesicle and are biseriate, with the metulae twice as long as the phialides. Conidia are 3.5–4.5 μm in diameter, rough, and dark.

See Table 2.22 (p. 329) for differentiation of species most commonly encountered in the clinical laboratory.

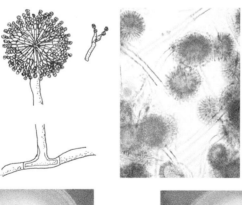

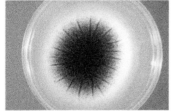

Aspergillus niger. SDA, 30°C, 4 days. Surface of colony.

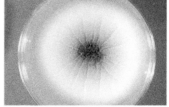

Aspergillus niger. SDA, 30°C, 4 days. Reverse of colony.

For further information, see
Nargesi et al., 2022

Aspergillus flavus species complex

For general information about the genus *Aspergillus*, see p. 327.

TAXONOMY NOTES: The species complex includes *Aspergillus albertensis* (teleomorph, *Petromyces albertensis*), *A. alliaceus* (teleomorph, *P. alliaceus*), *A beijingensis*, *Aspergillus flavus sensu stricto*, *A. nomius*, *A. oryzae*, *A. parasiticus*, *A. qizutongi*, *A. sojae*, *A. tamarii*, *A. terricola*, and *A. toxicarius*. These species are difficult to differentiate phenotypically and most are rare in clinical specimens. Some have not been associated with human infection. These species are also grouped within *Aspergillus* section Flavi.

PATHOGENICITY: It is the second most common species of *Aspergillus* to cause invasive aspergillosis. *Aspergillus flavus* has a stronger propensity among the *Aspergillus* species to cause invasive sinus disease. It also is the most common species causing invasive sinusitis in immunocompetent patients in the area of Sudan and in the Middle East. It is the most commonly reported food-borne fungus; many of the isolates produce aflatoxins. Aflatoxins constitute a group of highly potent carcinogens and hepatotoxins that are formed in stored grains, corn, and legumes that are subsequently ingested by humans and farm animals.

RATE OF GROWTH: Rapid; mature within 5 days.

COLONY MORPHOLOGY: Surface yellow-green to olive, often with specks of yellow; white border may be present. Texture is velvety to cottony. Reverse usually yellowish to tan.

MICROSCOPIC MORPHOLOGY: Septate hyphae; the conidiophores are long (400–800 × 8–18 µm), and when fully mature, the walls are characteristically rough/spiny, especially at the apex, i.e., along the area just below the vesicle. Both uniseriate and biseriate phialides are formed over most of the vesicle; they are loosely radiate and may cluster to form columns of conidia with age. Conidia are 3–6 µm in diameter with smooth or slightly rough walls.

See Table 2.22 (p. 329) for differential characteristics of the most commonly encountered *Aspergillus* species.

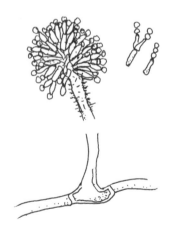
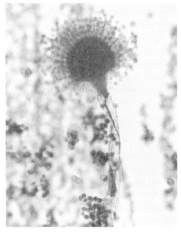

Aspergillus flavus **species complex** *(continued)*

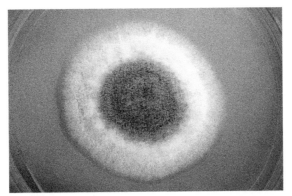

Aspergillus flavus. PDA, 30°C, 4 days. Surface of colony.

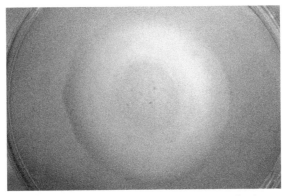

Aspergillus flavus. PDA, 30°C, 4 days. Reverse of colony.

For further information, see Amaike and Keller, 2011

Aspergillus versicolor species complex

For general information about the genus *Aspergillus*, see p. 327.

TAXONOMY NOTES: The species complex includes *Aspergillus creber, A. jensenii, A. protuberus, A. puulaauensis, A. sydowii, A. tabacinus,* and *A. versicolor sensu stricto.* These species are difficult to differentiate phenotypically and most are rare in clinical specimens. These species are also grouped within *Aspergillus* section Versicolores.

PATHOGENICITY: Occasionally involved in infections of various sites of the body, most commonly in the lung. The organism is widespread in the environment.

RATE OF GROWTH: Rapid; mature within 5 days.

COLONY MORPHOLOGY: Surface is suedelike, often having radial grooves; color varies, but most commonly green or tan with spots of yellow, orange, or pink. Reverse may be white, yellow, orange, or red. Colony diameter is relatively smaller than most other species of the genus.

MICROSCOPIC MORPHOLOGY: Septate hyphae; conidiophores smooth, medium length (200–500 × 4–7 μm); vesicles 9–16 μm in diameter. Biseriate, with metulae approximately the same size as the phialides, loosely covering half to all of the vesicle. Small conidial heads occasionally form, resembling penicilli. Conidia are round, slightly or clearly rough, and 2–3.5 μm in diameter. Hülle cells may occasionally be present.

See Table 2.22 (p. 329) for differential characteristics of the most commonly encountered *Aspergillus* species.

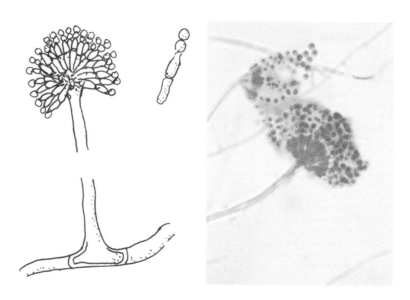

Aspergillus versicolor species complex *(continued)*

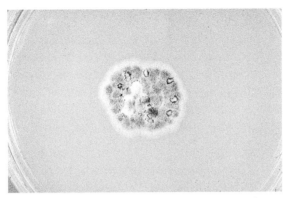

Aspergillus versicolor. SDA, 30°C, 4 days. Surface of colony.

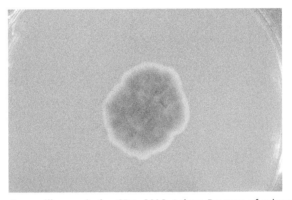

Aspergillus versicolor. SDA, 30°C, 4 days. Reverse of colony.

For further information, see
Géry et al., 2022
Siqueira et al., 2016

Aspergillus ustus species complex

For general information about the genus *Aspergillus*, see p. 327.

TAXONOMY NOTES: The species complex includes *Aspergillus calidoustus*, *A. granulosus*, *A. insuetus*, *A. keveii*, *A. pseudodeflectus*, *A. puniceus*, and *A. ustus sensu stricto* (*A. ustus sensu stricto* is currently recognized by the name *Emericella usta*. It is recommended *Aspergillus ustus* is reported). These species are difficult to differentiate phenotypically and most are rare in clinical specimens. Some have not been associated with human infection. These species are also grouped within *Aspergillus* section Usti.

PATHOGENICITY: Have been reported as an occasional etiologic agents of infection in various sites including heart, lung, ears, burn tissue, and skin. Present in low numbers in soil. Isolates of *A. calidoustus* tend to be resistant to the currently licensed antifungal triazoles but have low MICs to amphotericin B. *A. calidoustus* is more common in clinical specimens than *A. ustus sensu stricto*. *A. calidoustus* can be differentiated from *A. ustus sensu stricto* by its ability to grow well at 37°C.

RATE OF GROWTH: Rapid; mature within 5 days.

COLONY MORPHOLOGY: Surface light yellowish brown or dull grayish brown to olive-gray, occasionally with light yellow edges; may produce yellow-brown or purplish droplets on mycelium; texture velvety. Reverse yellowish brown.

MICROSCOPIC MORPHOLOGY: Septate hyphae; conidiophores smooth, brown when mature, short (130–300 × 4–7 µm); vesicles 9–15 µm in diameter. Biseriate, with metulae slightly shorter than the phialides, loosely covering upper half to three-quarters of vesicle. Conidia are rough walled and 3–4 µm in diameter. Hülle cells that are irregularly shaped, usually elongate, may be present.

See Table 2.22 (p. 329) for differential characteristics of the most commonly encountered *Aspergillus* species.

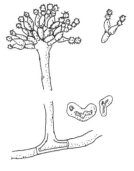
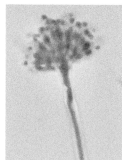
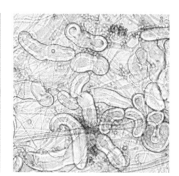

Hülle cells of *A. calidoustus*.
Courtesy of Deanna A. Sutton,
doctorfungus.org.

Aspergillus ustus species complex *(continued)*

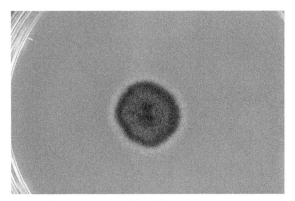

Aspergillus calidoustus. SDA, 30°C, 4 days.

For further information, see
Glampedakis et al., 2020
Glampedakis et al., 2021
Varga et al., 2008

Aspergillus tanneri

For general information about the genus *Aspergillus*, see p. 327.

PATHOGENICITY: This species causes potentially fatal chronic invasive pulmonary and disseminated aspergillosis in patients with chronic granulomatous disease. *A. tanneri* has also been found to have elevated MICs to amphotericin B, voriconazole, and itraconazole. These elevated MICs correlate with the fatal outcomes in the two initial patients reported with this organism, who had received antifungal therapy.

RATE OF GROWTH: Slow; mature after 10 days. Optimum growth temperature is 30°C; grows slower at 37°C. The preferred media for this organism are malt extract agar (MEA) and Czapek agar. It grows fastest on MEA, slightly slower on Czapek agar. Very slow growth on cornmeal agar; mature in 21 days.

COLONY MORPHOLOGY: The organism may appear initially on Sabouraud medium as white, nonsporulating colonies. When grown on MEA or Czapek agar, the surface is white when young and becomes yellow over time. Reverse remains colorless.

MICROSCOPIC MORPHOLOGY: Uniquely, this species of *Aspergillus* does not produce conidiophores when grown on most routine fungal media such as Sabouraud dextrose agar and potato dextrose agar; only septate hyphae are seen. When grown on MEA or Czapek agar, the conidiophores are smooth, long, slender, and 2–4 µm wide; vesicles are 5–7 × 7–10 µm. It is biseriate with metulae shorter than the phialides, each metula bearing two or more phialides covering one-half to two-thirds of the vesicle. The conidia are round, hyaline, smooth, and 2–3 µm in diameter. Conidiophores lacking vesicles, and bearing phialides of reduced size, are often found on trailing hyphae; these structures appear almost penicillate.

As most clinical laboratories may not have Czapek agar or MEA readily available, a non-sporulating hyaline mould that is thought to be clinically causing refractory pulmonary or disseminated infection should be submitted for molecular identification as early as possible to guide patient care.

A. tanneri is not included in Table 2.22, as it does not form conidia on routine media.

Aspergillus tanneri (continued)

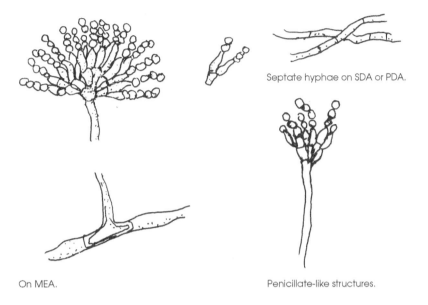

Septate hyphae on SDA or PDA.

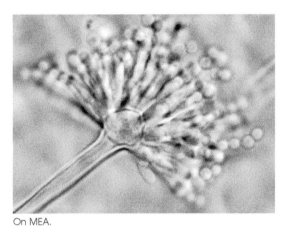

On MEA.

Penicillate-like structures.

On MEA.

Penicillate-like structure.

For further information, see Sugui et al., 2012

Aspergillus nidulans species complex

For general information about the genus *Aspergillus*, see p. 327.

TAXONOMY NOTES: The species complex includes *Aspergillus delacroxii*, *A. nidulans sensu stricto* (teleomorph, *Emericella nidulans*), *A. sublatus*, *A. tetrazonus*, and *A. unguis*. These species are difficult to differentiate phenotypically and most are rare in clinical specimens. These species are also grouped within *Aspergillus* section Nidulantes.

PATHOGENICITY: A soil organism with widespread distribution. Has been reported as the etiologic agent of infection in a variety of sites including lung, brain, bone, eyes, nasal sinus, and skin, as well as disseminated infection. It causes more lethal infections in patients with chronic granulomatous disease than do the other species of *Aspergillus*.

RATE OF GROWTH: Rapid; mature within 5 days.

COLONY MORPHOLOGY: Surface velvety, green; buff to yellow or purplish brown areas if cleistothecia are present; white border. Reverse buff, brownish orange, or deep reddish purple.

MICROSCOPIC MORPHOLOGY: Septate hyphae; conidiophores smooth, short (usually <200 μm long × 3–6 μm in diameter), and brown, darkening with age. Vesicles 8–12 μm in diameter. Phialides biseriate with the metula and phialide being equal in length, forming only on the upper half of the vesicle. Conidia are round, smooth or slightly rough, and 3–4 μm in diameter. Sexual state exhibits round cleistothecia (100–250 μm in diameter) producing red ascospores (3–4 × 4–6 μm) upon extended incubation (within 14 days). The cleistothecia are commonly surrounded by numerous round Hülle cells (10–25 μm in diameter).

See Table 2.22 (p. 329) for differential characteristics of the most commonly encountered *Aspergillus* species.

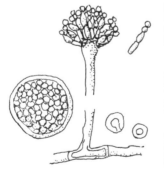
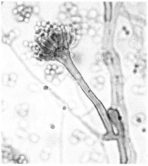
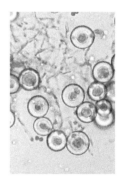

Hülle cells of *A. nidulans*.
Courtesy of Victoria
Ruppert.

Aspergillus nidulans **species complex** *(continued)*

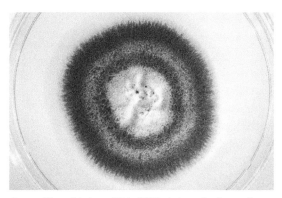

Aspergillus nidulans. SDA, 30°C, 4 days. Surface of colony.

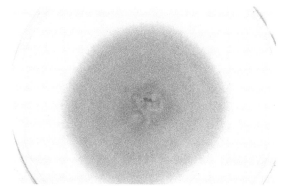

Aspergillus nidulans. SDA, 30°C, 4 days. Reverse of colony.

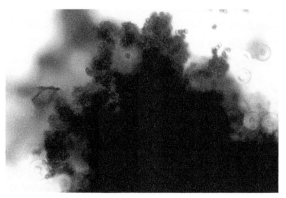

Aspergillus nidulans. Red ascospores and hyaline Hülle cells.

For further information, see
Chen et al., 2016
Henriet et al., 2012

Aspergillus glaucus

For general information about the genus *Aspergillus*, see p. 327.

PATHOGENICITY: Worldwide distribution, prefers dry environment; seldom encountered clinically. Occasional reports of infection of nails, ear, brain, and cardiovascular and visceral sites.

RATE OF GROWTH: Moderate (within 6–10 days) to slow (after 10 days). Species is osmophilic, so the growth rate is significantly enhanced by addition of 20% sucrose to the medium.

COLONY MORPHOLOGY: Surface feltlike, dull green with yellow areas of cleistothecia production. Reverse white to yellow.

MICROSCOPIC MORPHOLOGY: Septate hyphae; conidiophores smooth, medium length (300–700 × 8–15 µm). The phialides are uniseriate and may be loosely columnar or radiate, covering most of vesicle. Conidia rough, 5–8 µm in diameter. Sexual state exhibits round yellow cleistothecia, 60–150 µm in diameter. Ascospores mature slowly (~14 days), are 5–7 × 3–5 µm, with a central furrow/groove.

See Table 2.22 (p. 329) for differential characteristics of the most commonly encountered *Aspergillus* species.

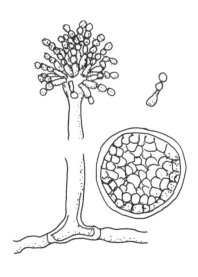
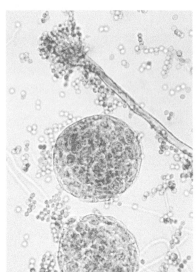

Aspergillus terreus species complex

For general information about the genus *Aspergillus*, see p. 327.

TAXONOMY NOTES: The species complex includes *Aspergillus alabamensis*, *A. citrinoterreus*, *A. floccosus*, *A. hortai*, *A. neoafricanus*, and *A. terreus sensu stricto*. These species are difficult to differentiate phenotypically and most are rare in clinical specimens. Some have not been associated with human infection. These species are also grouped within *Aspergillus* section Terrei.

PATHOGENICITY: Widespread in the environment. Known to regularly cause infection in a wide variety of body sites with possible dissemination. It is also an agent of allergic bronchopulmonary aspergillosis. It is unique among the *Aspergillus* spp. in its capability of *in vivo* adventitious conidiation and its intrinsic resistance to amphotericin B.

RATE OF GROWTH: Rapid; mature within 5 days.

COLONY MORPHOLOGY: Surface tan to cinnamon brown, texture velvety or powdery. Reverse yellow to tan.

MICROSCOPIC MORPHOLOGY: Septate hyphae; conidiophores smooth, relatively short (<300 μm long and 4–7 μm in diameter). Vesicles 10–20 μm in diameter. Phialides biseriate, with the metulae and phialide being equal in length, forming only on the upper half of the vesicle, compactly columnar. Conidia are round, smooth, 2–2.5 μm in diameter. Round solitary conidia are commonly produced along sides of hyphae submerged in medium.

See Table 2.22 (p. 329) for differential characteristics of the most commonly encountered *Aspergillus* species.

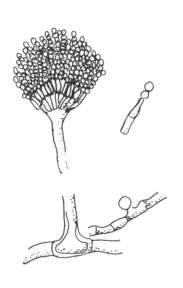 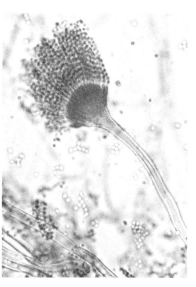

Aspergillus terreus species complex *(continued)*

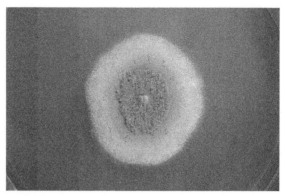

Aspergillus terreus. PDA, 30°C, 4 days. Surface of colony.

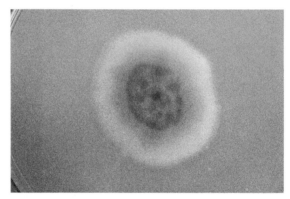

Aspergillus terreus. PDA, 30°C, 4 days. Reverse of colony.

For further information, see
Lass-Flörl et al., 2021
Posch et al., 2018

Aspergillus clavatus

For general information about the genus *Aspergillus*, see p. 327.

TAXONOMY NOTES: *Aspergillus clavatus* is currently recognized as *Neosartorya clavata*. It is recommended *A. clavatus* is reported.

PATHOGENICITY: A soil organism with widespread distribution. Seldom found in clinical specimens but has been implicated in diseases including allergic aspergillosis, pulmonary infections, endocarditis, infection of the external ear canal (otomycosis), and various toxic syndromes.

RATE OF GROWTH: Rapid; mature within 5 days.

COLONY MORPHOLOGY: Surface green with white border; densely packed with conidia that readily spread on agar to produce additional colonies. Reverse is white to tan.

MICROSCOPIC MORPHOLOGY: Septate hyphae; conidiophores smooth and large (500–2,000 μm × 10–30 μm). Phialides are uniseriate and closely packed on surface of extremely large club-shaped vesicle (usually 40–60 μm wide, up to 250 μm long). Conidia are smooth, round to oval (2.5–4 × 3–6 μm).

See Table 2.22 (p. 329) for differential characteristics of the most commonly encountered *Aspergillus* species.

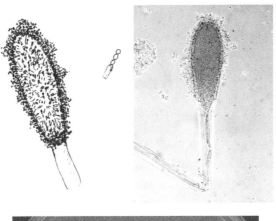

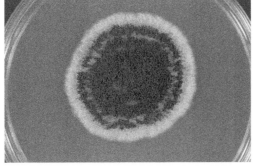

Aspergillus clavatus. PDA, 30°C, 4 days.

Penicillium spp.

TAXONOMY NOTES: The genus *Penicillium* and the teleomorphic genera *Talaromyces* and *Eupenicillium* have morphologically similar species and it may be necessary to incorporate molecular techniques to distinguish between species of these three genera.

PATHOGENICITY: Commonly considered contaminants but found in a variety of diseases in which their etiologic significance is uncertain. Among the wide range of multiple *Penicillium* spp., only a few have caused invasive disease; these include *P. chrysogenum* and *P. citrinum*. They have been known to cause corneal, cutaneous, external ear, respiratory, and urinary tract infections, as well as endocarditis after insertion of valve prostheses. Disseminated disease has been reported in severely immunocompromised patients. Many strains produce toxins. Identification of the exact species of a possibly pathogenic isolate of *Penicillium* is best accomplished with molecular methods. Recovery of *Penicillium* from a clinical specimen should still prompt the pursuit of other organisms that may be causing disease.

See also *Talaromyces marneffei* (formerly *Penicillium marneffei*) (p. 183).

RATE OF GROWTH: Rapid; mature within 5 days. Depending on the species, can be no or poor growth at 37°C.

COLONY MORPHOLOGY: Surface at first is white, then becomes very powdery and blue to slate gray to green with a white border. Some less common species differ in color and texture. Reverse is usually white, but may be red or brown. Some species produce a diffusible red pigment. If the isolate produces a red reverse and diffuse pigment in the agar, *T. marneffei* (p. 183) should be considered; this is especially relevant if the patient has recently visited Southeast Asia.

MICROSCOPIC MORPHOLOGY: Hyphae are septate (1.5–5 μm in diameter) with branched or unbranched conidiophores that have secondary branches known as metulae. On the metulae, arranged in whorls, are flask-shaped phialides that bear unbranched chains of smooth or rough, almost round conidia (2.5–5 μm in diameter). The entire structure forms the characteristic "penicillus" or "brush", or "skeleton hand", appearance. Moulds with similar microscopic appearance include *Paecilomyces variotii* (p. 350), *Rasamsonia argillacea* (p. 351), and *Purpureocillium lilacinum* (p. 352). Colony color can often help distinguish between these genera.

Penicillium **spp.** *(continued)*

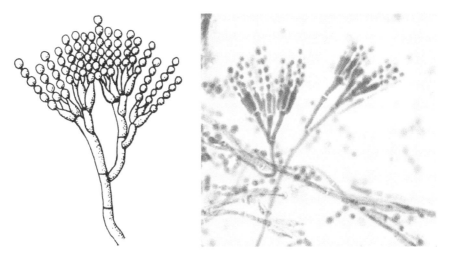

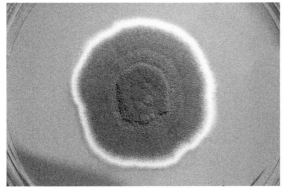

Penicillium sp. SDA, 30°C, 4 days.

For further information, see
Houbraken et al., 2020

Paecilomyces variotii

PATHOGENICITY: Associated with sinusitis and pneumonia in immunocompromised patients, as well as post-cataract endophthalmitis, wound infections, cerebrospinal fluid shunt infection, vascular catheter-associated infections, and keratitis.

RATE OF GROWTH: Rapid; mature within 5 days.

COLONY MORPHOLOGY: Surface is flat and powdery or velvety; yellowish brown or sand color, usually with a lighter border. Reverse is off-white, light yellow, or pale brown. Grows at 37°C; some isolates may also grow between 40 and 50°C.

MICROSCOPIC MORPHOLOGY: Resembles *Penicillium* spp. (p. 348), but the phialides of *P. variotii* are more elongated and taper to a long, slender tube, giving them the shape of drawn-out bowling pins; they bend away from the axis of the conidiophore and may appear singly along the hyphae. The conidia (~2–4 × 3–5 µm or more) are elliptical or oblong and occur in long, unbranched chains. Subspherical to pyriform chlamydospores (4–8 µm in diameter) may be present singly or in short chains.

For differentiation of *Paecilomyces variotii*, *Rasamsonia argillacea*, and *Purpureocillium lilacinum* see Table 2.23 (p. 354).

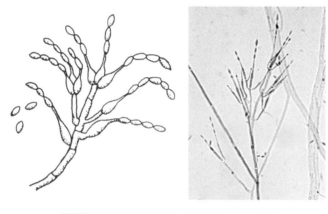

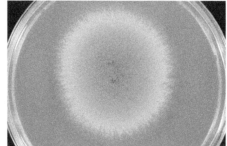

Paecilomyces variotii. SDA, 30°C, 4 days.

For further information, see
Barker et al., 2014
Sprute et al., 2021a

Rasamsonia argillacea species complex

TAXONOMY NOTES: The species complex includes *Rasamsonia aegroticola*, *R. argillacea sensu stricto*, *R. eburnea*, and *R. piperina*. These species are difficult to differentiate phenotypically. *R. argillacea* was formerly known as *Geosmithia argillacea*.

PATHOGENICITY: Causes invasive pulmonary infections in patients with risk factors such as chronic granulomatous disease, immunosuppressive treatment, or hematopoietic stem cell transplant; often with poor outcomes. Recovered from patients with cystic fibrosis; the clinical impact of airway colonization is variable. Isolates have low echinocandin MICs, while elevated azole MICs have been observed, in particular for isavuconazole and voriconazole. Human infections are rare; however, its close resemblance to *Paecilomyces variotii* has probably led to under reporting.

RATE OF GROWTH: Moderate; mature within 6–10 days. Growth is optimal at 36°C, and restricted at lower temperature (<28°C); good growth occurs at 42°C.

COLONY MORPHOLOGY: Surface is flat and powdery; may be cream to pale brown. Reverse is yellow to pale brown.

MICROSCOPIC MORPHOLOGY: Hyphae are septate. Conidiophores, metulae, and phialides are rough walled. Conidiophores are often branched, and metulae support cylindrical phialides with a short tapering tip. *R. argillaceae* conidia are smooth and cylindrical (boxcar-shaped) (~1.5–2.0 × 3.5–4.5 μm or more) and form chains. Mature conidia can appear ovoid. For differentiation of *Rasamsonia argillacea*, *Paecilomyces variottii*, and *Purpureocillium lilacinum*, see Table 2.23 (p. 354).

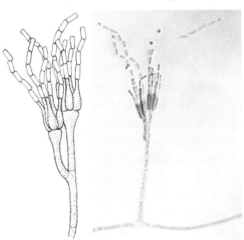

Reprinted from De Ravin SS et al. 2011. *Clin Infect Dis* 52:e136–143.

For further information, see
Abdolrasouli et al., 2018
De Ravin et al., 2011
Houbraken et al., 2012
Houbraken et al., 2013
Stemler et al., 2020

Purpureocillium lilacinum

TAXONOMY NOTES: This species was formerly known as *Paecilomyces lilacinus*.

PATHOGENICITY: Most commonly causes endophthalmitis (post-cataract surgery) and keratitis. It may also cause invasive sinusitis in immunocompetent and diabetic patients. Among immunocompromised patients, it most frequently causes subcutaneous infections and, less often, deep infection, including pneumonia and osteomyelitis.

RATE OF GROWTH: Rapid; mature within 5 days.

COLONY MORPHOLOGY: Surface is flat and powdery or velvety; may be pinkish, mauve, violet, or reddish gray; often has whitish border. Reverse is off-white or pinkish. Growth does not usually occur above 37°C.

MICROSCOPIC MORPHOLOGY: Conidiophores are long (400–600 μm), rough walled, branch, and form rough-walled metulae that support densely clustered phialides that are flask or short tenpin shaped (oval at their base and tapered to a short, narrow neck). The conidia are smooth or slightly rough walled, oval or fusiform (~2.0–2.2 × 2.5–3.0 μm) in swerving chains.

For differentiation of *Purpureocillium lilacinum*, *Paecilomyces variotii*, and *Rasamsonia argillacea* see Table 2.23 (p. 354).

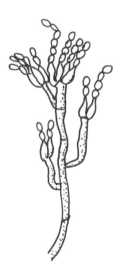
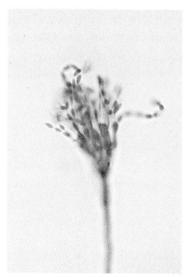

Purpureocillium lilacinum (continued)

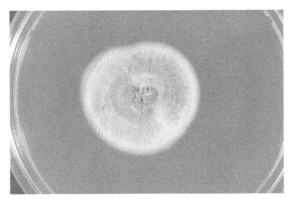

Purpureocillium lilacinum. PDA, 30°C, 4 days. (Courtesy of Victoria Ruppert.)

For further information, see

Barker et al., 2014
Pastor and Guarro, 2006
Sprute et al., 2021b

THERMALLY MONOMORPHIC MOULDS

TABLE 2.23 Differential characteristics of *Paecilomyces variotii*, *Rasamsonia argillacea*, and *Purpureocillium lilacinum*

Organism	Colony color	Conidiophores	Phialides	Conidia (µm)	Growth temperature
Paecilomyces variotii	Tan to yellowish brown	Smooth walled	Broadly spaced on each metula	Elliptical or oblong, smooth; ~2–4 × 3–5 (or longer)	Reported to grow well at 50°C, but many do not grow at >40°C
Rasamsonia argillacea	Cream to pale brown	Rough walled	Densely clustered on each metula	Cylindrical, smooth; ~1.5–2.0 × 3.5–4.5 (or longer)	Restricted at lower temperature (<28°C). Optimal at 36°C. Displays good growth at 42°C, with a maximum >50°C
Purpureocillium lilacinum	Pinkish, violet, or reddish gray	Rough walled	Densely clustered on each metula	Oval or fusiform, smooth or slightly rough; ~2.0–2.2 × 2.5–3.0	Restricted at 37°C

Scopulariopsis spp.

TAXONOMY NOTES: *Scopulariopsis brevicaulis* and *S. brumptii* are the species most often encountered in the clinical laboratory. *S. brumptii* is currently recognized as *Microascus paisii*. It is recommended *S. brumptii* is reported.

PATHOGENICITY: Known to infect the nails (usually toenail) and are associated with subcutaneous and invasive infection at various sites, including endocarditis, sinusitis, and disseminated infection, primarily in immunocompromised patients. Isolates of *S. brevicaulis* tend to be resistant *in vitro* to antifungal triazoles and have characteristically high MICs to amphotericin B that exceed safely achievable concentrations. *Scopulariopsis* spp. are also commonly encountered as contaminants.

RATE OF GROWTH: Rapid; mature within 5 days.

COLONY MORPHOLOGY: Surface is at first white and glabrous and then usually becomes powdery light brown with a light tan periphery. Some less frequently encountered species may be dark grayish, brown, or black. Reverse is usually tan with brownish center; occasionally darker.

MICROSCOPIC MORPHOLOGY: Septate hyphae with short, often branched conidiophores bearing annellides that may be cylindrical or bowling pin shaped (swollen at the base and narrowing to an extended apex). The annellides form in brush-like groups or singly. The conidia, in chains, are roundish (4–9 μm in diameter), thick walled, rough and spiny when mature, sometimes slightly pointed at the apex, and cut off at the base, forming a short neck. The conidia are larger, rough, and uniquely shaped by being cut off at one end and sometimes slightly pointed at the other.

For differentiation of *S. brevicaulis* and *S. brumptii*, see Table 2.24 (p. 357).

Scopulariopsis spp. *(continued)*

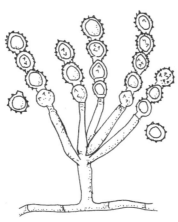

S. brevicaulis.

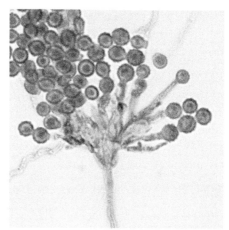

S. brevicaulis.

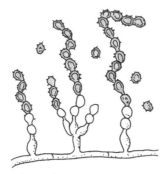

S. brumptii.

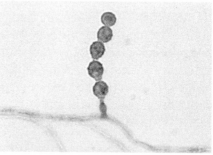

S. brumptii.

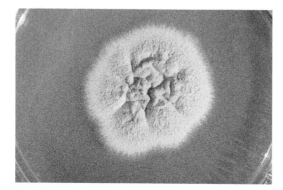

Scopulariopsis brevicaulis. SDA, 30°C, 5 days. Surface of colony.

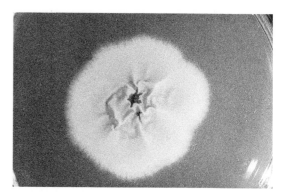

Scopulariopsis brevicaulis. SDA, 30°C, 5 days. Reverse of colony.

For further information, see
Pérez-Cantero and Guarro, 2020a

TABLE 2.24 Differential characteristics of *Scopulariopsis brevicaulis* versus *Scopulariopsis brumptii*

| Organism | Pathogenicity | Colony | Annellides | | | Conidia | |
			Shape	Size (μm)	Arrangement	Diameter (μm)	Color
S. brevicaulis	Frequently involved in nail infections; occasional reports of invasive disease	Light brown	Fairly cylindrical	2.5–3.5 × 9.0–25.0	Most in brushlike groups, some single	5.0–8.0	Hyaline or pale brown
S. brumptii	Occasionally found in pulmonary disease	Dark gray or grayish brown	Like tenpins; swollen at base, narrowing at apex	2.5–3.5 (at base) × 5.0–10.0	Most single, some in groups	3.5–5.5	Dark brown to blackish

Gliocladium spp.

PATHOGENICITY: Commonly considered contaminants; not known to cause disease.

RATE OF GROWTH: Rapid; mature within 5 days.

COLONY MORPHOLOGY: Surface is at first white. The center then becomes dark green; some strains may be pinkish. Fluffy growth spreads over plate in 1 week. Reverse is white.

MICROSCOPIC MORPHOLOGY: The hyphae, conidiophores, and phialides are similar to those of *Penicillium* spp. (p. 348); however, the conidia of *Gliocladium* do not remain in chains but clump together with the conidia of adjacent phialides to form large clusters or balls. Looks similar to a hand holding a ball by the fingertips.

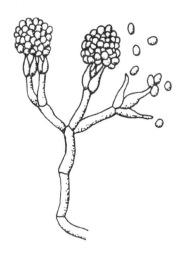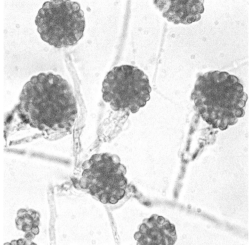

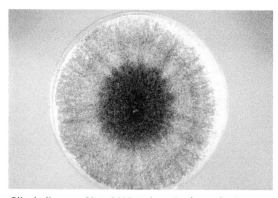

Gliocladium sp. SDA, 30°C, 5 days. Surface of colony.

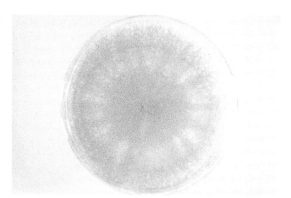

Gliocladium sp. SDA, 30°C, 5 days. Reverse of colony.

Trichoderma spp.

PATHOGENICITY: Commonly considered contaminants, but there has been an increasing number of reports of infections, particularly caused by *Trichoderma longibrachiatum*, in immunocompromised patients and cases of peritonitis in patients undergoing peritoneal dialysis.

RATE OF GROWTH: Rapid; mature within 5 days.

COLONY MORPHOLOGY: White fluff covers agar in a few days and then becomes more compact and woolly. Green patches are eventually produced due to formation of conidia (typically at the margin of the colony). Reverse is colorless or light orangey tan to yellow.

MICROSCOPIC MORPHOLOGY: Hyphae are septate. Conidiophores are short and often branched at wide angles; phialides are flask shaped and form at wide angles to the conidiophore, most often in pairs, one on either side of the conidiophore. Conidia are round (3–4 μm in diameter) or slightly oval (2–3 × 2.5–5.0 μm), single celled, and clustered together at the end of each phialide. Clusters are easily disrupted unless microscopic preparations are handled with exceptional care.

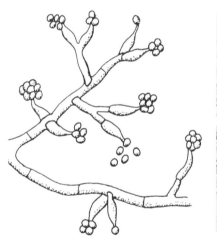 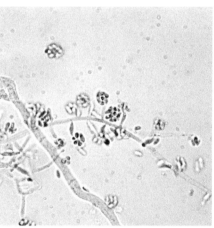

Trichoderma spp. *(continued)*

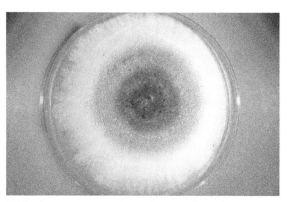

Trichoderma sp. SDA, 30°C, 5 days. Surface of colony.

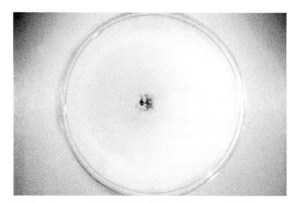

Trichoderma sp. SDA, 30°C, 5 days. Reverse of colony.

For further information, see
Sal et al., 2022
Sandoval-Denis et al., 2014

Metarhizium anisopliae species complex

TAXONOMY NOTES: The species complex includes *Metarhizium acridum*, *M. alvesii*, *M. anisopliae sensu stricto*, *M. baoshanense*, *M. brachyspermum*, *M. brittlebankisoides*, *M. brunneum*, *M. campsosterni*, *M. clavatum*, *M. globosum*, *M. guizhouense*, *M. humberi*, *M. indigoticum*, *M. majus*, *M. lepidiotae*, *M. kalasinense*, *M. pingshaense*, *M. robertsii*, *M. phasmatodeae*, *M. gryllidicola*, and *M. sulphureum*. These species are difficult to differentiate phenotypically.

PATHOGENICITY: Ubiquitous saprophytes that have a beneficial association with plant roots but are pathogenic to a wide range of insects and arthropods, which makes it useful as an insecticide. Rarely reported as the cause of human infection and no reports associated with mycoinsecticide use. Most cases are keratitis or sclerokeratitis in immunocompetent individuals following over-wearing contact lenses, exposure to farm soil, or ocular trauma with vegetable matter. Sinus infection has also been reported in immunocompetent patients. Skin lesions and disseminated infections have been reported in immunocompromised individuals.

RATE OF GROWTH: Moderate; mature within 6–10 days. Optimal growth temperature is 25°C with little or no growth at 37°C but some isolates are able to grow at low temperatures (5°C) or higher temperatures with 37°C as the maximum temperature.

COLONY MORPHOLOGY: Typically flat, compact, and velvety with a dense heaped center. Some isolates are thick and cottony. Initially white to buff and then typically turn olive green but may be dark green, light green, yellow-green, pale yellow, greyish yellow, white or brownish. Some isolates have different colors in the center and the margin or two colors in the center. May grow in dense concentric rings as conidia are produced in visible columns. Most isolates have a white fringe of variable width. Reverse is most often brownish orange but may be yellow or white.

MICROSCOPIC MORPHOLOGY: Hyphae are septate and hyaline. Conidiophores are of variable length and aggregate in tufts with verticillate branching. Phialides are characterized by a candelabrum-like dense parallel arrangement of cylindrical phialides. Conidia are produced in chains and are cylindrical or ovoid. *M. globosum* conidia are globose.

Metarhizium anisopliae species complex *(continued)*

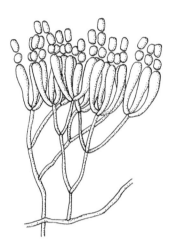

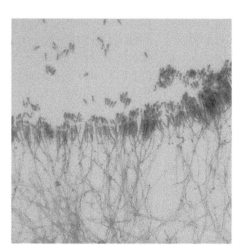

For further information, see
Brunner-Mendoza et al., 2022
Mongkolsamrit et al., 2020

Beauveria bassiana

PATHOGENICITY: Commonly considered a contaminant. Not often involved in human infection, but there have been reports of several cases of keratitis (corneal infection) and one disseminated infection in a leukemia patient. It is known to be pathogenic in insects, especially silkworms, where it has historical significance for one of the first known causes of fungal disease.

RATE OF GROWTH: Rapid; mature within 5 days.

COLONY MORPHOLOGY: Surface is white to cream, occasionally pinkish; fluffy to powdery. Reverse is white.

MICROSCOPIC MORPHOLOGY: Hyphae are septate, narrow, and delicate. Conidia-producing structures are flask shaped with a narrow zigzag terminal extension bearing a conidium at each bent point (sympodial geniculate growth). Conidia are small (2–4 µm in diameter), one celled, and round to oval, each forming singly on a tiny denticle. It is best to examine young cultures before dense clusters of conidiogenous cells form, making it difficult to observe the characteristic arrangement of conidia.

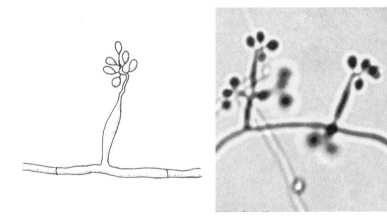

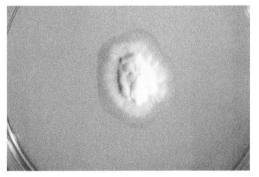

Beauveria sp. SDA, 30°C, 4 days.

For further information, see
Brunner-Mendoza et al., 2022

Verticillium spp.

PATHOGENICITY: Well known as important plant pathogens. They are also commonly known as contaminants in clinical laboratories. Reported as rare agents of keratitis, endophthalmitis post-cataract surgery, peritonitis, and cutaneous infection post-renal transplantation.

RATE OF GROWTH: Rapid; mature within 5 days.

COLONY MORPHOLOGY: Surface is at first white and then may become pinkish brown, red, green, or yellow; powdery or velvety in texture; spreading. Reverse is white or rust in color.

MICROSCOPIC MORPHOLOGY: Septate hyphae. Conidiophores are simple or branched at several levels and in whorls (i.e., verticillate); phialides are very elongate, having pointed apex, also arranged in whorls. Conidia are oval and single celled, appear singly or in clusters at ends of phialides, and remain in place only if slide preparations are handled with great care.

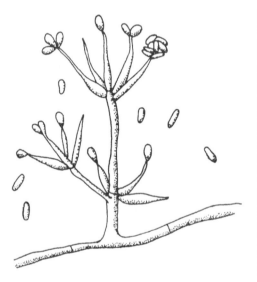
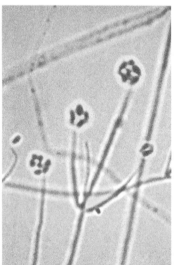

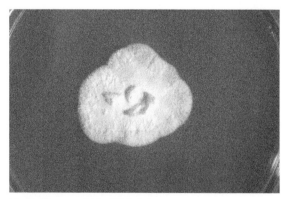

Verticillium sp. SDA, 30°C, 4 days.

Acremonium and *Sarocladium* spp.

TAXONOMY NOTES: *Sarocladium strictum* and *S. kiliense* were formerly known as *Acremonium strictum* and *A. kiliense*, respectively.

PATHOGENICITY: Most commonly known as etiologic agents of white grain mycetoma and localized infections of the nails and cornea. Disseminated infections have been reported in immunosuppressed patients. The organisms may also be encountered as contaminants.

RATE OF GROWTH: Rapid (mature within 5 days) to moderate (mature within 6–10 days).

COLONY MORPHOLOGY: At first compact, glabrous; later becomes feltlike, powdery, or waxy. May be white, yellowish, light gray, or pale rose in color. Colony does not spread. Reverse is colorless, pale yellow, or pinkish.

MICROSCOPIC MORPHOLOGY: Extremely delicate. Hyphae are septate. Phialides are erect, unbranched, tapering, have no conspicuous collarette, and form directly on the fine, narrow hyphae; most (but not all) have a septum at the base delimiting them from the hyphae. Conidia are oblong (2–3 × 4–8 μm) and usually one celled but occasionally two celled. The conidia form easily disrupted clusters at the tips of the phialides.

To differentiate *Acremonium* and *Sarocladium* spp. from similar genera, see Table 2.13 (p. 224).

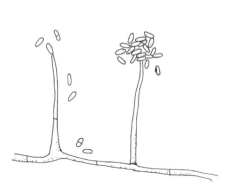 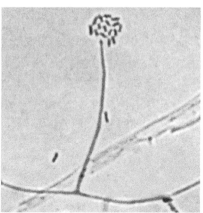

Acremonium and *Sarocladium* spp. *(continued)*

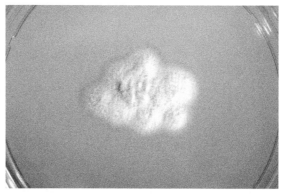

Acremonium sp. SDA, 30°C, 5 days. Surface of colony.

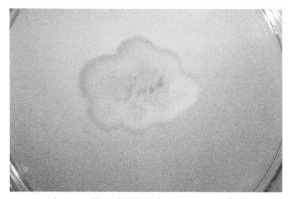

Acremonium sp. SDA, 30°C, 5 days. Reverse of colony.

For further information, see
Pérez-Cantero and Guarro, 2020b
Summerbell et al., 2011

Fusarium spp.

TAXONOMY NOTES: *Fusarium* is a genus in taxonomic flux. There are a number of species complexes pathogenic to humans. These species complexes include *F. solani* species complex, *F. oxysporum* species complex, *F. fujikuroi* species complex, *F. incarnatum equiseti* species complex, and *F. dimerum* species complex. Definitive identification of members of these species complexes requires molecular characterization.

PATHOGENICITY: Common worldwide causes of mycotic keratitis. Among immunocompetent patients, also cause mycetoma, sinusitis, septic arthritis, and onychomycosis. They are increasingly the cause of sinopulmonary and disseminated infections in profoundly neutropenic patients; in these cases, the organism can often be cultured from characteristic cutaneous lesions and from blood cultures. Additionally, lethal toxicoses, among which are fumonisins and trichothecenes, have been reported in individuals who ingested food prepared from grain that had been overgrown by toxin-producing species. The susceptibility profiles differ widely among species, with variably high MICs being observed for amphotericin B and triazoles. They are intrinsically resistant to echinocandins. Many are plant pathogens that can be traumatically inoculated into the cornea or subcutaneous tissues.

RATE OF GROWTH: Rapid; mature within 5 days.

COLONY MORPHOLOGY: At first white and cottony, but some species quickly develop a pastel pink or violet center with a lighter periphery. Some species, like *F. solani* species complex members, remain white, while others, like *F. oxysporum sensu stricto*, become tan or orangey. Reverse is usually light but may be deeply colored.

MICROSCOPIC MORPHOLOGY: Septate hyphae. There are two types of conidiation: (i) unbranched or branched conidiophores with phialides that produce large ($2-6 \times 14-80$ μm), sickle- or canoe-shaped macroconidia (with three to five septa); and (ii) long or short simple conidiophores bearing small ($2-4 \times 4-8$ μm), oval, one- or two-celled conidia singly or in clusters resembling those of *Acremonium* spp. (p. 365). Chlamydoconidia may be present in some species.

Fusarium spp. *(continued)*

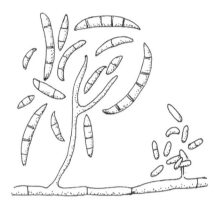

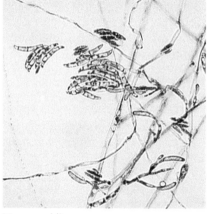

Macroconidia.

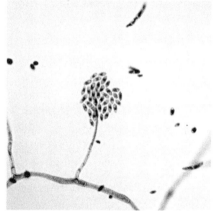

Microconidia.

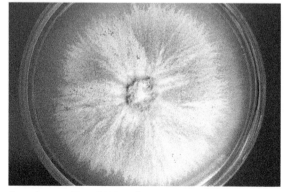

Fusarium sp. SDA, 30°C, 4 days.

For further information, see
DeLucca and Walsh, 2015
Nucci and Anaissie, 2007

Coniochaeta spp.

TAXONOMY NOTES: This genus was formerly known as *Lecythophora*.

PATHOGENICITY: Have occasionally been involved in subcutaneous abscess, keratitis, endophthalmitis, sinusitis, peritonitis, and endocarditis.

RATE OF GROWTH: Moderate; mature within 6–10 days.

COLONY MORPHOLOGY: At first flat, smooth, moist to slimy, somewhat yeastlike, pink to salmon or orange (one of the very few orange moulds causing human infection); may develop clumps of erect hyphal fuzz. If isolate produces chlamydospores, the center of the colony will become blackish brown. Reverse is pink or tan.

MICROSCOPIC MORPHOLOGY: Hyphae septate, hyaline, or very lightly pigmented. Phialides usually do not have a septum at the base; most are extremely short, volcano-shaped structures along the sides of the hyphae, but they may be larger and flask shaped or nearly cylindrical. Phialides have parallel-sided collarettes that may require oil immersion microscopy to be seen. Conidia are hyaline or almost so, single celled (1.5–2.5 × 3.0–6.0 μm), oval to cylindrical, and sometimes slightly curved. May form chlamydoconidia that are brown, ~4.5 × 7.0 μm, thick walled, broadly club shaped, and cut off at the base.

The two clinically encountered species of *Coniochaeta* differ in that *C. mutabilis* produces brown chlamydoconidia that eventually turn the colony brown, whereas *C. hoffmannii* does not produce chlamydoconidia and the colony therefore remains pink or salmon.

To differentiate *Coniochaeta* from similar genera, see Table 2.13 (p. 224).

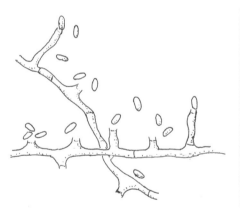
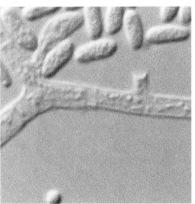

Courtesy of Wiley Schell.

For further information, see
Khan et al., 2013

Trichothecium roseum

PATHOGENICITY: Commonly considered a contaminant. Not known to cause infection.

RATE OF GROWTH: Rapid; mature within 5 days.

COLONY MORPHOLOGY: At first white and woolly and then becomes pink or peach colored. Reverse is white to cream.

MICROSCOPIC MORPHOLOGY: Septate hyphae. Conidiophores are long, slender, and mostly unbranched. Conidia (8–10 × 12–18 μm) are smooth, slightly thick walled, two celled, and pear or club shaped, with a well-marked truncate attachment point frequently off to one side, forming a "foot." The conidia are produced in alternating directions and remain side by side in an elongated group.

The long conidiophores and the smooth walls, attachment points, and arrangement of the conidia serve to distinguish this organism from *Nannizzia nana* (p. 297).

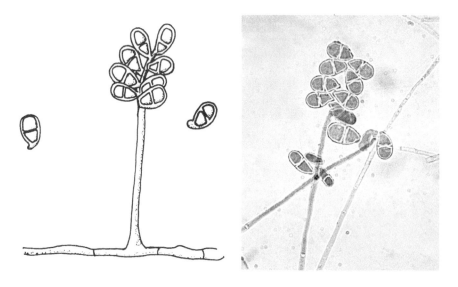

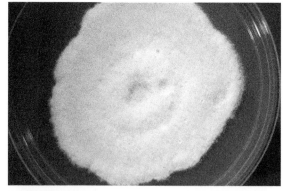

Trichothecium roseum. PDA, 30°C, 8 days. The extended incubation was required for pigment production.

Chrysosporium spp.

PATHOGENICITY: Commonly considered contaminants. Isolated from specimens of skin and nails, but their significance is often uncertain. There has been a report of systemic infection in a patient with chronic granulomatous disease and a cerebral infection in an HIV-positive patient. *Chrysosporium* spp. involved in skin infections of snakes, chameleons, crocodiles, and iguanas have been moved to the genus *Ophiomyces*.

RATE OF GROWTH: Moderate; mature within 6–10 days.

COLONY MORPHOLOGY: Varies greatly among the many species. May be spreading or compact; surface cottony or powdery; flat or raised; usually white, yellow, or tan but may be pink or slightly orange. Reverse is usually white, yellow, tan, or brown but may be another color.

MICROSCOPIC MORPHOLOGY: Septate hyphae. Conidia may form directly on the hyphae or at the ends of simple or branched, stalk-like, short or long conidiophores. Conidia are usually one celled (2–9 × 3–13 μm), clavate, with a rounded apex and broad flattened base; the walls may be thin or a bit thick and are most often smooth, occasionally rough. A fringe or remnant of supporting cell wall may stay on the base of the conidium after it matures and detaches. Intercalary conidia (referred to as alternating arthroconidia by some mycologists) are sometimes formed; they are cylindrical or barrel shaped or may bulge on only one side. Large sexual fruiting bodies (ascocarps) may occasionally be seen in culture.

- The morphology of *Chrysosporium* may resemble that of *Blastomyces parvus* (formerly *Emmonsia parva*), but yeast do not develop at 37°C; some species will not grow at 37°C.
- Young conidial formation may mimic that of *Blastomyces dermatitidis/gilchristii* (p. 177), but it will not display thermal dimorphism.
- Morphology may also resemble that of microconidium-producing *Trichophyton* spp., and some species of *Chrysosporium* will grow on dermatophyte test medium (p. 455) and turn it red.
- *Chrysosporium tuberculatum* produces tuberculated macroconidia which resemble *Histoplasma capsulatum*. It does not make microconidia and does not display thermal dimorphism.
- For differentiation of *Chrysosporium* from *Sporotrichum*, see Table 2.25 (p. 373).

Chrysosporium **spp.** *(continued)*

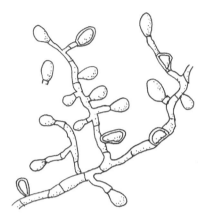
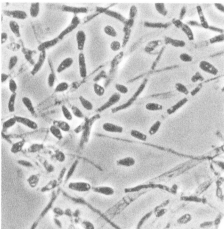

Courtesy of Lynn Sigler.

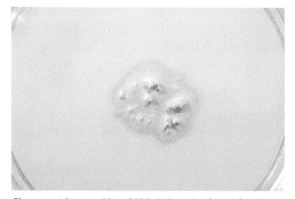

Chrysosporium sp. PDA, 30°C, 6 days. Surface of colony.

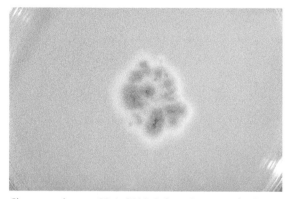

Chrysosporium sp. PDA, 30°C, 6 days. Reverse of colony.

TABLE 2.25 Differential characteristics of *Chrysosporium* versus *Sporotrichum*[a]

Organism	Colony	Media with cycloheximide[b]	Alternating arthroconidia	Urease[c]	Temp tolerance	Large[d] chlamydospores at 37°C
Chrysosporium (p. 371)	Usually discrete; may spread to cover entire plate	Growth	Remain in chains; may be rare or absent	+	Grows slowly or not at all at 37°C	0
Sporotrichum (p. 374)	Spreads, rapidly covers entire plate	No growth	Usually abundant; often break from hyphae and form clusters	0	Grows well at 37–40°C; some grow at 45°C	+

[a] Abbreviations: +, positive; 0, negative.

[b] Cycloheximide at 0.04%, as in Mycosel agar.

[c] Christensen's urea with 10 days of incubation.

[d] Chlamydospores up to 60 μm in diameter when isolate is subcultured.

Sporotrichum pruinosum

PATHOGENICITY: Commonly considered a contaminant. Has been found in sputa from patients with chronic respiratory disorders, but its significance is unclear.

RATE OF GROWTH: Rapid; mature within 5 days. Thermotolerant, grows well at 40°C; many strains can grow at 45°C. It is inhibited by cycloheximide.

COLONY MORPHOLOGY: Spreads rapidly to cover entire surface of plate. Colony is initially cottony, then powdery; at first white, may become cream, yellowish, tan, pinkish, or slightly orange. Reverse is white or light tan.

MICROSCOPIC MORPHOLOGY: Hyphae are broad, lightly pigmented, and septate with bridges known as clamp connections at the septa. Conidiophores form at acute angles to the hyphae and then branch at acute angles; each branch ends with a conidium, giving a tree- or candelabrum-like appearance. The conidia are single celled, ovoid (3–6 × 5–10 μm), typically somewhat pointed at the apex and abruptly flattened at the base. The conidia often retain a portion of attached conidiophore after separation. The conidial walls are fairly thick and are usually smooth. Alternating arthroconidia are often abundant; they may be cylindrical or barrel shaped.

Large (up to 65 μm in diameter), round to oval, thick-walled chlamydospores form when incubated at 37°C, and may also develop at 25°C.

To distinguish *Sporotrichum* from *Chrysosporium*, see Table 2.25 (p. 373).

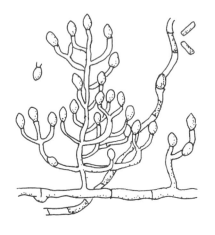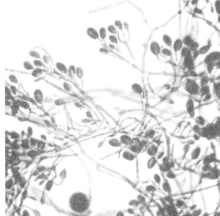

Sporotrichum pruinosum *(continued)*

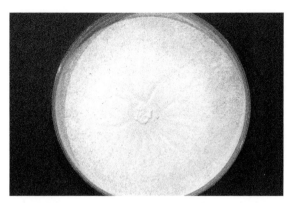

Sporotrichum pruinosum. SDA, 30°C, 6 days. Colony spreads to cover entire agar surface.

For further information, see
Chowdhary, 2014a

Sepedonium spp.

PATHOGENICITY: Commonly considered a contaminant; not known to cause disease.

RATE OF GROWTH: Moderate; mature within 6–10 days.

COLONY MORPHOLOGY: At 25–30°C, colonies are at first white and waxy, then become fluffy, and with age often turn yellow. At 37°C, there is little or no growth. Reverse is white.

MICROSCOPIC MORPHOLOGY: Hyphae are septate with simple or branched conidiophores. Conidia are large (7–17 μm), round, thick walled, and usually rough and knobby. Differs from *Histoplasma capsulatum* (p. 172) in not forming microconidia, not converting to a yeast at 35–37°C.

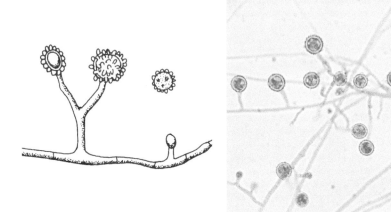

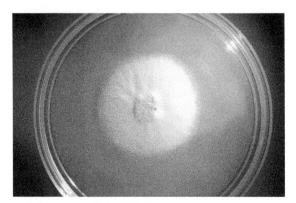

Sepedonium sp. SDA, 30°C, 6 days.

Chrysonilia sitophila

TAXONOMY NOTES: This species was formerly known as *Monilia sitophila*. The teleomorph of *C. sitophila* is *Neurospora sitophila*.

PATHOGENICITY: Commonly considered a contaminant; has rarely been involved in peritonitis, eye infections, and occupational asthma.

RATE OF GROWTH: Rapid; mature within 5 days.

COLONY MORPHOLOGY: White at first and then salmon colored. Thin, floccose mycelium rapidly spreads over surface of agar.

MICROSCOPIC MORPHOLOGY: Hyphae are septate; simple conidiophores produce branching chains of oval conidia (5–10 × 10–15 µm). The conidia are arthroconidia and are connected by narrow disjunctors. The older hyphae break up, forming thick-walled rectangular arthroconidia.

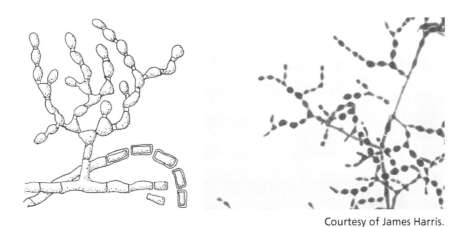

Courtesy of James Harris.

Schizophyllum commune

PATHOGENICITY: An environmental basidiomycetous fungus (shelf fungus), and a common invader of rotten wood. Human infections are rare, although it is probably the most common filamentous basidiomycete associated with human disease. Allergic bronchopulmonary mycosis and sinusitis represent the majority of cases. It can also cause invasive disease, especially in the setting of immunosuppression, with the lungs the most frequently involved organ. Skin, heart, eye, and brain infections have also been described.

RATE OF GROWTH: Rapid; mature within 5 days. Grows well at 25, 37, and 42°C. No growth on cycloheximide-containing media.

COLONY MORPHOLOGY: Surface is densely woolly, white to pale brown. Surface of monokaryotic isolates (characterized by a single nucleus in each cell) are flat and thinly cottony. Dikaryotic isolates (characterized by two nuclei in each cell) can produce characteristic macroscopic tube- or fan-shaped fruiting bodies (basidiocarps) when grown on some media (e.g., potato dextrose agar and Czapek agar) at 25°C. Fruiting bodies have split gills on the lower side and may take several weeks to develop; often requiring alternating light and dark conditions. Monokaryotic isolates do not form fruiting bodies. Reverse is pale brown. It produces a strong, unpleasant odor.

MICROSCOPIC MORPHOLOGY: Hyaline septate hyphae have varying widths (1.5–5 μm). Hyphae of dikaryotic isolates often have clamp connections and protruding lateral pegs (spicules). Conidia are absent. Monokaryotic isolates do not have clamp connections and spicules may be absent. White, rapidly growing sterile isolates that grow well at 37°C, are inhibited by cycloheximide, and produce a disagreeable odor should be suspected as *S. commune*.

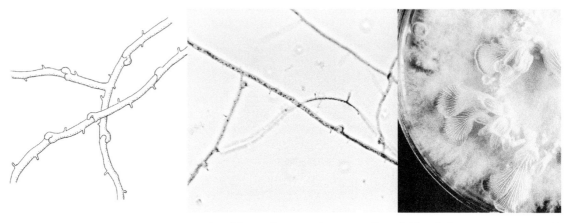

For further information, see
Cavanna et al, 2019
Chowdhary et al., 2014a
Rihs et al., 1996
Sigler et al., 1995
Sigler et al., 1999

Reprinted from Rihs JD et al. 1996. *J Clin Microbiol* 34:1628–1632.

Schizophyllum commune. Czapek agar, 25°C, 14 days. Surface of colony showing fruiting bodies.

PART III

Basics of Molecular Methods for Fungal Identification

Larone's Medically Important Fungi: A Guide to Identification, 7th Edition.
Lars F. Westblade, Eileen M. Burd, Shawn R. Lockhart, and Gary W. Procop.
© 2023 American Society for Microbiology. DOI: 10.1128/9781683674436.piii

Introduction

Phenotypic methods relying on colony morphology, microscopic observation, and in some instances biochemical reactions, remain the mainstay of fungal identification. However, molecular methods are increasingly being used for the detection and/ or differentiation of medically important fungi (Persing et al., 2016; Zhang et al., 2021). Molecular methods offer distinct advantages in their ability to

- Identify a mould that is not producing microscopic reproductive structures (conidia or spores) or produces only structures that are noncontributory to routine morphologic identification (e.g., chlamydoconidia); or identify a yeast or mould that is not represented in the database of the commercial identification system used in the laboratory.

- Accomplish the above point in a relatively rapid and objective manner as compared to the time and expertise often required for conventional identification, especially when the isolate does not grow rapidly and/or does not have familiar classic morphology.

- Definitively identify an organism whose characteristics closely resemble those of other fungi.

- Identify an organism directly in a clinical specimen that is seen on microscopic examination but does not grow in culture.

- Evaluate the similarities and differences between organisms for taxonomic classification and corrections in nomenclature.

- Determine the precise genotype of an isolate, an important factor in epidemiologic analyses.

The present downside of molecular identification of fungi includes (i) the lack of methods standardization, (ii) the lack of definitive information as to clinical relevance and anticipated antifungal response of organisms that have no history in the medical literature, and (iii) erroneous or incomplete data in reference databases.

Fungal Targets

The success of molecular identification of a fungal isolate depends on the choice of a reliable target sequence or gene. While the choice is commonly guided by the presumptive identification of the isolate, the technique being employed, and the level to which identification is being sought, optimal molecular targets possess several general characteristics.

- Present in multiple copies, in order to provide good PCR sensitivity
- Relatively conserved, to ensure amplification from a broad range of fungi when utilizing panfungal primers; following amplification, variable regions within the amplicon are desirable for species- and genus-specific identification
- An optimum size (~500 to 800 bp), short enough to be sequenced with ease in automated sequencers but long enough to provide adequate information for identification
- Presence of its sequence information in databases, for reliable comparison and accurate interpretation of results

The most successful molecular target that has been consistently used for molecular identification of fungi is the ribosomal DNA (rDNA) complex; it is a multicopy collection of genes that codes for ribosomal RNA. In eukaryotes, this gene complex comprises the 18S (small-subunit rDNA), a 5.8S subunit, and the 28S (large-subunit rDNA) genes. Interspaced between these three gene segments, and separating them from one another, are regions that have historically been called "spacers." Internal transcribed spacer 1 (ITS1) is the region between the 18S and 5.8S genes, and ITS2 is the region between the 5.8S and the 28S genes (Fig. 3.1).

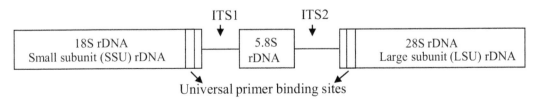

FIGURE 3.1 Ribosomal DNA (rDNA) gene complex.

The ITS1 and ITS2 regions are relatively variable among species, making them good targets for species identification (Schoch et al., 2012). The other regions of the rDNA are more conserved across the different species of a genus while being variable among genera; therefore, they are targeted for genus-level identification. In 2012, the International Fungal Barcoding Consortium formally recommended that the ITS regions be used as the primary targets for fungal identification since they show greater variation and have better discriminatory power than other regions. The entire ITS region is about 600 base pairs long. Universal primers for the majority of fungi have been designed to amplify the ITS1, ITS2, or the entire ITS region (Table 3.1). In some genera, such as *Aspergillus*, *Cladosporium*, *Fusarium*, *Penicillium*, and *Trichoderma*, the heterogeneity of the ITS1 and −2 regions between species is not sufficient to provide adequate species identification (Rath and Steinmann, 2018). In these instances, ITS can only provide an identification to species complex level. Often this is adequate but if discrimination to species level is clinically important for these closely related species, additional marker(s) are needed. Other markers may be needed in cases in which the ITS primers are unable to amplify the fungal isolate or if ITS sequences cannot be obtained due to intra-strain variability among the multiple copies of the ITS within the ribosomal RNA gene cluster (this can be overcome by analyzing longer amplicon fragments using next-generation sequencing technologies). Other molecular targets commonly used for fungal identification include β-tubulin, calmodulin, D1/D2 region of 28S rRNA, and elongation factor (Table 3.1). One strategy in which portions of multiple genes are sequenced (multilocus sequencing) is sometimes used but it is expensive and requires phylogenetic expertise for interpretation (Table 3.2).

TABLE 3.1 Frequently used fungal molecular targets and primers for sequence-based species identification

Molecular target	Acronym	Fungal genera identified	Primer	Primer sequence 5'–3' Forward Reverse	Approximate product size (base pairs)	Optimal annealing temperature °C	Reference
Internal tran-scribed spacer	ITS	All fungi	ITS-1 ITS-4	TCC GTA GGT GAA CCT GCG G TCC TCC GCT TAT TGA TAT GC	600	52	White et al., 1990
Large ribosomal subunit (28S)	D1/D2	All yeasts; many of the Mucorales	NL-1 NL-4	GCA TAT CAA TAA GCG GAG GA TTG GTC CGT GTT TCA AGA CG	620	52	Kurtzman and Robnett, 1991
β-tubulin	TUB	Penicillium	Bt2a Bt2b	GGT AAC CAA ATC GGT GCT GCT TTC ACC CTC AGT GTA GTG ACC CTT GGC	495–550	54	Glass and Donaldson, 1995
Intergenic spacer	IGS	Trichosporon	26SF 5SR	ATC CTT TGC AGA CGA CTT GA AGC TTG ACT TCG CAG ATC GG	200–700 depending on species	56	Sugita et al., 2002
Modified internal transcribed spacer	Modified ITS	Dermatophytes	LR1 SR6R	GGT TGG TTT CTT TTC CT AAG TAA AAG TCG TAA CAA GG	630	52	Gräser et al., 2000
Calmodulin	CAL	Alternaria	CALDF1 CALDR1	ACG AAG TCT CCG AGT TCA AGG	566–763	58.5	Lawrence et al., 2013
		Aspergillus	CMD5 CMD6	CTT CTG CAT CAT CAY CTG GAC G CCG AGT ACA AGG AGG CCT TC CCG ATA GAG GTC ATA ACG TGG	580	55	Alshehri and Palanisamy, 2020
Chitin synthase	CHS	Sporothrix	CHS-79F CHS-354R	TGG GGC AAG GAT GCT TGG AAG AAG TGG AAG AAC CAT CTG TGA GAG TTG	300	58	Rodrigues et al., 2015

TABLE 3.2 Examples of fungal molecular targets and primers for multilocus sequence-based species identification

Fungal genera amplified	Molecular targets	Acronym	Primers	Reference
Fusarium	Elongation factor 1α and RNA polymerase II subunit	*EF-1α* *RPB2*	EF1-F EF2-R 5F2-F 7cr-R	O'Donnell et al., 2007
Cladosporium	Internal transcribed spacer; translation elongation factor 1α, and the actin gene	ITS, *EF-1α*, and *ACT*	ITS5-F ITS4-R EF-728-F EF-986-R ACT-512F ACT-783R	Sandoval-Denis et al., 2015
Curvularia	Internal transcribed spacer and glycerol-3-phosphate dehydrogenase	ITS *GPDH*	ITS1-F ITS4-R gpd1-F gpd2-R	Manamgoda et al., 2012

Classic Molecular Identification Methods

Polymerase Chain Reaction

A considerable number of laboratory-developed real-time or endpoint PCR techniques have been developed for the identification of fungi and are reported in peer-reviewed literature. These methods are generally based on amplification with either broad-range or specific primers and hybridization with species-specific probes with or without high-resolution melting curve analysis. These approaches are not further described here because they are not standardized and are used only by a few clinical laboratories.

Multiplex real-time PCR assays designed to detect Mucorales and/or *Aspergillus* spp. directly in clinical specimens are commercially available in Europe but there are no FDA-approved tests available in the United States. The commercially available tests include PN-700 MucorGenius and AsperGenius (PathoNostics, Maastricht, The Netherlands), MycoGENIE *Aspergillus* species–Mucorales species (Ademtech, Pessac, France), MycAssay Aspergillus (Myconostica Ltd., Cambridge, UK), Myco-Real Aspergillus (Ingenetix GmbH, Vienna, Austria), RenDX Fungiplex (Renishaw Diagnostics Ltd., Glasgow, UK), MycoGENIE *Aspergillus* spp. (Ademtech, Pessac, France), LightCycler SeptiFast (Roche Molecular Diagnostics, Penzberg, Germany), GeneProof Aspergillus PCR (GeneProof, Brno, Czechia), Aspergillus spp ELITe MGB Kit (ELITechGroup, Puteaux, France), Aspergillus Real-time PCR Panel (Eurofins Viracor, Lenexa, KS), A. fumigatus Bio-Evolution (Bio-Evolution, Bry-sur-Marne, France), and Fungiplex Aspergillus (Bruker Daltonik GmbH, Bremen, Germany).

Several reference laboratories in the United States, including Eurofins Viracor, ARUP, and the University of Washington Department of Laboratory Medicine, offer PCR panels to detect *Aspergillus* in clinical specimens (Rath and Steinmann, 2018). The utility of molecular tests for the diagnosis of invasive aspergillosis and mucormycosis has not been fully defined and it is recommended that they be used in conjunction with other tests such as culture, galactomannan, β-D-glucan, histological examination of biopsy specimens, radiographic imaging, and clinical assessment of risk factors for assessment of prior probability of invasive fungal disease.

Non-Sequencing-Based Identification Methods

There are a wide variety of molecular methods that have been used for the detection and/or differentiation of medically important fungi. Matrix-assisted laser desorption ionization–time of flight mass spectrometry (MALDI-TOF MS) is a protein-based method that has revolutionized the identification of microorganisms in clinical microbiology, including fungi (Bizzini and Greub, 2010). Non-sequencing nucleic acid-based methods may be separated into signal amplification methods and nucleic acid amplification methods.

MALDI-TOF Mass Spectrometry

MALDI-TOF MS is unique among the methods covered in this section in that it assesses the protein composition of an organism, rather than the nucleic acids. It does not depend on analysis of genetic information for identification of an isolate but is instead based on analysis of a spectrum of organic biomolecules present in the isolate. In brief, the proteins from a small amount of a fungal isolate are extracted from the isolate and spotted onto a metal plate. The sample is overlaid with a defined organic matrix that stabilizes the molecules and, when dried, crystallizes the molecules in the isolate. The plate is then inserted into an instrument for mass spectrometry. The sample-matrix mixture is subjected to a pulsed laser beam of appropriate frequency that causes the sample-matrix to be partially ionized and vaporized, carrying intact biomolecules from the isolate into the vapor phase. The vaporized molecules are passed through a vacuum drift tube, where high voltage is applied to accelerate the charged particles toward a detector; the smaller ions reach the detector in a shorter amount of time than do the larger ions. The time required for the charged ions to reach the detector is the "time of flight," or TOF portion of the assay, which varies according to the mass-to-charge ratio of the individual molecules. The TOFs exhibited by the time-of-flight pattern from the various molecules are recorded and yield a unique mass spectrum (pattern) that is compared to a well-developed database for isolate identification.

There are presently two FDA-approved, commercial MALDI-TOF MS systems available in the United States: the Vitek MS (bioMérieux, Inc., Durham, NC) and the MALDI Biotyper CA (Bruker Daltonics, Billerica, MA). Although the initial capital investment in the instrumentation for these systems is moderately high, the return on investment is favorable, as the subsequent cost of materials is very low. The reagent cost is only a few cents for each organism identification and the time-to-identification is measured in minutes (~11 min if just one isolate is tested; 2.5 min per isolate if a batch of 96 isolates is run, with the average time per isolate in published reports being 4 to 6 min). MALDI-TOF MS identification has become the standard of practice in many laboratories for the identification of medically important yeasts (Bader et al., 2011; Buchan and Ledeboer, 2013; Walsh and McCarthy, 2019; Stevenson et al., 2010) and moulds (Hettick et al., 2008; Sanguinetti and Posteraro, 2017), largely replacing assimilation assays and microscopic morphology.

Signal Amplification Methods

The earliest commercially available molecular methods used in the clinical microbiology laboratory were signal amplification probes. These probes, which are being discontinued, were used on cultured fungi suspected to represent *Blastomyces dermatitidis*, *Coccidioides immitis*, or *Histoplasma capsulatum*. Additional signal amplification methods have been developed to rapidly identify fungi in positive blood cultures. These have included peptide nucleic acid fluorescent *in situ* hybridization (PNA FISH) methods, as well as microarray hybridization (Farina et al., 2012; Miller and Tang, 2009).

PNA FISH

A PNA FISH probe is a synthetic molecule that closely resembles DNA. PNA and DNA differ mainly in their structural backbones. The backbone of a DNA probe is composed of negatively charged alternating sugar phosphate moieties; when used in a FISH assay, these must overcome a natural destabilizing electrostatic repulsion associated with cellular penetration in order to hybridize with a complementary nucleic acid target. The backbone of a PNA probe is noncharged polyamides (peptides), affording superior penetration through cell walls and membranes. Additionally, PNA molecules are resistant to degradation by enzymes that can affect DNA probes.

FDA-approved PNA FISH kits, originally developed by AdvanDx (Woburn, MA) have been acquired by OpGen (Rockville, MD). These have been used for the direct identification of the most commonly encountered *Candida* spp. on preparations from blood cultures that contain yeasts (Radic et al., 2016; Rigby et al., 2002). rRNA abundantly produced by the growing yeast cells serves as a species-specific target for the PNA FISH probes. A variety of fluorescent-labeled individual probes and combination probes have been developed (Radic et al., 2016; Rigby et al., 2002).

Nucleic Acid Amplification Methods

T2 Magnetic Resonance

The T2 system (T2 Biosystems, Lexington, MA) is a self-contained, automated, sample-to-answer molecular detection system designed for direct detection of infectious pathogens from clinical samples without the requirement for culture

(Mylonakis et al., 2015). The T2Candida Panel is an FDA-cleared and CE-marked assay for the direct detection and identification of five common *Candida* species from peripheral whole-blood specimens. A specimen collection tube is loaded directly on the instrument with sequential automated steps of lysis to release pathogen nucleic acid, followed by PCR. Amplified products are then hybridized to their specific nucleic acid probes, which are tagged with paramagnetic particles. The detection of the amplified organisms occurs due to a change in the arrangement of these paramagnetic particles that provides a specific magnetic resonance signature. Positive results are reported as one of three categories that include five *Candida* species. The three result categories are based on Infectious Diseases Society of America guidelines for treatment of *Candida* bloodstream infection: *C. albicans* or *C. tropicalis* (A/T); *C. krusei* or *C. glabrata* (K/G); and *C. parapsilosis* (P). Hands-on processing time for the specimen is ~5 min, and a result is provided within ~4 h, with a reported analytic sensitivity of 1 CFU/ml. Clinical trials showed sensitivity and specificity compared to culture-based methods of ~91 and 99%. Subsequent work has suggested that in at least some populations, sensitivity may exceed that of culture.

Broad-Panel Molecular Testing and Other Emerging Sample-to-Answer Technologies

Technical advances in microfluidics and assay design have allowed the production of integrated systems that combine sample preparation (i.e., cellular lysis and nucleic acid extraction), amplification, and analysis. These so-called "sample-to-answer" platforms have vastly simplified molecular testing and may be categorized as moderate- or even low-complexity. The development of multianalyte panels affords the detection of 10–20 pathogens that cause a particular disease (e.g., meningitis). This has been referred to as syndromic testing. Although many of the targets are bacteria and viruses, some fungi and parasites are included when clinically relevant. The BioFire Blood Culture Identification 2 (BCID2) Panel (bioMérieux, Inc., Salt Lake City, UT) provides detection and identification of six *Candida* spp. (including *Candida auris*) and *Cryptococcus* (*C. neoformans*/ *C. gattii*) (Peri et al., 2022), and *C. neoformans*/*C. gattii* is included in the BioFire Meningitis/Encephalitis panel (Leber et al., 2016). Unfortunately, the *Cryptococcus* portion of the BioFire Meningitis/Encephalitis panel has not been without challenges (Liesman et al., 2018). The ePlex BCID-FP Panel, originally developed by GenMark Diagnostics (Carlsbad, CA) but acquired by Roche (Indianapolis, IN) is another option for the rapid identification of fungi in positive blood cultures. This product detects 11 *Candida* spp. (including *C. auris),* *C. neoformans, C. gattii, Fusarium,* and *Rhodotorula* (Bryant et al., 2020).

Numerous other products are in the pipeline and promise increased options for the rapid diagnosis of fungal infections. An automated FISH-based assay for the detection and identification and rapid phenotypic susceptibility testing of several common bacteria, together with detection and identification of two common *Candida* spp. (Accelerate Diagnostics, Tucson, AZ) is also available (Pancholi et al., 2018). It can be anticipated that the number of such products available will continue to increase, with detection of an increasing variety of fungal pathogens.

Sequencing-Based Identification Methods

Sanger Sequencing

There exists within microorganism groups conserved genetic sequences that flank variable DNA sequences, the latter of which contains taxonomically important information. When PCR primers are designed to hybridize with the conserved genetic sequences within a group, then a "broad-range" PCR has been produced. This PCR would be expected to amplify a portion of DNA from all of the organisms within the group to which it was designed (e.g., fungi). Typical targets for broad-range fungal PCR are conserved regions within the large ribosomal subunit gene and the ITS regions. Broad-range PCR is the first step in sequence-based identification of microorganisms. After nucleic acid amplification has been achieved, the intervening taxonomically important genetic information may be interrogated using DNA sequencing. Sanger sequencing, which is briefly described below, is the most common DNA sequencing method used in clinical laboratories today.

Sanger sequencing has also been termed "chain termination sequencing" or "cycle sequencing," and is a first-generation sequencing technology. In brief, this method uses an amplified nucleic acid substrate, which in this example is the end-product of a broad-range PCR. The nucleotide sequence of the target substrate DNA is determined by synthesizing a complementary strand of the DNA using DNA polymerase in a manner similar to PCR, but with some important differences. Unlike PCR, the forward and reverse primers are applied in separate reactions, so that only one strand is generated with each cycle. Another important difference is that unlike PCR, two chemically distinct sets of nucleotides are used. The commonly used deoxynucleotide triphosphates (dNTPs), which add bases to the elongating strand of DNA, are accompanied by one of four dideoxynucleotide triphosphates (ddNTPs), which when incorporated terminate chain elongation. Traditionally, Sanger sequencing is performed in eight separate sequencing reactions (Table 3.3), but may now be performed in fewer reactions using different reporter dyes. Each of the four types of ddNTP (ddATP, ddCTP, ddGTP, or ddTTP) is labeled with a different dye or reporter molecule. As the reaction proceeds, DNA synthesis is terminated randomly each

TABLE 3.3 Lane construction for traditional bidirectional Sanger sequencing[a]

	Forward primer	Reverse primer	ddATP	ddTTP	ddCTP	ddGTP
Lane 1	+	0	+	0	0	0
Lane 2	0	+	+	0	0	0
Lane 3	+	0	0	+	0	0
Lane 4	0	+	0	+	0	0
Lane 5	+	0	0	0	+	0
Lane 6	0	+	0	0	+	0
Lane 7	+	0	0	0	0	+
Lane 8	0	+	0	0	0	+

[a] Lanes 1 and 2 determine the position of every adenosine (A) nucleotide in the target DNA substrate, and so forth for the remaining nucleotides. This is done in a bidirectional manner (i.e., Lane 1 using the forward primer; Lane 2 using the reverse primer). Bidirectional sequencing helps to determine the accuracy of each nucleotide assignment in the DNA sequence determined. +, present; 0, absent.

time a ddNTP is incorporated. As each different ddNTP is labeled with a different-color dye, all terminated fragments contain a dye at their elongating end. Following a sufficient amount of time to allow for optimal generation of extended products, which are essentially DNA chains terminated at different lengths, the products are analyzed by capillary electrophoresis-based automated analyzers. The results are displayed as colored peaks (a sequencing chromatogram) indicating each differently colored ddNTP addition to the new complementary strand. Examination and analysis of the color and height of the peaks yield the nucleotide sequence of the target DNA.

One of the limitations of broad-range PCR and Sanger sequencing for the identification of microorganisms in primary specimens is that if more than one organism from the same group is present, identification may not be achieved. This is because DNA from both organisms (e.g., *C. albicans* and *C. neoformans*) will be amplified, and although the sequencing reaction was carried to completion, the resulting sequence consisting of a mix of the two originating sequences cannot be resolved or separated by this technology. Next-generation sequencing (see the following section) is able to resolve this problem.

For an extensively illustrated description of the basic and modified Sanger sequencing method, see: https://youtu.be/FvHRio1yyhQ

Massive Parallel or Next-Generation Sequencing

Massive parallel sequencing, also commonly referred to as deep sequencing or next-generation sequencing (NGS) (Goodwin et al., 2016; Slatko et al., 2018), is a DNA sequencing technology similar in principle to Sanger sequencing in that it provides DNA sequence information by synthesis of the target DNA. There are a variety of NGS applications, but for the purposes of this section we will concentrate on PCR-targeted NGS and metagenomic (i.e., "shotgun" or hypothesis-free) testing. PCR-targeted NGS is similar to multiplex PCR, except in this instance the various PCR products that can be generated by the multiplexed PCR reactions are resolved (i.e., sorted out) by NGS, rather than using detector probes or microarrays. This type of application affords the design of multiplex panels for syndromic testing, as described previously. In this approach, the assay contains primer sets for the pathogens of interest that cause a particular disease (e.g., bloodstream infections). Another application may be to include primer sets that detect a particular organism, as well as antimicrobial resistance genes and/or virulence factors of that organism.

Metagenomic applications open an entirely new field in medical diagnostics. In brief, everything in the clinical specimen is sequenced (i.e., human, microbial, and any other DNA present). For microbial detection, human sequences are bioinformatically subtracted from the dataset leaving non-human sequences for further analysis. This has been referred to as "hypothesis-free" testing since one does not have to consider the most likely causes of disease and test for them. Rather, one considers the microbial-associated sequences present and works to determine if any of these may explain the condition of the patient. Although a powerful new tool, contaminating microbes and normal microbiota will be detected by this method, so there is a possibility of overinterpretation of these as pathogens. For an illustrated description of the technologies in use, see: https://www.ebi.ac.uk/training/online/courses/functional-genomics-ii-common-technologies-and-data-analysis-methods/next-generation-sequencing/.

NGS of plasma microbial cell-free DNA (i.e., DNA liberated by microbial cells released into the bloodstream) to diagnose fungal infections has been described (Hoenigl et al., 2023). This testing should not be performed in the absence of culture, although it may offer an attractive option for patients that cannot tolerate invasive procedures to acquire specimens for culture, and its role in ruling out infection remains undefined. Ultimately, more studies are required to understand the broader clinical applications of plasma microbial cell-free DNA NGS for diagnosing invasive fungal infections, including bloodstream and anatomically remote (e.g., pulmonary) infections. NGS use is well established for outbreak investigation, such as the multistate *C. auris* outbreak (Vallabhaneni et al., 2016). An extensive critical review of the existing technologies and their advantages can be found in Goodwin et al. (2016).

Applications of DNA Sequencing

The following describes the common uses for nucleotide sequence information of an isolate.

Accurate Molecular Identification

In many circumstances, sequencing has proved to be more precise than phenotypic methods (Hibbett et al., 2016; Lücking et al., 2021). This is largely because there are many fungi within a complex that are morphologically identical, but represent genotypically distinct species. There are other instances wherein unrelated fungi are morphologically similar and may be mistaken for one another. Sequence-based identification has also been used as an alternative method for identifying commonly encountered fungi (Normand et al., 2018). DNA sequencing methods, like any other assay used in the clinical laboratory, must undergo a thorough validation prior to use (Pont-Kingdon et al., 2012).

The DNA substrate, usually obtained from a broad-range PCR targeting a taxonomically important gene (e.g., ITS region), is submitted for DNA sequencing. This sequence information, obtained from the patient's isolate, is then compared with curated sequences in a reputable database of known, confirmed fungal nucleotide sequences. This method is known as comparative sequence analysis. It is the most widely used method and currently considered the gold standard for molecular identification of fungi, and most other microorganisms. There are several databases that contain libraries of defined sequences from around the world. Some databases are curated (i.e., all sequences have been confirmed with reliable isolates and maintenance of entries is ongoing), whereas other databases accept submissions without further examination/confirmation. Beware of the latter as when a misidentified fungus is added to a non-curated database, future sequence-based misidentifications are sure to occur. Some databases may be freely accessed, whereas others charge a usage fee, which is understandable given the effort necessary for high-quality curation. A list of commonly used databases is provided in Table 3.4.

Comparison of the sequence of the test isolate to the library sequences in the database is performed by a software analysis tool known as BLAST (Basic Local Alignment Search Tool); it is a feature of all sequence databases. In BLAST search,

TABLE 3.4 Commonly used databases for identification of medically important fungi

Database	URL	Fungal genome region(s) represented
GenBank (NCBI Blast)	http://www.ncbi.nlm.nih.gov https://blast.ncbi.nlm.nih.gov/Blast.cgi	All
European Nucleotide Archive (ENA)	https://www.ebi.ac.uk/ena/browser/home	ITS
DNA Data Bank of Japan	http://www.ddbj.nig.ac.jp/	ITS
Barcode of Life Database (BOLD)	http://www.boldsystems.org/index.php/IDS_OpenIdEngine	ITS
Westerdijk Fungal Biodiversity Institute (formerly CBS-KNAW Fungal Biodiversity Centre or Centraalbureau voor Schimmelcultures)	https://wi.knaw.nl/	ITS, some β-tubulin
User-friendly Nordic ITS Ectomycorrhiza Database (UNITE)	https://unite.ut.ee/	ITS
FUSARIOID-ID	https://www.fusarium.org	ITS, D1/D2, *ACT*, *CAL*, histone H3, *RPB1*, *RPB2*, *TEF1*, *TUB2*
Fusarium-MLST	https://fusarium.mycobank.org	*TEF1*, *RPB1*, *RPB2*, *CAL*, β-tubulin, histone H3, IGS, ITS, 28S, and mitochondrial small subunit
Fungal MLST database Q-Bank	http://www.q-bank.eu/Fungi/	Partial actin, *TUB2*, *RPB1*, *RPB2*, *TEF1*, and others
The International Society for Human and Animal Mycology (ISHAM) Database	http://its.mycologylab.org	ITS
Naïve Bayesian Classifier	http://rdp.cme.msu.edu/classifier/classifier.jsp	28S, ITS

the sequence of the patient's isolate, or "query sequence," is run against the reference database to generate a list of matches, or "hits." A rank-ordered list of sequences, from the most similar to the least similar, is generated and displayed along with the percent similarity scores. A diagram of a pairwise alignment of the query sequence with each match is also provided. A score of ≥99% indicates that the query sequence is essentially the same as the sequence of the "hit." The lower limit of the score required for species-level identification of fungal isolates is not strictly defined, but it is generally agreed that <97% is too low for a match. It is also recognized that no single cutoff score can resolve species variability in certain fungal genera. Not surprisingly, the choice of the genetic target is important for highly precise discrimination. Although the commonly used ITS region may accurately define the genus of a fungus, there are many instances wherein the sequencing of an alternate gene is necessary for the ultimate identification of the species, should that degree of differentiation be necessary (Table 3.2).

Obviously, sequence-based identification relies on the number, accuracy, and general quality of the sequences being utilized; depending on the level of quality control, these attributes vary between databases. Errors in fungal sequences available at one of the most popular databases, GenBank (which is not curated), are known to be as high as 14 to 20%.

Laboratories that use sequencing for identification are responsible for validating the entire process, which includes sample preparation, generation of sequence data, and analysis and interpretation of sequencing results. Protocols for validation of laboratory-developed sequencing assays may vary between laboratories. General guidance for validation and ongoing quality monitoring is available from several resources including the Clinical and Laboratory Standards Institute (CLSI) and the Association for Molecular Pathology (AMP) (Clinical and Laboratory Standards Institute MM09, 2014; Association for Molecular Pathology, 2014).

A commercial system that uses comparative sequence analysis, the MicroSeq D2 rDNA Fungal Identification Kit (Applied Biosystems, Foster City, CA), provides a protocol, reagents required for amplification and sequence determination, and a curated database for identification of fungi (>1,000 species) covered by the system. Smartgene (Raleigh, NC) is an example of a commercially available, curated database.

Phylogenetic Analysis

The evolutionary relationships between organisms can be ascertained through the comparison of DNA sequences (Gregory, 2008; Hall, 2007; Sleator, 2011). Through molecular characterization of fungal isolates, it has become evident that even some morphologically indistinguishable fungi may be considered separate species, and in some instances may be placed into different clades. The former are commonly referred to as species complexes, since they are morphologically identical and cause similar diseases.

There are numerous computer programs available for phylogenetic analysis; a list can be found at http://evolution.genetics.washington.edu/phylip.html. The programs are based on statistical principles that evaluate the differences in the nucleotide sequences among the isolates being characterized and calculate the probability of the isolates being related to one another from a common ancestor. A phylogenetic or evolutionary tree, usually in the form of a cladogram or a phylogram, is generated to graphically demonstrate the percent of genetic similarity and the probability of the isolates being related. Although there are a variety of ways to depict a phylogenetic tree (Hall, 2007), common representations show a tree with isolates on branches that diverge, and the distance between the branched lines provides an estimate of the relative separation from their common ancestor (see Fig. 3.2 for a simplified sample tree). A sequence similarity of 99–100% clusters isolates on the same branch, essentially indicating that they belong to the same species; strains on very close branches may also be included in that species. A lower level of similarity places an isolate on a more distant branch, often resulting in the designation of a new species name or even transfer to a different genus. This is the major basis of the nomenclature and taxonomy changes seen throughout the recent mycology literature.

The molecular identification of members of species complexes is important for a number of reasons. Foremost, from a pure biological perspective it is important to understand the true nature of an organism and its appropriate classification.

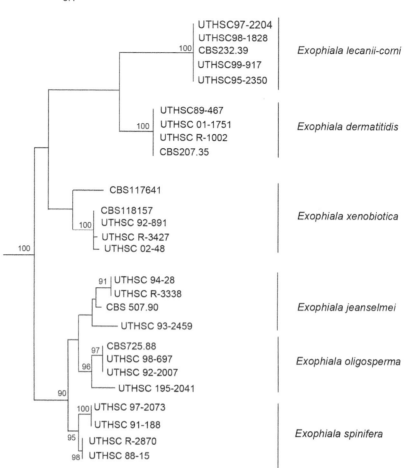

FIGURE 3.2 Sample phylogenetic tree of select *Exophiala* spp. Strain designations are shown at the end of each branch. (Condensed and adapted from Zeng et al., 2007.) To comprehend the evolutionary branching of the isolates, the tree should be viewed from the left to the right. Each bifurcation (branching) of the tree indicates likely evolutionary divergence. The number (known as the bootstrap value) at the point of bifurcation is a percentage based on numerous repeat sequence analyses and indicates the mathematical strength of the grouping; bootstrap values of >90 are shown at the branches. As the tree branches to the right, more closely related isolates ultimately cluster on the same or neighboring branches and are designated in the phylogram as one species. Nucleotide changes that exist are expressed as distance and are shown by the scale bar.

From a more practical perspective, it is important to understand if all members of a species complex cause the same type of disease (i.e., the pathophysiology of infection) and if these fungi have similar antifungal susceptibility patterns. For example, there are slightly different epidemiological cutoff values (ECVs) for members of the *C. parapsilosis* species complex; whether these are clinically meaningful enough to demand species-level differentiation remains to be determined (Clinical and Laboratory Standards Institute M57S, 2022; Lockhart et al., 2017).

Organism Typing

The same type of sequence information that is used for phylogenetic analysis can be used to type individual isolates that are involved in an outbreak or are repeatedly recovered from the same patient (Litvintseva et al., 2015). Typing of isolates has traditionally been performed by pulsed-field gel electrophoresis, but is now more commonly performed by DNA sequencing-based applications, such as multilocus sequence typing (MLST). MLST compares the nucleotide sequences of multiple points (loci) within housekeeping genes of the isolates. The combination of variations in the sequences of these loci within a species characterizes and classifies the isolates into separate subtypes. Isolates are characterized as distinguishable or indistinguishable, with the latter implying that the isolates may be the same strain (i.e., from the same parent).

Detection of Genetic Determinants of Resistance

There has been a significant expansion of information concerning the genetic alterations that are associated with the resistant phenotypes of medically important fungi. An understanding of these has served to explain intrinsic and acquired resistance that is seen in certain fungi. How these markers will be used in clinical medicine remains to be determined. However, one can envision the use of rapid molecular methods to detect genetic alterations that are responsible for acquired resistance in isolates from patients with serious fungal infections. Additionally, the detection of resistance-associated genetic elements would be useful to guide therapy in instances wherein an infecting fungus was detected by molecular methods in a histologic preparation, but corresponding tissues were not submitted for culture and subsequent susceptibility testing.

When massive parallel sequencing methods are used and large portions of the genome are available for analysis, then genetic signatures that provide taxonomic information, as well as those that provide information regarding resistance, may be present in the same analysis, thereby simultaneously identifying the pathogen and providing guidance regarding potential resistance to antifungal agents.

PART IV
Laboratory Technique

PART IV Laboratory Technique

Larone's Medically Important Fungi: A Guide to Identification, 7th Edition.
Lars F. Westblade, Eileen M. Burd, Shawn R. Lockhart, and Gary W. Procop.
© 2023 American Society for Microbiology. DOI: 10.1128/9781683674436.piv

Laboratory Procedures

PART IV Laboratory Technique

LABORATORY PROCEDURES

Collection and Preparation of Specimens

No matter how experienced the mycologist, isolation and identification of fungi from clinical specimens are not likely to be accomplished unless the specimen is properly collected and sent immediately to the laboratory. Tissue and fluids are the best specimens. Swabs should be avoided whenever possible; however, their use is required for certain specimens (e.g., collection of purulent material in the setting of conjunctivitis). Specimens should be transported in leakproof sterile containers, but anaerobic transport media or containers should not be used for transporting specimens for fungal culture. A label appended to the specimen container must contain a minimum of two patient identifiers; e.g., patient name and unique identification number. Transport at room temperature is recommended, particularly as dermatophytes are sensitive to cold temperatures. Optimal time for transportation is within 2 h of specimen collection and should occur less than 24 h after collection. Correctly collected, labelled, and transported specimens should be processed as soon as possible upon receipt in the laboratory. If processing immediately is not possible the specimen should be held at ambient temperature. When the quantity of the specimen is insufficient, the laboratory should contact the ordering physician to determine prioritization of testing. In some situations, specimens may be combined to ensure sufficient material for testing (e.g., tissue specimens collected from the same anatomic site). If a specific fungus is suspected by the physician, the laboratory should be notified as special media and culture procedures may be needed, and the information will be helpful for the safety of laboratory personnel. Refer to Table 4.1 for a list of anatomic sites associated with recovery of various pathogenic fungi.

All information associated with the disease process and specimen must be communicated on the requisition form that accompanies the specimen. This information includes

- Patient's name
- A unique patient identification number
- Patient's age
- Patient's sex
- Patient's location (patient's location in the hospital, if hospitalized)
- Physician's name and contact information
- Specific anatomic site cultured
- Date and time of specimen collection

If available, the patient's clinical diagnosis, medical history, underlying conditions, and any antifungal agents or other relevant treatment the patient has recently received should be provided. A thorough patient history documenting animal exposure, recent travel, or outdoor activities is extremely helpful.

Culture accuracy is highly dependent upon the specimen's condition. When unacceptable specimens are received, they should not be processed. They should be held under optimal conditions and the ordering physician contacted immediately to convey the potential for misleading results from culturing unacceptable specimens.

Ideally, unacceptable specimens should be rejected but for certain specimens, such as surgically obtained tissue, the decision to reject can be discussed with the ordering provider on a case-by-case basis. Specimens placed in formalin must not be processed for culture. If a specimen is rejected, rejection must be documented.

Specimens from the following anatomic sites and/or sources should not be sent for fungal culture

- Colostomy discharge materials
- Foley or urinary catheter tips
- Lochia
- Stool (including gastric contents and washings). Note, if fungal infection of the gastrointestinal tract is suspected, biopsy specimens of tissue are usually required for diagnosis.
- Vomitus

Specimens can be rejected in any of the following scenarios

- The specimen is collected from an inappropriate anatomic site and/or source
- The specimen is unlabeled. Irretrievable specimens (e.g., surgically obtained specimens) require special consideration and, if at all possible, should not be rejected. Rather, the institutional policy for reconciliation should be followed.
- There is a discrepancy between the requisition and the specimen label
- The information on the requisition is incomplete
- The transport time is greater than specified by laboratory procedure (typically, transport times greater than 72 h warrant rejection of the specimen)
- The specimen is received in an improper container or transport media
- The specimen is improperly collected (e.g., urine collected from a Foley bag)
- The container is leaking
- Multiple specimens for the same request collected on the same day. If appropriate, consider combining multiple specimens from the same anatomic site.

ABSCESSES AND WOUNDS (EXUDATES, PUS, AND DRAINAGE). Specimens are collected from closed abscesses by aseptic aspiration or from the active peripheral edge of an open abscess. Specimens <2 ml are directly inoculated to media, while specimens >2 ml should be centrifuged at $2,000 \times g$ for 10 min to concentrate the specimen prior to inoculating media with the sediment. Very mucoid specimens can be treated with a mucolytic agent (e.g., N-acetyl-L-cysteine or dithiothreitol) and centrifuged ($2,000 \times g$ for 10 min) to concentrate the specimen prior to inoculating the media with the sediment. Exudates, pus, and drainage are examined for granules using a dissecting microscope. If granules are present, the color is noted, and then a portion of the specimen is teased apart gently, crushed between two glass slides, and examined microscopically; the remainder is washed several times in sterile distilled water, crushed with a sterile glass rod or similar appliance, and inoculated onto appropriate media (granules may be bacterial and should be plated accordingly).

BLOOD. As recovery of fungi increases with the volume of blood tested, and since fungemia may be intermittent, at least two blood samples should be separately collected for culture.

Automated, continuous-monitoring blood culture systems (BacT/Alert [bioMérieux, Inc., Durham, NC], BACTEC [Becton, Dickinson and Company, Sparks, MD], and VersaTREK [Thermo Fisher Scientific, Waltham, MA]) are now used in the majority of clinical microbiology laboratories. Using standard blood culture media, studies have shown their acceptability to detect fungemia caused by yeasts, including most *Candida* spp., and incubation >5 days seldom is required (extending incubation to 10 days has been shown in some studies to provide increased recovery of *Candida glabrata* and *Cryptococcus neoformans*).

Moulds can sometimes be recovered using automated, continuous-monitoring blood culture systems and standard blood culture media, but often require special broth media or lysis-centrifugation for detection. The lysis-centrifugation Isolator system (Abbott, Scarborough, ME) was highly recommended for moulds, and was considered essential for the recovery of the dimorphic fungus *Histoplasma capsulatum*, but has been discontinued. Myco/F Lytic culture medium (Becton, Dickinson and Company) is a nonselective, specialized culture medium used with the automated BACTEC system developed for the recovery of fungi, including *H. capsulatum*, from blood and sterile body fluids. Cultures are monitored 7 days for yeast and 30 days for other fungi. If only an automated standard broth culture is performed, *H. capsulatum* can be recovered after the routine 5-day incubation of the bottle by removing a 5-ml aliquot, centrifuging it, streaking the sediment onto a supportive agar medium, and incubating it for up to 4 weeks; 2 weeks' incubation of the subculture is sufficient to detect all of the positives (James Snyder, University of Louisville, personal communication).

If a manual method is to be used, biphasic blood culture medium consisting of broth with an agar slant is significantly better than broth alone. A commercially available example of this method is the SEPTI-CHEK blood culture system (Thermo Fisher Scientific). Conventional broth blood cultures may require 20–30 days before becoming positive and must be subcultured at regular intervals regardless of gross appearance.

For the recovery of most *Malassezia* spp. from conventional broth blood cultures, it is advisable to add palmitic acid or olive oil to make final concentrations of 3 and 5%, respectively. Adding fatty acids to commercial blood culture bottles of the automated systems does not always seem to be necessary. Alternatively, automated Myco/F Lytic broth culture can be performed. Positive blood culture broths suggestive for *Malassezia* spp. should be subcultured to agar plates with sterile olive oil applied to the surface, or if available, complex media such as Leeming-Notman agar should also be inoculated.

Advances in nonculture methods for identification of organisms from blood include antigen detection, quantification of $(1{\rightarrow}3)$-β-D-glucan, and PCR. Antigen detection in serum includes capsular polysaccharide antigen for *Cryptococcus* spp. and galactomannan for *Aspergillus* spp. Serum for $(1{\rightarrow}3)$-β-D-glucan detects the presence of *Candida* spp., *Aspergillus* spp., and other fungi through a fluorescent signal assay. Whole blood and serum may be used as samples for PCR detection of a wide range of fungi, depending on the

TABLE 4.1 Common clinical sites for laboratory recovery of pathogenic fungi[a]

Agent/Disease	Blood	Bone	Bone marrow	Brain	CSF	Eye	Hair	Nails	Joint fluid	Prostate fluid	Lower respiratory tract	Sinus/nasal cavity	Skin/mucous membranes	Tissue	Urine
Aspergillus spp.		x		x		x		x			x	x	x	x	x
Blastomyces spp.		x		x	x				x	x	x	x	x	x	x
Candida spp.	x	x	x	x	x	x		x	x	x	x	x	x	x	x
Chromo-blastomycosis				x								x	x	x	
Coccidioides spp.	x	x	x	x	x				x	x	x	x	x	x	x
Cryptococcus neoformans/ gattii	x	x	x	x	x	x					x		x	x	x
Fusarium spp.	x	x	x	x		x		x	x		x	x	x	x	x
Histoplasma capsulatum	x	x	x	x	x	x					x	x	x	x	
Mucormycosis/ entomoph-thoromycosis		x		x		x					x	x	x	x	
Paracoccidioides brasiliensis	x		x	x	x					x	x	x	x	x	
Talaromyces marneffei	x	x	x	x					x				x	x	x
Scedosporium spp.	x		x	x	x	x					x	x	x	x	
Sporothrix schenckii	x	x	x	x	x						x	x	x	x	
Trichosporon and Cutaneotri-chosporon spp.	x	x	x	x	x	x			x	x	x	x	x	x	x

aPartially reproduced from Berkow and Sexton, 2023.

PART IV Laboratory Technique

LABORATORY PROCEDURES

assay, and the T2 assay detects the presence of *Candida* in whole blood using a combination of PCR and magnetic resonance. More detailed discussion of molecular methods for fungal identification may be found in Part III.

BODY FLUIDS. Body fluids (e.g., pleural, peritoneal, or joint fluids) are aseptically aspirated. They must sometimes be collected with heparin to prevent clotting. Specimens <2 ml are plated directly. For specimens >2 ml, the fluid is centrifuged at $2,000 \times g$ for 10 min and the sediment used to inoculate media; any clotted material should be minced with a sterile scalpel and combined with the concentrated fluid. At least 0.3 ml of inoculum is placed onto each medium. Alternatively, automated broth culture using Myco/F Lytic medium can be performed.

BONE MARROW. Samples of bone marrow should consist of at least 0.5 ml of aspirated marrow. The pediatric lysis-centrifugation Isolator system (Abbott) was well designed for this small-volume culture, but has since been discontinued. However, specimen can be collected in a heparinized syringe and inoculated onto appropriate fungal media at the bedside. Many laboratories use the same bottled-broth methods used for fungal blood cultures (see above), but the blood-to-broth ratio is not optimal; a Myco/F Lytic culture bottle (or pediatric blood culture bottle) is best in this instance. The specimen should also be smeared and stained with Giemsa or Wright stain if the presence of *H. capsulatum* is a possibility. A bone marrow biopsy may be acquired surgically. The biopsy should be placed in a sterile container with at least 1 ml of sterile, preservative-free saline and processed as described for tissues (see "Tissues").

CEREBROSPINAL FLUID (CSF). CSF collected by needle aspiration must be immediately transported to the laboratory at room temperature. If only 1 tube is received, it is processed by microbiology first. If multiple tubes are collected, microbiology should receive tube 2 or 3 (the less bloody of the two). If <2 ml of CSF is received, it is inoculated directly onto the media. If >2 ml is received, the CSF is centrifuged at $2,000 \times g$ for 10 min. The supernatant fluid is not decanted unless a portion is needed for cryptococcal antigen testing. With a sterile pipette, the sediment is removed and used to inoculate the medium and prepare smears for microscopic examination. Any remaining sediment is resuspended, and the medium is reinoculated with fairly large amounts of the whole specimen. Clots in the fluid should be minced before plating.

CUTANEOUS SPECIMENS. A sample of skin, nail, or hair is best placed on clean, strong paper; black paper is often best in order to see tiny particles of scrapings. The paper is folded and taped to form a leakproof packet and transported in an envelope. Commercial transport package systems are available, e.g., Dermapak (distributor in the United States: Key Scientific Products, Stamford, TX). It is advised to refrain from the use of tubes, as they may accumulate moisture that enhances growth of bacterial contaminants that may be in the specimen, as well as plastic bags or containers, as static electricity can cause specimen to adhere to the plastic. Cutaneous specimens should never be refrigerated because dermatophytes are sensitive to cold temperatures.

Skin. Specimens of skin are taken from an area previously cleansed with 70% alcohol. The active, peripheral edge of a lesion is scraped with a scalpel or the end of a microscope slide, and the scales are placed in an appropriate packet as described above. When sporotrichosis is suspected, pus aspirated from chancres and kerions is the superior material.

Nails. When fungal infection is suspected in nails, they should be cleansed with 70% alcohol and then scraped deeply enough to obtain recently invaded nail tissue. The most rewarding samples are usually from under the nail, close to the nail bed. If the infection is on the surface of the nail plate, scrapings are taken from that area. Initial scrapings that are likely to be contaminated should be discarded and only the deeper samples sent to the laboratory in a packet as described above.

Scalp and hair. Invaders of the scalp and hair are best isolated by culturing the basal portion of the infected hair. Infected hairs (>10) may be selected by placing the patient under a UV light (Wood's lamp; wavelength 365 nm) in a dark room; hairs infected with specific dermatophytes fluoresce under UV light. Hairs that are fluorescent, distorted, or fractured should be chosen for culture and collected using forceps.

EAR. Specimen is collected by firmly rotating a swab in the outer ear canal. The swab is transported at room temperature in the associated transport device, and media are directly inoculated based on the swab manufacturer's instructions.

EYE. Eye infections often require collection of specimens by ophthalmologists and direct inoculation of media at the site of collection. When collection is performed outside of the laboratory, the point of inoculation on the medium should be confirmed and the medium's expiration date checked upon receipt.

Conjunctiva. Purulent material is collected using a swab rotated to collect the exudate. The swab is transported at room temperature in the associated transport device, and media are directly inoculated based on the swab manufacturer's instructions.

Contact lenses. Contact lenses are submitted in a sterile container with 1 to 5 ml of sterile, preservative-free saline. The entire contact lens is vortexed in sterile fluid and the fluid is directly inoculated on media. Direct microscopic examination is not recommended.

Corneal scrapings. Corneal scraping cultures for fungi are most successful when the medium is directly inoculated by the ophthalmologist. Corneal scrapings are transferred from a platinum spatula to a noninhibitory agar plate (blood agar plates are the most commonly used in order to simultaneously culture for bacteria) by making a series of C-shaped streaks on the medium. Scraped material should also be smeared on precleaned slides. The labeled agar plate is kept at room temperature and immediately transported with the slide to the laboratory.

Vitreous humor (also known as vitreous fluid). Collected by aspiration. During the collection process vitreous is often diluted with irrigation fluid. It should be concentrated by centrifugation and the sediment used to inoculate media and prepare smears. Media containing cycloheximide should be avoided. However, because the volume obtained is often low, direct inoculation of media by the physician is frequently performed.

LOWER RESPIRATORY TRACT SPECIMENS. Yeast (other than *Cryptococcus neoformans/gattii*), when recovered from bronchial washings, bronchoalveolar lavage, and sputum specimens, represents colonization and is generally clinically insignificant. However, due to its emergence, laboratories may consider reporting *Candida auris* from respiratory specimens (indeed, any specimen) to inform colonization status of the patient.

Bronchial washings and bronchoalveolar lavage. Specimens are collected by bronchoscopy. Bloody or purulent material is directly inoculated to media. If >2 ml is received, the fluid can be centrifuged at 2,000 × g for 10 min and the concentrate used for plating. Excessively viscous specimens can be processed with a mucolytic agent, centrifuged (2,000 × g for 10 min), and the sediment plated.

Sputum. Sputum should be collected as a first early-morning sample after the patient's teeth are brushed and the mouth is well rinsed; 24-h specimens are not satisfactory, as they easily become overgrown with bacteria and saprobic fungi. Saliva is also unacceptable for fungal culture. Flecks containing pus, blood, or caseous material should be sought and used in culture and smears. Sputum decontaminated for culturing acid-fast bacilli is not acceptable, because the sodium hydroxide in the procedure destroys a large number of fungi; a mucolytic agent without sodium hydroxide (e.g., N-acetyl-L-cysteine or dithiothreitol) may be used with very viscous specimens. Screening for epithelial cells, as performed for bacterial cultures, does not apply.

MEDICAL DEVICE (STENTS, SURGICAL IMPLANTS). These are collected surgically and submitted in a sterile container with sterile, preservative-free saline to keep the device moist. The device is examined for vegetative growth and biofilms. If observed, the surface is scraped using a sterile scalpel to directly inoculate solid media and broth. Media with cycloheximide should be avoided. If vegetative growth or biofilm are not obvious, the device can be incubated in broth at 30°C.

NASAL AND SINUS SPECIMENS. Nasal swabs are discouraged; nasal tissue and sinus aspirate collected using surgical procedures or endoscopic aspiration are the optimal specimens. The advancing edge of lesions or ulcers in the nasal passages should be collected, and the resultant specimen prepared as described for tissues (see "Tissues"). Sinus aspirate is directly inoculated to media, but can be treated with a mucolytic agent, followed by centrifugation (2,000 × g for 10 min) and plating of the sediment for very viscous specimens.

PROSTATIC FLUID SECRETIONS. Prostate fluid (secretions of the testes, seminal vesicles, prostate, and bulbourethral glands) is collected by needle biopsy or prostatic massage after the bladder is emptied. This specimen is often positive for thermally dimorphic/endemic moulds in males with a history of chronic urinary tract infections but negative urine cultures. The secretions are collected in a sterile container for direct inoculation and microscopic evaluation. The secretions can be directly inoculated by the physician and a smear prepared. If inoculation is performed by the physician, the specimen's location on the medium and the medium's expiration date must be checked. To increase diagnostic yield, after the prostate fluid is obtained the next urine specimen can be collected for fungal culture (see "Urine").

TISSUES. Tissue is sent in a sterile container with a minimum of 1 ml of sterile, preservative-free saline to keep the specimen moist. Fungi are best recovered when tissue is minced, not ground, with a scalpel. The minced pieces of tissue are pressed into the agar until partially embedded. If infection with a mucormycete is suspected, the tissue must not be minced, ground, or homogenized, as these procedures destroy the hyphae and decrease the viability of the organisms. However, when *H. capsulatum* is suspected it is essential the tissue is ground with a mortar and pestle or tissue grinder in order to release the intracellular yeasts and enable their growth on the culture media. If necessary, a small amount of sterile saline or broth may be added to facilitate grinding. Therefore, it is advisable to grind or homogenize one portion of the tissue and mince another portion, and then to inoculate media with a mixture of the two preparations. Direct microscopic examination of tissue is best accomplished with thin paraffin sections stained with Gomori methenamine silver (commonly performed in the anatomic pathology laboratory). The mycology lab should still perform a calcofluor white stain (p. 434) on the minced/ground material. Subcutaneous tissue should be carefully examined for granules; if granules are present, they are handled as described above (see "Abscesses and Wounds [Exudates, Pus, and Drainage]").

URINE. Clean-catch, catheterized, suprapubic aspirate urine specimens are collected in a sterile container as a first morning specimen. Twenty-four-hour urine specimens are not acceptable. Large volumes (10 to 50 ml) are optimal. Boric acid preservative transport tubes are only appropriate for suspected cases of candidiasis. Upon reaching the laboratory, the urine is centrifuged at $2,000 \times g$ for 10 min, the supernatant is decanted, and ~0.5 ml of thoroughly mixed sediment is placed on each medium to be used. The sediment can also be used for smears. If quantitation is required, a calibrated loop is used to streak uncentrifuged urine onto a plate of appropriate medium. However, quantification is not useful for fungi. The clinical presentation of the patient must be given prime consideration in the determination of the significance of *Candida* spp. in urine. Yeast in urine may be a sign of dissemination in severely immunocompromised patients.

VAGINAL SPECIMENS. Vaginal specimens are primarily collected to screen for vaginal candidiasis. Specimens are collected using a swab and inoculated to antibacterial media or, preferably, a *Candida* spp. chromogenic agar according to the swab manufacturer's instructions.

For further information, see
Abdolrasouli and Howell, 2023a
Abdolrasouli and Howell, 2023b
Berkow and Sexton, 2023
Clinical and Laboratory Standards Institute M54, 2021
Miller et al., 2018

Methods for Direct Microscopic Examination of Specimens

Any specimen submitted for fungus culture can be examined microscopically for fungal elements. This examination is made in addition to, not instead of, a culture. As well as providing the physician with early information regarding the possible need for treatment, it may be helpful in determining the significance of the organism that will later be identified on culture. For a guide to interpreting direct microscopic examinations of clinical specimens, see Part I (pp. 33–38).

POTASSIUM HYDROXIDE (KOH) PREPARATION

Most organic substances that might be confused with fungi when viewed microscopically are converted to an almost clear background in the presence of moderately strong alkaline solutions. The fungi remain unaffected and are therefore more easily demonstrated.

Reagent (Clearing And Staining Agent)
1. Make a 10% KOH solution in Parker Super Quink Ink, permanent blue-black (50 ml of ink + 5 g of KOH pellets). The ink is readily available from a variety of vendors.
2. Centrifuge KOH-ink solution at 2,000 × g for 10 min.
3. Pour supernatant into plastic (not glass) sterile tube. Store at room temperature.

Slide Preparation
1. Place a portion of the specimen on a labeled slide.
2. Add 1 drop of KOH-ink solution to the slide; mix.
3. Put a coverslip over the preparation.
4. Heat gently. Do not boil. Portions of nails may demand repeated and prolonged heating for the necessary degree of chemical softening so that the material can be pressed out to afford good visibility; alternatively, submerge the nail in the KOH-ink overnight for complete softening and clearing.
5. The slide must be carefully examined microscopically to detect hyphal segments, spores or conidia, budding yeasts, spherules, or sclerotic bodies. Cotton swabs should not be used in preparing these slides, as the cotton strands may resemble hyphae.

KOH preparations are not permanent; the reagent will eventually destroy the fungi. The addition of a small amount of glycerol to the preparation will preserve it for several days.

KOH combined with calcofluor white (p. 434) is a more sensitive method, but a fluorescence microscope with appropriate filter is required.

INDIA INK PREPARATION
1. Place a small drop of India ink on a glass slide.
2. Mix with an equal amount of centrifuged (2,000 × g for 10 min) spinal fluid sediment or a suspension of isolated yeast. Sputum or pus can be cleared with KOH and heat and then mixed with India ink.
3. Coverslip, and examine the slide for encapsulated yeast cells.

If the India ink is too dark, dilute it by placing a drop of sterile distilled water on the slide next to the edge of the coverslip and allowing the water to slowly diffuse into the ink.

Capsular material is exhibited by the appearance of a clear, well-demarcated halo around a yeast cell. When seen in CSF, it is suggestive of *Cryptococcus neoformans* or *Cryptococcus gattii*, but identification must be confirmed by culture and biochemical testing of the isolate. Other species and genera also produce capsules. The capsules of cryptococci vary from 2–10 μm or more in width; they tend to be small in specimens from immunodeficient patients. Leukocytes may also appear haloed due to leakage of the cytoplasm, but the halo has a fuzzy, irregular appearance at the periphery, and the cell within the halo has a much paler cell wall than does *Cryptococcus* (see Fig. 4.1).

Cryptococci often lose their ability to produce capsules when grown on artificial media.

Several antigen detection systems, including the cryptococcal latex antigen test, enzyme immunoassay, and lateral flowthrough device, have been proven to be significantly more sensitive than the India ink preparation and are therefore recommended for the initial diagnosis of cryptococcal disease.

STAINED PREPARATIONS

Calcofluor white, Blankofluor, and Uvitex (p. 434) are different terms for an excellent fluorescent stain that binds to the fungal cell wall for detection of fungi in specimens. It can be combined with KOH (p. 414) if clearing is required. It is a valuable tool and is highly recommended.

Gram stain (p. 438) is most useful in the mycology laboratory for examining specimens for the presence of aerobic actinomycetes. It is commonly used in bacteriology laboratories and may demonstrate mycelial elements and yeast cells, but it does not allow for the best observation of morphologic features. Hyphae, pseudohyphae, and yeast cells of *Candida* spp. in direct exam and in tissue are well stained by Gram stain.

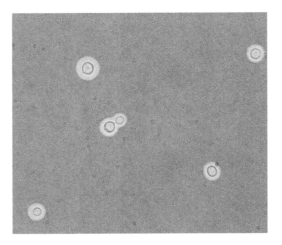

FIGURE 4.1 Cryptococci capsules.

A modified Kinyoun acid-fast stain (p. 432) is used to detect the partially acid-fast filaments of *Nocardia* spp. The routine Kinyoun method is used to stain ascospores.

Wright stain (commonly performed in hematology laboratories) or Giemsa stain (p. 435) is used for detecting intracellular yeast forms of *H. capsulatum* in blood and bone marrow.

The periodic acid-Schiff (PAS; customarily performed in histology laboratories) and Gomori methenamine silver (GMS) (p. 435) stains are considered the best for demonstrating fungi in tissue.

Primary Isolation

Specimens to be cultured for fungus must be inoculated onto media that in combination will ensure the growth of all fungi that may be clinically significant. A variety of possible batteries of media can be used, and the ultimate choice often depends on factors such as patient population, fungi endemic in the area, cost, availability, and personal preference. In any case, the battery should include media that have different factors and that complement each other.

There are a few major points to be considered when selecting a battery of fungal media.

- Chloramphenicol and/or gentamicin or other antibiotics are commonly employed to inhibit bacterial contamination. The antibiotics are likely to also prevent the growth of aerobic actinomycetes; therefore, if *Nocardia* or any other filamentous bacteria are suspected, it is necessary to inoculate media lacking the antibiotics commonly used in fungal media (see p. 111).

- Cycloheximide is incorporated in media to inhibit the rapidly growing saprobic fungi that could overgrow slow-growing primary pathogens. It is necessary to simultaneously use media lacking cycloheximide to grow the organisms that are commonly considered saprobes or contaminants but can also act as opportunistic pathogens. In addition, cycloheximide is known to inhibit the growth of some significant pathogens, e.g., *Aspergillus* spp., many *Candida* species, *C. neoformans/C. gattii*, *Fusarium* spp., *Lomentospora prolificans*, most mucormycetes, *Neoscytalidium dimidiatum*, and *Talaromyces marneffei*.

- It is also generally recommended that an enriched medium be used to ensure the growth of very fastidious thermally dimorphic fungi. An enriched medium containing an antibacterial agent(s) can serve a double purpose by eliminating contaminant bacteria while supporting fastidious fungal pathogens. Blood enrichment may promote the growth of fastidious dimorphic fungi, but it inhibits conidiation in the mould form.

Media that are commonly used for primary isolation of fungi from specimens are separated into five groups in Table 4.2 (p. 417). One medium each can be selected from as many groups as necessary, but cost containment dictates the use of as few media as possible while still guaranteeing recovery of possibly significant fungi. In earlier days, one battery of media for all fungal cultures was commonly used. This

TABLE 4.2 Media for primary isolation of fungi

Type of medium[a]	Properties/purpose
A. *Without antimicrobial agents* SDA (p. 463) PDA or PFA (p. 460) BHI agar (p. 449) SABHI agar (p. 462)	SDA provides classic pigment and morphology, but not necessarily the best primary growth or sporulation; it is poor for the recovery of dermatophytes and other groups of organisms (see Scognamiglio et al., 2010) PDA and PFA enhance production of reproductive structures and colony color BHI enhances the growth of the fastidious dimorphic fungi SABHI has some of the ingredients of both SDA and BHI
B. *With antibacterial agent(s)* SDA, BHI, or SABHI (usually with chloramphenicol, but may be gentamicin, or penicillin with streptomycin) IMA (p. 457) (usually contains chloramphenicol; some formulations contain gentamicin)	Inhibit bacteria while allowing fungi to grow IMA, BHI, and SABHI are enriched media and provide better recovery of fastidious fungi than does SDA
C. *With antibacterial and antifungal agents* Mycosel agar (p. 459) (contains chloramphenicol and cycloheximide) SDA, BHI, or SABHI (with any antibacterial agent in group B plus cycloheximide)	Chloramphenicol (or other antibacterial agent) inhibits bacterial growth Cycloheximide inhibits saprobic fungi that could otherwise overgrow pathogens Opportunists and true pathogens may also be inhibited by cycloheximide
D. *For dermatophytes* DTM (p. 455)	Partially selective and differential for dermatophytes Contain antibiotics to inhibit bacteria and cycloheximide to inhibit many nondermatophytes Contain indicator to demonstrate rise in pH, consistent with growth of dermatophytes
E. *Selective and differential for yeasts* CHROMagar Candida (p. 452) CHROMagar Candida Plus (p. 453) CHROMID Candida (p. 453) Chromogenic Candida Agar (p. 454)	Chloramphenicol inhibits bacteria Differentiation of yeast species is possible due to chromogenic substrates in the agar CHROMagars are able to yield discrete identification of more species of *Candida* than ChromID All are useful in detecting mixed cultures of yeasts

[a] Abbreviations: SDA, Sabouraud dextrose agar; PDA, potato dextrose agar; PFA, potato flake agar; BHI, brain heart infusion; SABHI, combination of Sabouraud and BHI; IMA, inhibitory mould agar; DTM, dermatophyte test medium.

approach usually increased the number of media utilized. A more efficient system is to establish batteries according to the source of the specimen or the specific organism suspected. It may also be beneficial to use media that have different bases; for example, if using Sabouraud dextrose agar (SDA) without antibiotics, use a different base medium containing antibiotics (e.g., inhibitory mould agar [IMA]). In a comparative study, IMA was found to be significantly superior to SDA in recovery of fungi on primary isolation (Scognamiglio et al., 2010). Nonetheless, SDA or other antibiotic-free medium is still required for recovery of *Nocardia* and other aerobic actinomycetes.

The following are suggested batteries consisting of a minimum number of media.

- Sterile body sites: one choice from group A and one from group B (or two from group A)
- Respiratory tract: one from group A, one from group B, and one from group C
- Skin, hair, and nails: one from group B and one from group C or D
- Throats, urines, and genitals ("TUGs"): one from group E (it has been shown that CHROMagar Candida can be used as the sole primary medium for these specimens; see Murray et al., 2005)

Some special situations require specific media.

- If *H. capsulatum* or *Blastomyces dermatitidis/gilchristii* is suspected, an enriched medium (e.g., BHI agar with antibacterial agent[s]) must be one of the choices (and remember, the yeast phase of these organisms is inhibited by cycloheximide).
- If an aerobic actinomycete (e.g., *Nocardia* spp.) is suspected, a medium without the antibacterial used in fungal media must be included. Buffered charcoal-yeast extract (BCYE) agar with and without antimicrobials (p. 450) is the medium of choice for *Nocardia* spp.

Whenever possible, and unless otherwise indicated, at least 0.5 ml of specimen should be inoculated onto each agar surface. Petri plates are the preferred media over tubes. Plate media provide a larger surface area allowing a greater volume of specimen to be inoculated, improved air exchange, and better observation of mixed culture and colony characteristics. However, for safety reasons tubes are preferred over plates when fungi are shipped to other laboratories. If plates are used, they should contain 40 ml of medium and be surrounded by a shrink seal to prevent dehydration; the shrink seal also prevents unintentional opening. Plates should NOT be used if *Blastomyces* spp., *Cladophialophora bantiana*, *Coccidioides* spp., or *H. capsulatum* are suspected.

If tubes are used, the media should be slanted in wide tubes (at least 20 mm in diameter) and optimally left in a horizontal position (on a culture rack designed for acid-fast bacilli) for 24 h after inoculation in order for the inoculum to remain dispersed rather than accumulating at the bottom of the slant. The tubes can then be stood vertically for subsequent incubation. The screw caps must be kept partially loosened to ensure proper atmospheric conditions.

The optimal temperature and atmosphere for growth of most clinically encountered fungi is 30°C. If a 30°C incubator is not available, cultures should be incubated at room temperature (~25°C). There is no advantage to simultaneously incubating routine primary cultures at 37°C; this should be reserved for when there is reason to suspect the presence of thermally dimorphic organisms or one of the few fungi that prefer the higher temperature. If the incubator is not well humidified, it is essential to place pans of water near the cultures.

Most cultures should be incubated for 4 weeks before being considered negative for fungus. Cultures for yeasts in oral thrush, vaginitis, or urine on chromogenic medium should be incubated according to manufacturer recommendations (typically 24 to 72 h); if on routine media, they are held for 10 to 14 days (however, most will grow within 7 days). Cultures suspected of containing thermally dimorphic systemic fungi should be incubated for 8 weeks before being reported as negative.

Macroscopic Examination of Cultures

After initial inoculation and incubation, cultures should be examined for growth every 2–3 days (daily for nonautomated blood cultures) during the first week and at least weekly thereafter. Rapid growers will appear by the first or second time the cultures are checked, whereas slow-growing fungi may not be evident for 2–3 weeks or longer. It is imperative that any yeast, mould, or actinomycete that grows on a primary medium be subcultured immediately to ensure the viability and isolation of the organism. When mature growth develops, the texture and surface color of the colony should be carefully noted. The color of the reverse (underside) of the colony must also be recorded, along with any pigment that diffuses into the medium. It is also helpful to observe whether or not the fungus grows on medium containing cycloheximide.

To ensure the cultivation of all fungi in a specimen (especially the slower-growing pathogens), it is advisable in many cases to hold the cultures for at least a month, even though some fungi may have been isolated. When more than one fungus is seen on the primary culture, a carefully streaked plate is usually necessary for isolation. The lid may be taped closed in several places for safety and prevention of dehydration, but care must be taken not to create anaerobic conditions. Shrink seals are perfect for this situation. As previously mentioned, to prevent dehydration of the plates, it is best if they contain 40 ml of agar, and a pan of water should be placed in the incubator. If *Blastomyces* spp., *C. bantiana*, *Coccidioides* spp., or *H. capsulatum* are suspected, plates should NOT be used.

Microscopic Examination of Growth

It is best to examine a fungus microscopically when the culture first begins to grow and form conidia or spores and again a few days later. In many instances the manner of conidiation or sporulation, which is so important to identification, is obscured in old cultures. Potato flake or potato dextrose agar often promotes conidiation or sporulation better than does SDA. Manipulation of mould growth must always be carried out in a Class II biological safety cabinet.

There are several methods for microscopically examining a fungus culture.

TEASE MOUNT. Place a drop of lactophenol cotton blue (LPCB) (p. 439) on a clean glass slide. With a sterile bent dissecting needle or sterile loop, remove a small portion of the colony from the agar surface and place it in the drop of LPCB. With two dissecting needles or sterile applicator sticks, *gently* tease apart the mycelial mass of the colony on the slide, cover with a coverslip, and observe under the microscope with low-power (100×) and high-dry (400×) magnifications. Unfortunately, this method does not always preserve the original position and structure of the conidia, spores, and other characterizing elements, but it is a very rapid method and is always worth performing. All moulds should be examined with a wet mount before setting up a slide culture.

CELLOPHANE TAPE MOUNT. Another rapid method of studying the microscopic morphology of a mould is with the aid of clear cellophane tape. Loop back on itself a 1.5-in. (~4-cm) strip of clear tape, sticky side out, and hold the tip of the loop securely with a forceps. Press the lower, sticky side very firmly to the surface of the fungal colony, and then pull the tape gently away; aerial hyphae will adhere to the tape. Then, with the tape strip opened up, place it on a small drop of LPCB on a glass slide so that the entire sticky side adheres to the slide, and examine it under the microscope. This method is usually successful in retaining the original positions of the characteristic fungal structures but has the drawback of requiring the organism to be grown on plated medium.

An alternative method has been described. It utilizes frosted tape on an applicator stick. The frosted tape is generally more readily available, more pliable, and easier to tear than is clear tape; the use of an applicator stick better permits sampling of fungi in tubed cultures (Harris, 2000).

SLIDE CULTURE. The best method for preserving and observing the structure of a fungus is the slide culture. It is not a rapid technique, but it is unsurpassed as a routine means of studying the fine points of the microscopic morphology of fungi. Always do a tease mount or cellophane tape mount before a slide culture; organisms suspected of being *Blastomyces* spp., *C. bantiana*, *Coccidioides* spp., or *H. capsulatum* should NOT be set up on slide culture.

The procedure is carried out as follows.

1. Cover the inside bottom of a 100-mm-diameter sterile petri plate with a piece of filter paper.
2. Place a bent glass rod, two pieces of plastic tubing (about 6 cm long, 5 cm apart), or the bending end of a flexible drinking straw in the petri plate.
3. Place a clean, labeled, sterilized glass microscope slide on the glass rod, plastic tubing, or bent straw.
4. From a plate of potato dextrose agar (or other agar when desired; e.g., potato flake agar) poured 4 mm deep, cut a 1-by-1-cm block with a sterile scalpel. Transfer the block to the center of the glass slide (see Fig. 4.2).
5. With a heavy nichrome wire needle (22 gauge), plastic inoculating needle, or sterile applicator stick, inoculate the fungus onto the centers of the four sides of the agar block.
6. Place a sterilized coverslip over the block, and apply slight pressure to ensure adherence.

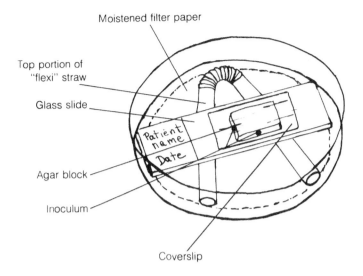

Top portion of "flexi" straw

Moistened filter paper

Glass slide

Patient name
Date

Agar block

Inoculum

Coverslip

FIGURE 4.2 Slide culture method schematic.

7. Place ~1.5 ml of sterile water on the filter paper on the bottom of the petri plate, replace the cover, and incubate the plate at room temperature, preferably in the dark (this can be accomplished by stacking plates in a wire basket and incubating in a designated cabinet with the door closed, but not airtight).

8. Examine periodically for growth, and add water if the plate begins to dry out. The fungus will ordinarily grow on the surface of the slide and also on the undersurface of the coverslip. The closed petri plate can be placed on the microscope stage, and the slide culture can be examined with the low-power (10×) objective.

9. When reproductive structures are well developed, use forceps to carefully remove the coverslip and place it on a drop of LPCB on a second slide.

10. With a heavy needle or applicator stick, gently flip the agar block off the original slide into a container of antifungal disinfectant. Put a drop of LPCB on the slide, and place a new coverslip over it.

11. Both microscopic preparations from steps 9 and 10 can be sealed around the edges with clear nail polish or mounting fluid and kept for further study or as teaching aids. These slide preparations have been found to last longer if they are stored in a flat position rather than standing on their sides. Huber's modified LPCB with polyvinyl alcohol (p. 439) is now widely used and is definitely the best method available for preserving slide preparations for long periods; it is the only acceptable method if the slide is to be shipped to another laboratory.

Procedure for Identification of Yeasts

The extent to which a yeast needs to be identified depends primarily on the body site from which it is isolated and the clinical relevancy of full identification. The particular needs of the patient population and economic issues in the laboratory also play major roles. The following is a scenario that meets minimum requirements while being cost-effective. More detailed discussion of molecular methods for identification of yeasts may be found in Part III.

Traditionally *Candida albicans*, at least, is differentiated from the other species of *Candida*, but even that level of identification is not usually necessary for isolates from the lower respiratory tract. *Candida* spp. are seldom of clinical significance in the lower respiratory tract, and diagnosis of *Candida* pneumonia is based on histologic examination, not culture. *Cryptococcus neoformans* and *Cryptococcus gattii* are typically the only yeasts of concern in such specimens (aside from the yeast forms of the thermally dimorphic fungi). *C. neoformans*/*C. gattii* can usually be rapidly ruled out by colony and microscopic morphology, with further testing only occasionally needed (see below), and the result reported as "yeast, not *Cryptococcus*."

When appropriate, screening any specimen for only *C. albicans* (not differentiated from *Candida dubliniensis*) on nonchromogenic agar can be rapidly accomplished by the germ tube test (p. 425), by commercial chromogenic enzyme tests, or by simply examining the colonies (on blood agar or chocolate agar; especially useful method in the bacteriology laboratory) for mycelial projections, commonly called "feet" (p. 123).

If throat, urine, and genital ("TUG") specimens and blood cultures smear-positive for yeasts have been inoculated directly onto CHROMagar Candida, isolates of *C. albicans*, *Candida tropicalis*, and *Candida krusei* will typically be identifiable within 48 h. Isolates resembling *Candida glabrata* on CHROMagar Candida can be identified in 1 h with the rapid assimilation of trehalose (RAT) test (p. 460) (Murray et al., 2005). Health care facilities with patients suspected of having a *C. auris* infection should consider identifying and reporting *C. auris* from all clinical specimens obtained from the patient, including specimens where species-level identification of yeast is not typically performed. *C. auris* can be misidentified by some biochemical platforms and only accurately identified using nucleic acid or proteomic (MALDI-TOF MS) methodologies, which may not be available to all laboratories. A new chromogenic agar, CHROMagar Candida Plus (p. 453), intended for the direct detection and presumptive identification of *Candida* spp., including *C. auris*, could facilitate recognition of *C. auris* in laboratories without *C. auris*-specific identification platforms.

The decision on how far to go with species identification of isolates from various body sites lies with each laboratory, the primary factors being the patients' needs and the clinical relevancy of the results.

With the above in mind, proceed.

IF THE COLONY IS MUCOID

Determination should immediately be made as to whether the isolate may be *C. neoformans*/*C. gattii*; this can be accomplished by

- a simple wet prep in sterile water or saline; *C. neoformans*/*C. gattii* appear as round cells of various sizes

- addition of India ink (p. 414) to the wet prep; will exhibit capsules (may be small), if present
- a urease slant (p. 467), inoculated especially heavily at the top of the slant (that area will turn positive more rapidly than the rest of the agar)

If any of the tests listed above suggest *Cryptococcus*, the isolate should be

- inoculated to cornmeal-Tween 80 (or analogous agar that shows microscopic morphology and is glucose free)
- from the cornmeal agar, tested for phenoloxidase with the caffeic acid disk test (p. 426); the caffeic acid test can be performed directly from the primary isolation medium, but a false negative may result if the medium contains dextrose

The first isolate of *Cryptococcus* from a patient should be confirmed with one of the commercial yeast identification kits or MALDI-TOF MS. If the isolate is shown to be *C. neoformans* or *C. gattii*, it is reasonable to do only the caffeic acid disk test on subsequent isolates. Differentiation of *C. neoformans* and *C. gattii*, if needed, is attainable with CGB agar (p. 450).

IF THE COLONY IS NOT MUCOID

1. Perform a germ tube test (p. 425). Only *C. albicans* (and *C. dubliniensis*) will produce germ tubes in serum within 3 h, and they can be differentiated (if desired) by the characteristics in Table 2.4 (p. 128).
2. If the germ tube test is negative and the colony is small and relatively slow growing, and the wet prep shows small, oval cells, perform the RAT test (p. 460) for the identification of *C. glabrata*.
3. If the isolate is not *C. albicans* or *C. glabrata* and further identification is desired, use a pure culture to perform biochemical tests or proteomic analysis (MALDI-TOF MS) for yeast identification; this is most commonly done with the use of a commercially prepared system, such as one of the following:

   Biochemical analysis:
   API 20C AUX (bioMérieux, Inc., Durham, NC)
   Rapid Yeast ID (Beckman Coulter, Brea, CA)
   RapID Yeast Plus (Remel, Lenexa, KS)
   Sherlock Microbial ID System (MIDI, Newark, DE)
   VITEK 2 YST (bioMérieux, Inc., Durham, NC)

   Proteomic analysis:
   Bruker MALDI Biotyper (Bruker Daltonics, Billerica, MA)
   VITEK MS (bioMérieux SA, Marcy l'Etoile, France)
4. Using the Dalmau method (p. 454), inoculate a plate of cornmeal-Tween 80 agar (p. 454) or another yeast morphology agar; this should accompany all biochemical identification systems.

IF AN ACCEPTABLE IDENTIFICATION IS NOT OBTAINED

After the purity of the isolate is rechecked, subsequent tests may be required for

- fermentation (p. 456)
- assimilation of potassium nitrate or additional carbohydrates (p. 444–448)
- appearance of isolate in Sabouraud broth (p. 464)
- inhibition of isolate by cycloheximide (p. 459)
- urease activity, if not included in the commercial system (p. 467)
- phenoloxidase (caffeic acid disk test [p. 426])

Consult Tables 2.2–2.10 (pp. 124, 126, 128, 134, 139, 150, 151, and 165) for identification of genus and species.

If the isolate remains unidentified and identification is required, nucleic acid methods, as described in Part III, can be employed. Whenever complete identification is not performed, it is advisable to hold the isolate for at least 7 days after reporting and to add a note to the report that is similar to "If further identification is required, please call Microbiology, extension *xxxx*."

Isolation of Yeast When Mixed with Bacteria

Yeasts may grow mixed with bacteria on primary culture. It is absolutely essential that only pure cultures be used in assimilation, fermentation, and other biochemical tests for identification.

Careful streaking of the organisms onto plated medium with or without antibiotics often yields isolated colonies. Likelihood of isolation is increased with the use of a chromogenic yeast agar (pp. 452, 453), inhibitory mould agar (p. 457), or similar media containing antibacterial(s). Cycloheximide (the antifungal in Mycosel agar) inhibits some yeasts.

Persistent bacterial contamination may be eliminated with the following acidification method.

1. Place 10 ml of Sabouraud dextrose broth in each of four tubes.
2. To tube no. 1, add 1 drop of 1 N HCl.
3. To tube no. 2, add 2 drops of 1 N HCl.
4. To tube no. 3, add 3 drops of 1 N HCl.
5. To tube no. 4, add 4 drops of 1 N HCl.
6. Make a suspension of the yeast-bacterium mixture in sterile water. Add a drop of the suspension to each of the four Sabouraud dextrose broth-HCl tubes. Incubate at 25–30°C for 24 h.
7. Subculture a loopful of broth from each tube to plated media and incubate for 48 h.

In most instances, there will be an acid concentration at which the bacteria are inhibited and the yeast is allowed to grow.

Germ Tube Test for the Presumptive Identification of *Candida albicans*

1. Make a very light suspension of a yeast in 0.5–1.0 ml of sterile serum in a 12-by-75-mm test tube. The optimum inoculum is 10^5–10^6 cells per ml; an increased concentration of inoculum often causes a significant decrease in germ tube production and false-negative results. Very few yeast cells should be seen per microscopic field when results are read. Pooled human sera is an excellent medium for production of germ tubes, but it must be negative for hepatitis and HIV and free of antifungal agents. Fetal bovine serum, rabbit serum, and other animal sera are also commonly utilized. A Pasteur pipette tip can be used to inoculate the serum and can be left in the tube during incubation.

2. Incubate at 35–37°C for no longer than 3 h.

3. Place 1 drop of the yeast-serum mixture on a slide with a coverslip. Examine microscopically for germ tube production.

A known strain of *C. albicans* should be tested with each new batch of serum.

Germ tubes are the beginnings of true hyphae and appear as filaments that are NOT constricted at their points of origin on the parent cell. If the filaments are constricted and septate at their points of origin, they are pseudohyphae, not germ tubes (see Fig. 4.3). The germ tube test is also positive with *C. dubliniensis,* and further testing may be performed if required; for epidemiological purposes, for example (see Table 2.4 [p. 128]).

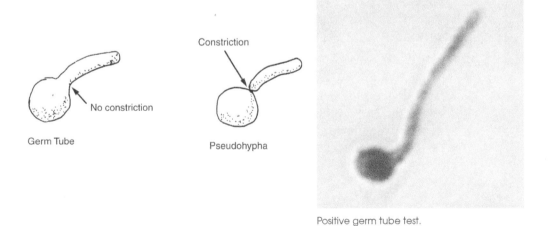

Positive germ tube test.

FIGURE 4.3 Germ tube test.

Rapid Enzyme Tests for the Presumptive Identification of *Candida albicans*

Several systems are commercially available for the rapid (5–30 min) presumptive identification of *C. albicans* in culture. Each system utilizes two substrates, one for the detection of β-galactosamidase and the other for the detection of l-proline aminopeptidase. Of the clinically encountered yeasts, only *C. albicans* produces both of these enzymes. Evaluations of the systems show them to be rapid, acceptable alternatives to the germ tube test (Heelan et al., 1996). Manufacturers' instructions must be followed.

Caffeic Acid Disk Test

Caffeic acid is one of several good substrates for the detection of phenoloxidase enzyme activity. When phenoloxidase is present, the caffeic acid is broken down to melanin, resulting in a dark brown to black color. As *C. neoformans*/*C. gattii* are the only clinically encountered yeasts that produce phenoloxidase, the test is extremely useful for identification and/or confirmation of these organisms (species separation can be accomplished with CGB agar [p. 450]). Although birdseed agar may also be used to detect phenoloxidase activity, the advantages of the disk test are speed and improved reliability.

1. Culture the isolated yeast on cornmeal-Tween 80 agar. Because phenoloxidase is inhibited by glucose, it is essential that the growth medium be glucose free; cornmeal-Tween 80 agar is usually the most readily available medium to meet this requirement.
2. Place a caffeic acid disk (available from Remel [Lenexa, KS] and from Hardy Diagnostics [Santa Maria, CA]) on a glass slide. Moisten the disk with 30–40 μl of water.
3. Inoculate the disk with several colonies of the isolated yeast.
4. Incubate the disk at 22–35°C in a moist chamber.
5. Read for development of brown to black pigment. Most positive reactions are seen within 30 min, but the test should be held at least 4 h before being considered negative. On rare occasions, an organism may require several generations of growth on cornmeal agar before the enzyme can be detected. (Image Appendix Figure 40.)

Olive Oil Disks for Culturing *Malassezia* spp.

(K. McGowan, Children's Hospital of Philadelphia, personal communication)

Malassezia spp. other than *M. pachydermatis* (p. 160) require long-chain fatty acids for growth. This need is usually met in the laboratory by overlaying an agar plate surface with sterile olive oil. As an alternative method, olive oil-saturated paper disks can be used.

1. Place large (½-in. [~13-mm]-diameter) blank disks (BBL, Sparks, MD) in a screw-cap sterile flask or jar (a urine specimen container is suitable).

2. Pour in enough sterile olive oil to reach a depth of 10–20 mm. Olive oil can be autoclaved.

3. Place disks (no more than can be easily covered by the oil) in the container and allow to soak in the olive oil; add oil and disks to container as needed. They can be kept for many months without deterioration.

4. When screening for *Malassezia* spp., streak specimen or aliquot of blood culture broth (after ~48 h of incubation) onto mycology agar without cycloheximide.

5. Remove a saturated disk from the olive oil, using a swab or forceps (allow excess oil to drip down the side of the container).

6. Place the disk on the area of initial inoculation of the plate.

7. Incubate at 35–37°C.

Malassezia spp., if present, often grow well in the area surrounding the disk. Special media for recovery of *Malassezia* spp., i.e., Leeming-Notman agar (p. 458), may be required.

Conversion of Thermally Dimorphic Fungi in Culture

A mycelial colony that is morphologically suggestive of a thermally dimorphic fungus at room temperature is classically grown in its yeast form at 35–37°C to confirm its identification. This or another confirmation method is essential, as there are several monomorphic moulds that resemble the filamentous phase of thermally dimorphic fungi. In addition, the mould forms of some dimorphic fungi may not be definitive microscopically, and the yeast phase can serve to identify them.

These organisms MUST be handled in a biological safety cabinet. To test for the ability of a mycelial form to convert to a yeast phase, proceed as follows.

1. Inoculate mycelial growth onto a fresh, moist slant of brain heart infusion agar in a screw-cap tube. A small amount of brain heart infusion broth added to the tube ensures sufficient moisture. After the fragment of mould inoculum has been emulsified in the moisture, pull it up and place it on the agar slant.

2. Incubate the slant at 35–37°C, preferably in carbon dioxide. Keep the screw cap closed tightly to retain the moisture, but loosen it daily to allow the colony to "breathe."

3. Periodically examine the slant, and make a wet preparation of any yeastlike area.

4. If only a mycelial form grows, transfer it to another moistened brain heart infusion slant and incubate it again at 35–37°C. It may be necessary to make several serial transfers to attain complete conversion to the yeast phase.

In some instances, *in vitro* conversion is exceedingly difficult or slow, and exoantigen tests or molecular methods may be preferred or required to confirm identification.

Sporulation Inducement Method for *Apophysomyces* and *Saksenaea*

This procedure (Padhye and Ajello, 1988) is recommended for use in identifying all nonsporulating mucormycetes isolated from clinical specimens. The growth on SDA at 25°C should consist of broad, pauciseptate, branched, hyaline hyphae without sporangial formation. The manipulations must be carried out in a biological safety cabinet.

1. Grow the isolate on an SDA plate at 25°C for 1 week.
2. Aseptically cut out a 1-cm² agar block permeated with the hyphal growth.
3. Transfer the block to a petri plate containing 20 ml of sterile distilled water and 0.2 ml of filter-sterilized 10% yeast extract. Shrink-seal the plates to prevent spillage.
4. Incubate the blocks in the water solution at 35–37°C (lower temperature will yield fewer or no sporangia). After 5 days of incubation, a thin film of growth should appear over the surface of the water.
5. Make wet preparations (with lactophenol cotton blue) of portions of the film on days 5, 10, and 15 of incubation. Examine microscopically for sporangia. See pp. 204 and 206 for descriptions of *Apophysomyces* and *Saksenaea*, respectively.

In vitro Hair Perforation Test (for Differentiation of *Trichophyton mentagrophytes* and *Trichophyton rubrum*)

1. Place 1-cm-long fragments of healthy human hair in a petri plate or tube. Sterilize by autoclaving at 15 lb/in² for 15 min. The clearest and fastest results are obtained with light-colored hair from a child (<12 years old). Adult hair will give correct results if the hair has not been exposed to hair spray or a combination of bleach and permanent wave (Salkin et al., 1985).
2. In a sterile 50-ml screw-cap tube, place 8–10 of the sterile hair fragments; add 20–25 ml of sterile distilled water and 0.1 ml of 10% filter-sterilized yeast extract. Plastic conical tubes used for concentrating specimens for acid-fast bacilli work well; tubes have proven safer to handle than petri plates when doing this test.
3. Place several fragments of the fungal culture in the tube.
4. Incubate at room temperature for 4 weeks or until a positive reaction is seen (average, 8–10 days). Examine at weekly intervals by placing one or two hairs from the culture onto a slide with a drop of lactophenol cotton blue and a coverslip. Look for wedge-shaped perforations caused by hyphae that penetrate the hairs perpendicularly (Fig. 4.4).

The hair is perforated by *T. mentagrophytes* but not by *T. rubrum* (see Table 2.19 [p. 302]).

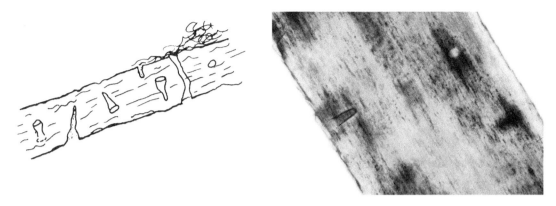

FIGURE 4.4 Positive *in vitro* hair perforation test schematic (left) and micrograph (right).

Temperature Tolerance Testing

When determining at what temperatures an organism can grow, it is important that the inoculations are equivalent. This is best attained by making an evenly dispersed suspension of the organism in sterile saline and placing the same amount on each slant or plate that will be incubated at various temperatures. One culture must be at optimum temperature (usually 30°C) as a control.

Maintenance of Stock Fungal Cultures

No single method is best for all types of fungi. Regardless of the method employed, a young, actively growing culture is essential for the first step.

WATER CULTURE TECHNIQUE

Rub a sterile moistened swab over the surface of an actively conidiating or sporulating fungus colony; wash the swab off into a screw-cap tube containing ~4 ml of sterile distilled water. To conserve space, isolates can be inoculated into a screw-cap microfuge tube containing ~1 ml of sterile distilled water. Tighten the cap, and store at room temperature. Add sterile distilled water periodically if any evaporation occurs. This technique will also work well for most yeast species where a large loopful of a young reproductive isolate is resuspended in water.

To prepare a subculture, shake the water culture to resuspend the fungus. With a sterile Pasteur pipette aseptically transfer 2–3 drops of the suspension to a slant or plate of a supportive fungal medium. Incubate the agar at 25–30°C.

FREEZING TECHNIQUE

Freezing can be accomplished by suspending a young reproductive isolate using a sterile moistened swab for moulds or an inoculating loop for yeasts in a cryovial containing 10–15% glycerol and freezing at −70°C. To subculture, remove the cryovial from the freezer and chip off some of the frozen glycerol stock and inoculate directly to a fresh plate or slant. Alternatively, and for cultures that produce few conidia, small squares of agar (4 to 5 mm) with fungal growth may be cut out from an agar plate of a culture and placed in a cryovial containing 10–15% glycerol. The cryovial is frozen at −70°C. To subculture, the cryovial is thawed and one (or more) agar block is inoculated directly to a fresh plate or slant. The tube may be refrozen. The organisms to most likely fail to survive are *C. dubliniensis* and the dermatophytes (see Espinel-Ingroff et al., 2004).

Controlling Mites

Mites are tiny arachnids (0.05–0.15 mm long, barely visible to the naked eye) that graze on fungi if given the opportunity. Their most common means of entry into the mycology laboratory is on specimens of hair, skin, or nails or in cultures received from other laboratories that have a mite problem. These tiny creatures can cause enormous problems as they walk from one culture to another, contaminating the cultures with the bacteria and fungi they carry on their bodies.

The very best system of mite control is to prevent their initial entry into the laboratory. If there is a risk of mites, culture plates and tubes should be sealed with parafilm or shrink seals. If mites are detected and have spread, it is advisable to autoclave and discard all of the cultures that are not absolutely essential to save and to thoroughly clean the laboratory with an effective disinfectant. An attempt to save indispensable cultures can be made by transferring them to slants of media containing 0.1% hexachlorocyclohexane or by exposing the mite-infested fungi to naphthalene (mothball) crystals. Exposure can be attained by placing the cultures in a plastic bag along with naphthalene (or other chemicals poisonous to mites); if the fungi are in tubes, the caps must be loosened. Alternatively, a gauze plug containing the crystals can be put in the neck of each tube. By placing petri plates of naphthalene in incubators and refrigerators for at least a week, those areas can be cleared of mites.

Do not conduct yeast assimilation tests in the vicinity of the chemicals; the vapors may be used as a carbon source by the yeasts, yielding false-positive results.

Another method for salvaging cultures relies on the fact that mites are rapidly killed by freezing, while their eggs can survive for 48–72 h at −20°C. Therefore, a culture might be saved by placing it at −20°C for more than 72 h and then subculturing an area that appears to be unaffected by the mites. A dissecting microscope is useful in this instance to select the best colonies.

For further information on mites, see
McGinnis, 1980
Pitt and Hocking, 2009

Staining Methods

Positive and negative controls must be run on new lots of stain and periodically thereafter as need dictates. If the stain is not frequently used, it is advisable to run controls each time the staining procedure is performed.

Acid-Fast Modified Kinyoun Stain for *Nocardia* spp.

The filaments of *Nocardia* spp. are partially acid fast, and will stain pink-to-red with this procedure. Other partially acid-fast bacteria, such as *Gordonia, Rhodococcus,* and *Tsukamurella* stain similarly. It is important to remember that mycobacteria, which are fully acid fast (i.e., Ziehl-Neelsen or Kinyoun), also stain with this staining procedure. In contrast, partially acid-fast organisms do not stain with the full acid-fast stain.

Procedure
1. Make a smear and fix with heat.
2. Flood slide with Kinyoun carbol-fuchsin for 5 min.
3. Pour off excess stain.
4. Flood slide with 50% alcohol and immediately wash with water.
5. Decolorize with 1% aqueous sulfuric acid (see alternative decolorizer below).
6. Wash with tap water.
7. Counterstain with methylene blue or brilliant green for 1 min.
8. Rinse with water, dry, and examine under oil immersion objective.

Negative and positive controls should be included each time this method is used.

Reagents

Kinyoun carbol-fuchsin (same as for staining mycobacteria)

Basic fuchsin	4 g
Phenol	8 ml
Alcohol, 95%	20 ml
Distilled water	100 ml

Dissolve the dye in the alcohol, and then add the water and phenol.

1% aqueous H_2SO_4 (see alternative decolorizer below)

Concentrated H_2SO_4	1 ml
Distilled water	99 ml

Be sure to add the acid to the water, not vice versa.

Counterstain

Methylene blue	2.5 g
Ethanol, 95%	100.0 ml

or

> Brilliant green ....0.5 g
> Distilled water .... 100.0 ml

Alternative decolorizing agent

The following decolorizing agent, commonly used in the fluorochrome method for acid-fast bacilli, may be successfully used to substitute for steps 4 and 5 of the above procedure.

> Concentrated HCl..0.5 ml
> Ethanol, 70% .... 99.5 ml

Acid-Fast Stain for Ascospores

When staining for ascospores, the classic Kinyoun method is used (as for mycobacteria), i.e., decolorize with solution of:

> Concentrated HCl.. 3 ml
> Ethanol, 95% ....97 ml

Add acid to alcohol; mix well.
The ascospores will stain red; other cells will take the counterstain.

Ascospore Stain

1. Culture the fungus on a medium that promotes ascospore formation (see p. 443).
2. Make thin smear and fix with heat.
3. Stain with 5% aqueous malachite green (filter before using) containing Tergitol 7 (Sigma-Aldrich, St. Louis, MO) for 3 min.
4. Wash with tap water.
5. Decolorize with 95% ethyl alcohol for 30 sec.
6. Wash with tap water.
7. Counterstain with 5% aqueous safranin for 30 sec.
8. Wash with water, allow to dry, and examine under oil immersion objective.

Ascospores stain green, and vegetative cells stain red.

The acid-fast stain (above) is also useful for observing ascospores. It should be noted that ascospores may be observed in simple aqueous wet mounts without any stain.

Calcofluor White Stain

Calcofluor white (CFW), which also is known in Europe as Blankofluor and Uvitex, has become a valuable and routine reagent in the clinical mycology laboratory. It binds to β-(1→3) and β-(1→4) polysaccharides, such as cellulose and chitin (present in fungal cell walls), and fluoresces when exposed to long-wave UV light. It is exceedingly useful for direct microscopic examination of specimens, as the fungal elements are seen much more easily than with the older traditional plain potassium hydroxide (KOH) preparations. Additionally, it is exceptional for exhibiting certain morphologic structures of fungi that have been isolated on culture.

Preparation of Stain Solution

CFW M2R (Fluorescent Brightener 28)................ 100 mg
Evans blue .... 50 mg
Distilled water.. 100 ml

Note: The powder form of CFW M2R is available from Sigma-Aldrich (St. Louis, MO). Several other companies produce prepared solutions of various formulations and names. It is imperative to follow manufacturers' instructions for use; excitation wavelengths may vary and require filters other than those described below.

Mix well. Store at room temperature in a dark bottle.

Procedure

1. Smear specimen onto glass slide. The specimen may be stained while wet or allowed to dry on the slide and rehydrated with the CFW solution. If the slide is to be subsequently reprocessed with another stain, it must first be allowed to dry and then heat fixed before applying the CFW.
2. Add 1 drop of CFW solution. One drop of 10% KOH may also be added if clearing is required.
3. Apply coverslip. Allow slide to sit at room temperature at least 5 min, since it often takes a few minutes for the CFW to penetrate the organism.
4. Examine slide with a UV (fluorescent) microscope equipped with an excitation filter that transmits wavelengths between 300 and 412 nm (the optimum wavelength for excitation of CFW M2R is 365 nm) and a barrier filter (530 nm) that removes UV and blue light while transmitting longer wavelengths.

The required light source is a mercury vapor lamp. Quartz halogen bulbs are usually not suitable, as the energy output is too low.

Fungal elements will stand out as bright apple green on a red background; the barrier filters that allow transmission of shorter wavelengths and yield white elements on a blue background are no longer recommended for eye safety reasons.

Quality control must be performed on a routine basis to ensure the quality of the reagent, procedure, and microscope.

Positive control is a suspension of a yeast or mould, e.g., *Candida* sp. or *Aspergillus* sp.

Negative control is a solution without fungi.

If the slide is to be saved or restained, remove the coverslip, rinse the slide briefly with distilled water, and air dry. The slide can later be restained with CFW or other stains, such as Gomori methenamine silver, Gram, etc.

For further information, see
Harrington and Hageage, 2003

Giemsa Stain

The Giemsa stain is used for the detection of fungi in bone marrow or blood smears, and body fluids (e.g., cerebrospinal fluid). Intracellular *Histoplasma capsulatum* may be seen in bone marrow aspirates or in peripheral blood smears of patients with disseminated histoplasmosis. Blood smears prepared with blood from the bottom of the tube, where heavily infected cells are often found, or buffy coat preparations from centrifuged citrated blood increase the yield. *H. capsulatum* appears as small, oval yeast cells that stain light to dark blue with a hyaline halo due to the unstained cell wall (see p. 172). There is often a clear space surrounding *Cryptococcus* spp. due to the mucopolysaccharide capsule. Both *Candida* spp. and *Malassezia* spp. have been seen in peripheral blood smears of patients with intravenous access catheter-associated fungemia. Giemsa stain is commercially available.

Procedure
1. Place slide in 100% methanol for 1 min (to fix smear).
2. Drain off methanol.
3. Flood slide with Giemsa stain (freshly diluted 1:10 with distilled water) for 5 min.
4. Wash with water; air dry.

Gomori Methenamine Silver (GMS) Stain

Of the special stains for fungi in histologic sections, methenamine silver nitrate is considered by many to be the most useful for screening clinical specimens. It provides better contrast and often stains fungal elements that may not be revealed by other procedures. Fungi are sharply delineated in black against a pale green background. The inner parts of hyphae are charcoal gray. Certain bacteria (including *Nocardia* spp.), as well as some tissue elements, also take the stain, so it must be remembered that all that is gray or black is not necessarily a fungus.

Histology laboratories routinely perform some method of GMS staining. The following are simpler and faster methods that may be used on smeared material or deparaffinized tissue.

METHENAMINE SILVER STAIN (METHOD OF MAHAN AND SALE [1978])

Note: Prepared reagents for an equally rapid method that employs a microwave oven are commercially available from Sigma-Aldrich (St. Louis, MO).

Solutions Required (All Are Aqueous Solutions)

10% chromic acid (chromium trioxide)
5% silver nitrate
3% methenamine (hexamethylenetetramine)
5% borax (sodium borate)
1% gold chloride
1% sodium metabisulfite
5% sodium thiosulfate

Preparation of Stains

Methenamine silver nitrate solution

3% methenamine .... 40 ml
5% silver nitrate .... 2 ml
5% borax .... 3 ml
Distilled water .... 35 ml

This solution must be freshly prepared before use; it can be used only once. The other solutions may be reused for up to 1 month provided fungal contamination does not occur.

Light green stock solution

Light green SF-yellowish .... 0.2 g
Distilled water .... 100.0 ml
Glacial acetic acid .... 0.2 ml

Solution is stable for 1 year.

Working solution

Stock light green solution .... 10 ml
Distilled water .... 40 ml

Solution is stable for 1 month.

Procedure

Before starting, heat Coplin jar of methenamine silver nitrate solution in oven or water bath until the solution becomes a deep golden brown (~95°C). Then, proceed as follows.

1. If slide to be stained is paraffin fixed, rehydrate (see procedure, p. 440); other slides must be fixed by heating or submerging in alcohol. Positive-control slides must be included each time the staining procedure is performed.
2. Rinse slides with water.

3. Place slides in reagents in Coplin jars as follows.
   a. Chromic acid (discard after use).........................10 min
   b. Running tap water .... 5 sec
   c. 1% sodium metabisulfite.......................................1 min
   d. Hot tap water (57-60 °C)......................................1 min
   e. Methenamine silver nitrate solution, ~95°C .... 5–10 min

   Periodically remove the control slide, wash with water, and observe microscopically to determine when optimal staining has been achieved. The color should never be so intense as to obscure the morphologic detail of a fungus. Prolonged staining time may be required when old and nonviable fungal elements or filaments of actinomycetes are suspected.

   When control shows optimal staining, rinse all slides in hot tap water and then in gradually cooler water.
   f. Distilled water ....Rinse
   g. 1% gold chloride ....10 sec
   h. Distilled water ....Rinse
   i. 5% sodium thiosulfate .... 3 min
   j. Running tap water ....30 sec
   k. Light green working solution ....30 sec

4. Rinse twice with each increasing concentration of ethanol: 70%, 95%, and absolute alcohol.
5. Dip slides twice in xylene.
6. Place drop of mounting medium on slide, and cover with coverslip.

MORE RAPID METHENAMINE SILVER STAIN (METHOD OF SHIMONO AND HARTMAN [1986])

The solutions and procedure for the Shimono-Hartman method are identical to those for the method of Mahan and Sale (see above), except that the methenamine solution is not preheated and the slides are stained while on a heating platform.

1. Begin staining procedure as for Mahan and Sale's method above, steps 3.a–d.
2. At this point, place slides on a 70°C heating platform or hot plate. The slides can be placed directly on the heated surface or in a large (150-mm-diameter) glass petri plate to handle any spillage.
3. Layer the methenamine silver solution onto the slides.
4. When the control tissue becomes golden brown (~1 min if slide is directly on heating plate, 4–5 min if slide is in a petri plate), remove slides from heat.
5. Continue from step g to completion as in Mahan and Sale's method.

   The advantages of this system are that the time required to heat the methenamine solution in volume is eliminated along with the general manipulations and handling of the hot solution. Additionally, a smaller volume of methenamine solution is usually required, resulting in cost saving.

Gram Stain (Hucker Modification)

Fungi are Gram positive but often stain poorly.

Procedure

1. Fix the smear with heat or with 100% methanol for 1 min (drain off methanol after 1 min).
2. Place crystal violet solution on the slide for 20 sec.
3. Wash gently with tap water.
4. Apply Gram iodine solution to the slide for 20 sec.
5. Wash gently with tap water.
6. Decolorize quickly in solution of equal parts acetone and 95% ethanol.
7. Wash gently with tap water.
8. Counterstain with safranin for 10 sec.
9. Wash with tap water; air dry or blot dry.

Reagents

Crystal violet solution

a. Crystal violet, 85% dye content............................2 g
   Ethyl alcohol, 95% .... 10 ml
   Dissolve the dye in alcohol.
   Add distilled water...100 ml
b. Ammonium oxalate...4 g
   Distilled water ....400 ml

Dissolve the ammonium oxalate in the water.
Mix the crystal violet-alcohol solution (a) with the ammonium oxalate solution (b).

Gram iodine solution

   Iodine..1 g
   Potassium iodide...2 g

Dissolve the iodine and potassium iodide completely in 5 ml of distilled water.

   Add distilled water............................240 ml
   Sodium bicarbonate,
   5% aqueous solution..........................60 ml

(i.e., 3 g of $NaHCO_3$ + 57 ml of distilled water)
Mix well; store in amber glass bottle.

Counterstain

   Safranin O 1g
   Ethyl alcohol, 95% ....40 ml

Dissolve the dye in the alcohol.

Add distilled water..400 ml

Mix well.

Note: A slide that has been Gram stained can be decolorized by flooding it with acetone for 30–60 sec and rinsing it well with water. Special fungus-staining procedures can then be performed on the slide.

Lactophenol Cotton Blue

Lactophenol cotton blue is used as both a mounting fluid and a stain. Lactic acid acts as a clearing agent and aids in preserving the fungal structures, phenol acts as a killing agent, glycerol prevents drying, and cotton blue gives color to the structures.

Lactic acid ....20 ml
Phenol crystals.....................................20 g
(or phenol, concentrated ....20 ml)
Glycerol (or glycerine) ....40 ml
Distilled water.....................................20 ml
Cotton blue ....0.05 g
(or 1% aqueous solution.................2 ml)

1. Dissolve the phenol in the lactic acid, glycerol, and water by gently heating (if crystals are used).
2. Add cotton blue (Poirrier's blue and aniline blue are analogous to cotton blue).
3. Mix well. For use, see p. 419.

Lactophenol Cotton Blue with Polyvinyl Alcohol (PVA) (Huber's PVA Mounting Medium, Modified)

This modification of Huber's plastic mount (Huber and Caplin, 1947) is excellent for making permanent mounts of fungal wet preparations or slide cultures. Upon drying for at least 24 h on a flat surface, these mounts are permanent and will not be dissolved in ether, xylene, or alcohols, and the fixed fungal structures remain picture-perfect for years.

Reagents
PVA; molecular weight, 70,000–100,000
Phenol, purified grade
Lactic acid, ACS reagent
Aniline blue, certified. This is analogous to cotton blue.

Preparation

1. Add 7.5 g of PVA powder to 50 ml of cold deionized water in a beaker.
2. Transfer beaker to a heated stirring plate; add a magnetic rod for mixing.
3. Place a thermometer in the beaker to monitor temperature.
4. Add 22 g of lactic acid (BEFORE adding phenol).
5. Add 22 g of phenol crystals (or 22 ml of melted phenol).
6. Add 0.05 g of aniline blue.
7. Heat and stir the solution until the temperature reaches 90°C. Do not boil or go over 100°C. Remove from hot plate.
8. Dispense into small dropper bottles. Tighten dropper bottle caps, and store at room temperature.

Procedure

Place 1 drop of PVA mounting fluid on a slide with a sample of fungal growth. Apply coverslip. Allow to dry on a flat surface.

Huber's modified PVA mounting medium may be used as a replacement for lactophenol cotton blue. Care must be taken to avoid coverslip runover or droppings on the benchtop, since they are difficult to remove. While the solution is in liquid form, it can be cleaned from surfaces with water; after it dries, a razor blade is required to remove the hardened material.

Slides can be examined microscopically at low or high dry power as soon as the slides are prepared. After adequate drying time (2–4 days), the slides can be examined under oil immersion, cleansed in xylene, decontaminated by dipping in disinfectant, or shipped (without risk of leakage) to a reference laboratory.

The solution is available in prepared form as MycoPerm Blue from a variety of vendors.

Rehydration of Paraffin-Embedded Tissue (Deparaffination)

Treat slides as follows.

> Xylene (in Coplin jar) ....12 min

Repeat, using two more jars of xylene.

> Absolute ethanol...................................... Rinse twice
> 95% ethanol .... Rinse twice
> 70% ethanol .... Rinse twice
> Distilled water .... Rinse twice

Proceed with staining procedure.

Media

PART IV Laboratory Technique

MEDIA

MEDIA

PART IV Laboratory Technique

Many of the media prepared for mycology are used relatively rarely in the typical clinical microbiology laboratory. Freshness during long storage may be maintained by dispensing agar medium into screw-cap tubes, autoclaving it, allowing it to cool as butts, and storing it (with caps tightly closed) in the refrigerator. The media must be labeled with the name of the medium, the date of preparation, and the date of expiration. When needed, the appropriate number of butts are melted in a boiling-water bath and allowed to cool as slants or cooled slightly and poured into petri plates.

Most of the media can be purchased in dehydrated form. Commercially prepared tubes or plates are also available for most, but not all, of the formulations.

Whenever a new batch of medium is placed in use, positive- and negative-control organisms must be tested. If the medium is not often used, it is advisable to run controls each time an unknown organism is tested.

Ascospore Media

ACETATE ASCOSPORE AGAR

Potassium acetate	5.00 g
Yeast extract	1.25 g
Dextrose	0.50 g
Agar	15.00 g
Distilled water	500.00 ml

1. Dissolve by boiling for 1 min; dispense in screw-cap tubes.
2. Autoclave (15 lb/in^2) for 15 min.
3. Allow tubes to cool in slanted position or as butts to be melted and slanted as needed.

GORODKOWA MEDIUM

Dextrose	1.25 g
NaCl	2.60 g
Beef extract	5.00 g
Agar	5.00 g
Distilled water	500.00 ml

1. Dispense into screw-cap tubes.
2. Autoclave (15 lb/in^2) for 15 min.
3. Allow to harden as slants or as butts to be melted and slanted as needed.

V-8 MEDIUM FOR ASCOSPORES (AND INDUCTION OF SPORULATION, ESPECIALLY DEMATIACEOUS MOULDS)

V-8 vegetable juice .... 500 ml
Dry yeast..10 g
Agar..20 g
Distilled water .... 500 ml

1. Dissolve agar in water by boiling.
2. Mix vegetable juice and dry yeast, adjust to pH 6.8 with 20% KOH, add to agar-water mixture, and mix well.
3. Dispense into screw-cap tube.
4. Autoclave (15 lb/in^2) for 15 min.
5. Allow to cool as slants or as butts to be melted and slanted as needed.

Assimilation Media (for Yeasts)

Assimilation is the utilization of a carbon (or nitrogen) source by a microorganism in the presence of oxygen. A positive reaction is indicated by the presence of growth or a pH shift in the medium. For identification of yeasts, see Tables 2.3, 2.8, and 2.9 (pp. 126, 150, and 151, respectively).

Wickerham Broth Method

Carbon assimilation medium

Yeast nitrogen base ....6.70 g
Appropriate carbohydrate ....5.00 g
Distilled water .... 100.00 ml

1. If necessary, heat to dissolve.
2. Sterilize by Seitz or membrane filter.
3. Add 0.5 ml of the solution to 4.5 ml of sterile distilled water in screw-cap tubes.

These tubes may now be stored in the refrigerator, ready for use, for 1 month.

Note: Care must be taken to ensure that carbon compounds are pure and not mixed with other carbohydrates. It is advisable to check each new lot of a carbon compound with control yeasts that can and cannot assimilate it before using the material in assimilation studies.

Nitrate assimilation medium

Yeast carbon base ....11.70 g
Potassium nitrate (KNO$_3$)..............................0.78 g
Distilled water .... 100.00 ml

1. Warm gently to dissolve.
2. Sterilize by Seitz or membrane filtration.
3. Add 0.5 ml of medium to 4.5 ml of sterile distilled water in screw-cap tubes.

These tubes may be stored in the refrigerator for 1 month.

Tubes of yeast nitrogen base without sugar and yeast carbon base without KNO_3 should be prepared and used as controls to check "carryover" of nutrients that may have been stored within the yeast cell when grown on the previous medium.

Note: The carbon and nitrate assimilation media can be distributed in 150-μl aliquots into 96-well microplates. In that instance, prepare a suspension of the yeast adjusted to an optical density of 0.21–0.29. Inoculate each well with 50 μl of the suspension (resulting in a final inoculum of 2×10^5 to 2×10^6 CFU/ml). Incubate at 25–30°C.

Test Procedure

1. Make a suspension of the yeast in sterile distilled water. This suspension should not exceed the turbidity of McFarland no. 1 standard (prepared by mixing 0.1 ml of 1% barium chloride with 9.9 ml of 1% sulfuric acid).
2. Add 0.1–0.2 ml of the yeast suspension to each tube of medium. Include a tube of yeast nitrogen base without any carbon source and a tube of yeast carbon base without KNO_3 as controls for carryover.
3. Incubate tubes at the yeast's optimal temperature. If the organism grows at 35–37°C, positive reactions are usually more rapid at this temperature. Shaking the culture tubes will also enhance growth.
4. Examine cultures over a period of 7–14 days for dense turbidity caused by growth.
5. The negative-control tubes without a carbon or nitrogen source should show no growth. If growth is present, the test is invalid because of carryover. In such cases, a small amount of growth from each tube should be transferred to another tube of the same medium and the test should be repeated.

AUXANOGRAPHIC PLATE METHOD (HALEY AND STANDARD MODIFICATION)

For carbon assimilation tests

Yeast nitrogen base .... 0.67 g
Noble or washed agar .... 20.00 g
Distilled water .... 1,000.00 ml

1. Dispense in 20-ml quantities into 18-by-150-mm screw-cap tubes.
2. Autoclave (15 lb/in²) for 15 min.
3. Allow to harden as butts. Store in refrigerator.

Test Procedure

1. Melt a tube of nitrogen base medium in a boiling-water bath; allow to cool to 47–48°C.
2. With a sterile cotton-tipped applicator, make a heavy suspension of a 24- to 72-h yeast culture in 4 ml of sterile distilled water. The density should equal that of a McFarland no. 4 or 5 standard.

3. Pour the yeast suspension into the tube of molten yeast nitrogen base agar. Mix very thoroughly by inverting tube several times.
4. Pour the yeast-agar mixture into a sterile 15-by-150-mm petri plate. Allow to solidify at room temperature.
5. Place carbohydrate disks, evenly spaced, on the plate.
6. Incubate at 30°C for 18–24 h; examine for growth around each disk. Any amount of growth around a disk indicates that the yeast assimilates that sugar. The plates may be reincubated for an additional 24 h, but reincubation is usually not necessary.

For nitrate assimilation tests

Medium

Yeast carbon base	12 g
Noble or washed agar	20 g
Distilled water	1,000 ml

Tube in 20-ml aliquots and autoclave at 15 lb/in² for 15 min. Store in refrigerator.

Peptone solution for growth control

Peptone	10 g
Distilled water	100 ml

Sterilize by filtration; store in refrigerator.

Test Procedure

1. Melt a tube of yeast carbon base medium in a boiling-water bath; allow to cool to 47–48°C.
2. Make an aqueous suspension of the yeast to a density equal to a McFarland no. 1 standard.
3. Add 0.1 ml of the yeast suspension to the tube of medium. Mix thoroughly.
4. Pour the yeast-agar mixture into a sterile 15-by-100-mm petri plate. Allow to solidify at room temperature.
5. Place ~1 mg of KNO_3 crystals on agar surface away from the center of the plate.
6. Place ~0.1 ml of peptone solution (growth control) on agar surface opposite the KNO_3 site.
7. Incubate at 30°C for 48–96 h. Growth must occur in the "peptone area" for test to be valid. If growth is seen in the peptone area, examine for growth in the KNO_3 area (growth indicates assimilation of KNO_3).

AGAR WITH INDICATOR METHOD

For carbon assimilation tests

This modification of the Wickerham medium was devised by Adams and Cooper (1974). It is easier to read than the conventional methods, yet it is equally reliable.

The medium is in the form of agar slants with an indicator added. It is less troublesome than other formulations, as it can be sterilized by autoclaving after the carbohydrates have been added. The quality of each batch of medium should be tested with standard reference strains of yeasts.

Basal medium

Bromcresol purple (1.6%)	0.2 ml
0.1 N NaOH	1.0 ml
Noble agar	2.0 g
Deionized water	90.0 ml

Heat to dissolve.

Stock carbohydrate solution

Carbohydrate	1.00 g
(if using raffinose	2.00 g)
Yeast nitrogen base	0.67 g
Deionized water	10.00 ml

Mix to dissolve; gently heat if necessary.

Preparation

1. Add each stock carbohydrate solution to a separate portion of the melted agar base; leave one portion free of carbohydrate for use as negative controls.
2. Mix well.
3. Adjust to pH 7.0.
4. Dispense in 5-ml amounts in 16-by-125-mm screw-cap tubes.
5. Sterilize by autoclaving at exactly 10 lb/in^2 for 10 min.
6. Allow to solidify in a slanted position.
7. Store in refrigerator at 4°C.

Inoculation and Incubation

1. Suspend a 2-mm loopful of pure culture in 9 ml of sterile water.
2. Inoculate each assimilation slant with 0.1 ml of the suspension.
3. Incubate at 25–30°C, examining at 7 and 14 days for abundant growth and acid production (yellow).

Assimilations are considered negative when there is no significant difference between the growth of the organism on the carbohydrate medium and that on the control medium without carbohydrate.

MODIFIED POTASSIUM NITRATE ASSIMILATION TEST

(Pincus et al., 1988)

Potassium nitrate .... 1.4 g
Yeast carbon base .... 1.6 g
Bromothymol blue .... 0.12 g
Noble agar .... 16.0 g
Distilled water .... 1,000 ml

1. Adjust final pH to 5.9–6.0.
2. Dispense into screw-cap tubes.
3. Autoclave at 15 lb/in^2 for 15 min.
4. Cool tubes in slanted position.

Test Procedure

1. Inoculate the surface of the slant with yeast isolate.
2. Incubate at 25–30°C.
3. Examine daily; most positive results are seen within 24 h.

Interpretation

Positive: Slant becomes blue-green or blue.
Negative: Slant remains greenish yellow.

Birdseed Agar (Niger Seed Agar; Staib Agar)

Guizotia abyssinica seed .... 50 g

(Commonly known as niger seed; it is available at most stores that sell bird feed.)

Distilled water .... 100 ml

1. Pulverize in blender.
2. Add 900 ml of distilled water.
3. Boil for 30 min.
4. Cool and filter through four layers of gauze, and then add enough distilled water to make volume 1,000 ml.
5. Add:

KH_2PO_4 .... 1 g
Creatinine .... 1 g
Agar .... 15 g

Note: Glucose, 1 g, is added in the formulation for identification of *Candida dubliniensis* (p. 125), but it can inhibit pigment production by *Cryptococcus neoformans* and *Cryptococcus gattii*. Chloramphenicol, 1 g, may be added in the formulation for pigment production and isolation of *C. neoformans* and *C. gattii* (pp. 147 and 149).

6. Mix well. Autoclave (15 lb/in²) for 15 min.
7. Pour into tubes and cool in slanted position or as butts to be melted and slanted or plated as needed.

Test Procedure

A. For pigment production by *C. neoformans*/*C. gattii*

Inoculate with suspected *Cryptococcus* sp. (fresh isolate) and incubate at 25–30°C for no more than 7 days.

Only *C. neoformans* and *C. gattii* produce phenoloxidase, which breaks down the substrate, resulting in the production of melanin and the development of dark brown to black colonies. Colonies of other yeasts are cream to beige; see p. 148).

Chemically defined tests such as the caffeic acid disk test also detect phenoloxidase and have the advantage of rapidity and sensitivity; see p. 426.

B. For differentiation of *C. dubliniensis* versus *Candida albicans*

1. Inoculate a plate of the medium with a 48-h-old colony; streak for isolation.
2. Incubate at 30°C for 48–72 h. Examine macroscopic morphology of colonies (see Table 2.4 [p. 128]).

Brain Heart Infusion (BHI) Agar

BHI agar is classically recommended for the cultivation of fastidious pathogenic fungi, such as *Blastomyces* spp. and *Histoplasma capsulatum*. The ingredients are listed here for ease of comparison with other enriched fungal media that are commonly used.

BHI	8.0 g
Peptic digest of animal tissue	5.0 g
Pancreatic digest of casein	16.0 g
Sodium chloride	5.0 g
Dextrose	2.0 g
Disodium phosphate	2.5 g
Agar	13.5 g
Distilled water	1,000 ml

Antibiotics are often added to inhibit bacteria, and sheep blood is added to further enrich the medium and enhance the growth of fastidious pathogenic fungi.

Buffered Charcoal-Yeast Extract (BCYE) Agar

This medium is best known for cultivation of *Legionella* spp., but it has also proved useful in the recovery of *Nocardia* spp.

Excellent recovery occurs on nonselective and selective BCYE agars. The formulation containing vancomycin (BCYE-PAV) is preferred over the formulation with cefamandole (PAC) for the primary isolation of *Nocardia* spp. from specimens likely to contain other organisms. The media are commercially available. The contents of BCYE media (BBL, Sparks, MD) are

Yeast extract	10.0 g
L-Cysteine HCl	0.4 g
Ferric pyrophosphate	0.25 g
ACES [N-(2-acetamido)-2-aminoethanesulfonic acid] buffer	10.0 g
Charcoal, activated	2.0 g
α-Ketoglutarate	1.0 g
Agar	15.0 g
Purified water	1,000.0 ml

BCYE Selective Agar with PAV has added:

Polymyxin B	40,000 units
Anisomycin	80.0 mg
Vancomycin	0.5 mg

Canavanine Glycine Bromothymol Blue (CGB) Agar

(Klein et al., 2009; Kwon-Chung et al., 1982)

CGB agar is used for the differentiation of *C. gattii* versus *C. neoformans*.

Solution A

Glycine	10 g
KH_2PO_4	1 g
$MgSO_4$	1 g
Thiamine HCl	1 mg
L-Canavanine sulfate	30 mg
Distilled water	100 ml

1. Dissolve ingredients; adjust to pH 5.6.
2. Filter sterilize the solution using a 0.45 (or 0.22)-μm filter.
3. Store in refrigerator if not used same day.

Solution B

Bromothymol blue ....0.4 g
0.01 N NaOH..64 ml
Distilled water...36 ml

1. Dissolve the bromothymol blue in the NaOH.
2. Add the water.

Medium Preparation

Distilled water..880 ml
Solution B...20 ml
Agar...20 g

Mix in flask and autoclave at 25 lb/in^2 for 15 min. Cool to ~50°C. Add

Solution A...100 ml

Mix well and dispense into plates or into tubes for slants.

CGB agar can be stored in the refrigerator for at least 3 months without losing its efficacy.

Inoculate agar with a small amount of the isolate. Incubate at 25–30°C for 48 h.

Interpretation

C. gattii yields a positive reaction. The medium turns from greenish yellow to cobalt blue; this is due to the organism's ability to grow in the presence of L-canavanine and utilize glycine as its sole source of carbon and nitrogen, causing an increase in pH. Some *C. gattii* isolates may take up to 5 days to yield a positive reaction.

C. neoformans yields a negative (or very weak) reaction. The medium remains greenish yellow, as the organism is inhibited by canavanine and does not utilize glycine. If the inoculum is too heavy, a weak reaction may occur; this should be interpreted as negative.

Casein Agar

For characterization of some dematiaceous fungi.

Solution A

Skim milk (dehydrated or
instant nonfat dry milk) ....10 g
Distilled water..90 ml

Add milk with constant stirring to avoid lumping.

Solution B

Agar...3 g
Distilled water..97 ml

1. Autoclave each solution separately at 15 lb/in² for 10 min.
2. Cool both solutions to 45–50°C, and then combine solutions and mix well.
3. Pour into petri plates (or into screw-cap tubes and allow to solidify as butts to be melted and poured as needed).

Inoculate an area approximately the size of a dime (15-mm diameter) heavily with a pure culture. Include positive- and negative-control cultures. Three or four organisms can be tested on one 100-mm-diameter plate if they are evenly spaced. Incubate at 30 or 37°C for 2 weeks. Examine every few days for clearing (hydrolysis) of casein around or directly beneath the colony.

For results with "black yeasts," see Table 2.16 (p. 246).

CHROMagar Candida Medium

CHROMagar Candida medium (Becton, Dickinson and Company, Sparks, MD; CHROMagar, Paris, France) is for the isolation of all, and the definitive differentiation of a few, of the most commonly encountered yeasts in the clinical laboratory. (Image Appendix Figure 38.) It has proven acceptable for use as the sole primary fungal medium for specimens in which yeasts are the primary concern, i.e., throats, urines, and genitals (so-called "TUG" specimens) and blood cultures smear-positive for yeast. It is extremely effective in detecting mixed yeast populations in clinical specimens.

Chromogenic substrates produce unique and specific colors for the identification of

C. albicans (light to medium green)

Candida tropicalis (dark blue to metallic blue-purple)

Candida krusei (light rose with a whitish border; rough)

Studies have shown that further identification tests for these three species are not necessary.

Other yeasts (cream color or light to dark mauve; *Candida glabrata* forms pink colonies but cannot be reliably distinguished on this basis from other yeasts)

Candida rugosa (unique blue-green with whitish border; slightly rough)

Trichosporon spp. (dark pink to purple; rough)

Lodderomyces elongisporus (turquoise)

Filamentous fungi (colors that may differ from those exhibited on routine mycology agar, but their microscopic morphology does not change)

Notes:

- Plates produce the best color development in the colonies when incubated at 37°C (they should NOT be incubated below 30°C).

- Incubate in atmospheric air, not in CO_2, for 36–48 h.

- It is advisable to minimize exposure of the plates to light both before and during incubation.

- All yeasts and filamentous fungi will grow, while bacteria are inhibited by chloramphenicol. The moulds may not have their typical colony color, but they will retain their characteristic microscopic morphology (Morhaime et al., 2004).

CHROMagar Candida Plus Medium

CHROMagar Candida Plus medium (CHROMagar, Paris, France) consists of a proprietary chromogenic substrate for detection and identification of *C. auris*, and other *Candida* spp., by colony color (de Jong et al., 2021; Mulet Bayona et al., 2022). This formulation was specifically developed for the detection of *C. auris*, especially in mixed cultures. There are a few rare species that have the same phenotype as *C. auris* so results should be considered preliminary.

    C. auris (light blue with a light blue halo)

CHROMID Candida Agar

CHROMID Candida agar (bioMérieux, Inc., Durham, NC) is a chromogenic medium for the culture and isolation of yeasts, the identification of *C. albicans*, and the separation of other yeast species into two groups. Most filamentous fungi will also grow. Bacteria are inhibited. It can be useful in detecting mixed yeast populations in clinical specimens. The plates are incubated in ambient air for 48 h at 35–37°C; some organisms require 30°C for optimal growth.

    The colony colors indicate the following.

    Blue = *C. albicans* or *C. dubliniensis* (some strains of *Trichosporon* spp. can be blue, but the colony morphology is very different from that of the *Candida* spp.; *C. dubliniensis* is often turquoise)

    Pink = *C. tropicalis*, *Candida kefyr*, *Candida lusitaniae*, or *Candida guilliermondii*

    White, dry, downy = *C. krusei*

    White or cream, smoother = other yeasts and some filamentous moulds (*Cryptococcus* spp. may be white, pink, or blue)

    Note: Plates must always be stored and incubated in the dark.

Chromogenic Candida Agar (Brilliance Candida Agar)

Chromogenic Candida Agar (Brilliance Candida Agar) (Oxoid, Basingstoke, UK) consists of a proprietary chromogenic substrate for detection and identification of the following *Candida* spp. by colony morphology and color: *C. albicans*, *C. tropicalis*, and *C. krusei*.

  C. albicans/*C. dubliniensis* (light to medium green)

  C. tropicalis (dark blue)

  C. krusei (pink-brown with a whitish border)

  C. glabrata and other yeasts (beige, yellow, brown)

Cornmeal Agar

Cornmeal	40 g
Agar	20 g
Tween 80 (polysorbate 80)	10 ml
Distilled water	1,000 ml

1. Mix cornmeal well with 500 ml of water; heat to 65°C for 1 h.
2. Filter through gauze and then paper until clear; restore to original volume.
3. Adjust to pH 6.6–6.8; add agar dissolved in 500 ml of water.
4. Add Tween 80; autoclave (15 lb/in²) for 15 min.
5. Dispense into petri plates or into screw-cap tubes to form butts to be melted and poured as needed.

Cornmeal with Tween 80 is used in distinguishing the different genera of yeasts and the various species of *Candida* and can also be useful in slide cultures, as it stimulates conidiation in many fungi.

If 10 g of dextrose is added to the medium in place of the Tween 80, the medium can be used to differentiate *Trichophyton mentagrophytes* from *Trichophyton rubrum* on the basis of pigment production (see Table 2.19 [p. 302]).

For studying the morphology of yeasts, the **Dalmau method** is recommended. It is performed by using one-fourth or one-third of a cornmeal-Tween 80 agar plate for each organism. (Image Appendix Figure 41.)

1. Make one streak of a young, actively growing yeast down the center of the area (do not cut the agar); make three or four streaks across the first to dilute the inoculum.
2. Cover with a 22-by-22-mm coverslip.
3. Incubate at room temperature, in the dark, for 3 days.
4. Examine by placing the plate, without its lid, on the microscope stage and using the low-power (×100) and high-dry (×400) objectives. The most characteristic morphology (especially the terminal chlamydospores of *C. albicans*) is often found near the edge of the coverslip.

C. albicans should be included as a control for production of chlamydospores and blastoconidia.

Dermatophyte Test Medium (DTM)

Specimens from hair, skin, or nails may be inoculated directly onto DTM and incubated at room temperature with the cap of the culture tube loose. Dermatophytes change the color of the medium from yellow to red within 14 days. Care must be taken in specimen collection and interpretation of results, as many contaminants and other fungi increase the number of false-positive changes in color. DTM does not interfere with macroscopic morphology and microscopic characteristics of the dermatophytes, but it cannot be used to study pigment production because of the intense red color of the indicator. (Image Appendix Figure 42.)

Phytone	10.0 g
Dextrose	10.0 g
Agar	20.0 g
Phenol red solution	40.0 ml
0.8 M HCl	6.0 ml
Cycloheximide	0.5 g
Gentamicin sulfate	0.1 g
Chlortetracycline HCl	0.1 g
Distilled water	1,000.0 ml

1. Dissolve the phytone, dextrose, and agar by boiling them in the water.
2. While stirring, add 40 ml of phenol red solution (0.5 g of phenol red dissolved in 15 ml of 0.1 N NaOH made up to 100 ml with distilled water).
3. While stirring, add the 0.8 M HCl.
4. Dissolve cycloheximide in 2 ml of acetone, and add to hot medium while stirring.
5. Dissolve gentamicin sulfate in 2 ml of distilled water, and add to medium while stirring.
6. Autoclave at 12 lb/in² for 10 min, and cool to ~47°C.
7. Dissolve chlortetracycline in 25 ml of sterile distilled water in sterile container, and add to medium while stirring.
8. Dispense into sterile 1-oz (~30-ml) screw-cap bottles or screw-cap tubes; slant and cool. The final pH of the medium is 5.5 ± 0.1, and the medium should be yellow in color.
9. Store in refrigerator at 4°C.

Esculin Agar

Used in the differentiation of *Candida norvegensis* from similar *Candida* spp.

When esculin (a glycoside) is hydrolyzed, it yields esculetin; esculetin, in the presence of an iron salt, forms a brown-black complex that diffuses into the medium. The medium, containing esculin, ferric citrate, and supportive ingredients for growth, is commercially available (this formulation does not contain bile salts).

Test Procedure

1. Streak several actively growing isolated colonies onto the slanted medium.
2. Incubate tubes aerobically at 35–37°C (with caps loosened) for 24–72 h for *Candida* spp.
3. Observe for a black diffusing color in the medium surrounding the colonies.

Interpretation

Positive hydrolysis: Black color diffused in medium.
Negative: No black color in the medium.
For select *Candida* spp., see Table 2.6 (p. 134).

Fermentation Broth for Yeasts

Broth

Bromothymol blue	0.04 g
Powdered yeast extract	4.50 g
Peptone	7.50 g
Distilled water	1,000.00 ml

Stock carbohydrate solutions

Carbohydrate	6 g
Distilled water	100 ml

1. Filter sterilize through a 0.22-μm-pore-size filter.
2. Dissolve bromothymol blue in 3 ml of 95% ethanol. Add to other ingredients.
3. Dispense 2-ml aliquots into narrow screw-cap tubes.
4. Place Durham tube (mouth down) into each tube of broth.
5. Autoclave at 15 lb/in² for 15 min. Allow to cool.
6. Add 1 ml of each carbohydrate solution to separate tubes of broth. (After the carbohydrates have been added, the broths may be stored for 1 month in the refrigerator.)

Test Procedure

1. Inoculate each of the carbohydrate broths with a pure culture of the organism grown on a sugar-free medium. Be sure that the Durham tube is completely filled with broth before incubating.

2. Incubate at room temperature for 10–14 days, examining at 48- to 72-h intervals for production of gas (observed in Durham tube).

Gas production is the only reliable evidence of carbohydrate fermentation; acid production (color change in indicator) may simply indicate that the carbohydrate has been assimilated. All fermented carbohydrates will also be assimilated, but many carbohydrates that are assimilated are not necessarily fermented. For identification of yeasts, see Table 2.3 (p. 126) and Table 2.9 (p. 151).

Yeast fermentation broth is commercially available from Remel (Lenexa, KS) (with bromothymol blue) and from Becton, Dickinson and Company/BBL (Sparks, MD) (without bromothymol blue).

Inhibitory Mould Agar (IMA)

IMA is an enriched medium that contains chloramphenicol (some formulations also contain gentamicin) but no cycloheximide; bacteria are inhibited, while fungi grow well. When specimens are contaminated with bacteria, IMA is especially useful in recovering fungi that are inhibited by cycloheximide and would not grow on Mycosel agar, e.g., *C. neoformans/gattii*, *Lomentospora prolificans*, the mucormycetes, many species of *Candida* and *Aspergillus*, and most saprobic or opportunistic fungi. IMA has been shown to be superior to Sabouraud dextrose agar as a primary medium (Scognamiglio et al., 2010). IMA is commercially available in dehydrated and prepared form from many suppliers. The ingredients are listed below to allow comparison with other enriched fungal media.

Pancreatic digest of casein	3.0 g
Peptic digest of animal tissue	2.0 g
Yeast extract	5.0 g
Dextrose	5.0 g
Starch	2.0 g
Dextrin	1.0 g
Chloramphenicol	0.125 g
Sodium phosphate	2.0 g
Magnesium sulfate	0.8 g
Ferrous sulfate	0.04 g
Sodium chloride	0.04 g
Manganese sulfate	0.16 g
Agar	15.0 g
Distilled water	1,000.0 ml

Leeming-Notman Agar (Modified)

(Kaneko et al., 2007; Leeming and Notman, 1987)

For isolation of *Malassezia* spp. Provides better recovery of some *Malassezia* spp. than does Dixon agar. It is also a good medium for maintenance of *Malassezia* cultures.

Bacteriological peptone .... 10.0 g
Glucose.. 10.0 g
Yeast extract ....2.0 g
Ox bile, desiccated ....8.0 g
Glycerol.. 10.0 ml
Glycerol monostearate......................................0.5 g
Olive oil.. 20.0 ml
Agar.. 15.0 g
Deionized water....................................... 1,000.0 ml

1. Combine the above ingredients and let stand for ~10 min.
2. Adjust pH to 6.2 with 1 M HCl.

Tween 60 ....5.0 ml

3. Warm Tween 60 to 60–70°C before adding to mixture.
4. Boil mixture briefly to dissolve components.
5. Autoclave 15 lb/in^2 for 20 min.
6. Cool to ~50°C. (Add antimicrobial solutions if desired: chloramphenicol 50 µg/ml; cycloheximide 200 µg/ml.)
7. Pour into petri plates. Store in refrigerator.

Lysozyme Medium

For aerobic actinomycetes.

Basal glycerol broth

Peptone...1.0 g
Beef extract ....0.6 g
Glycerol.. 14.0 ml
Distilled water ....200.0 ml

1. Combine ingredients; mix well to dissolve.
2. Pour 95 ml of broth into a separate container.

3. Dispense the remainder into screw-cap tubes in 5-ml quantities. These will be used as control tubes.
4. Autoclave the tubes and the separate portion at 15 lb/in^2 for 15 min.

Lysozyme broth

Lysozyme	50 mg
0.01 N HCl	50 ml

1. Sterilize by filtration.
2. Aseptically add 5 ml of lysozyme solution to the 95 ml of basal glycerol broth.
3. Mix well.
4. Dispense 5-ml aliquots into sterile screw-cap tubes.
5. Store all tubes in the refrigerator.

Test Procedure

1. Inoculate a tube of control broth (glycerol broth without lysozyme) and a tube of lysozyme broth with the organism to be tested.
2. Incubate at 25–30°C until control tube shows good growth. The organism must grow in the control tube for the test to be valid. Growth in the lysozyme broth indicates resistance to the enzyme.

A known *Streptomyces* sp. should be used as a susceptible control organism; i.e., growth must occur in the control tube but not in the lysozyme tube to prove the lysozyme is active. See Table 2.1 (p. 110).

Mycosel Agar

Mycosel agar is a selective medium that is frequently part of the battery that is used for primary isolation of fungi. It contains chloramphenicol to inhibit the growth of bacteria and cycloheximide to inhibit fungi that are commonly considered saprobes. However, cycloheximide also inhibits the growth of some known pathogens, e.g., *C. neoformans/C. gattii, Aspergillus fumigatus, L. prolificans, Talaromyces marneffei,* some species of *Candida,* and most mucormycetes, as well as many other opportunistic fungi.

The medium is also used to test an organism's ability to grow in the presence of cycloheximide; the interpretive information may state the level of cycloheximide against which the reference organisms were tested. Mycosel agar contains 0.04% cycloheximide.

Mycosel is produced in prepared and dehydrated form from many suppliers; the formulations may vary slightly.

Papaic digest of soybean meal	10.0 g
Dextrose	10.0 g
Agar	15.5 g

Cycloheximide...400.0 mg
Chloramphenicol... 50.0 mg
Distilled water .... 1,000.0 ml

Potato Dextrose Agar and Potato Flake Agar

Potato dextrose agar and potato flake agar are available commercially prepared or in dehydrated form and should be prepared according to manufacturers' instructions. They support the growth of most clinically encountered fungi, and some laboratories use one of them as a primary medium. They can sometimes stimulate the production of conidia and pigment when other media fail to do so and are therefore often recommended for slide cultures or for inducing an isolate to exhibit a characteristic pigment.

Rapid Assimilation of Trehalose (RAT) Broth

(Stockman and Roberts, 1985, and personal communication)

The RAT test is used for the rapid identification of *C. glabrata*. It is ONLY for yeasts that

- form colonies that are relatively slow growing and small
- are microscopically small and oval and have terminal budding
- form neither germ tubes nor pseudohyphae in the germ tube test
- are suggestive of *C. glabrata* on CHROMagar Candida agar

The RAT test is based on the utilization of trehalose in the presence of a protein inhibitor, cycloheximide. This broth contains more nitrogen and carbohydrate than the traditional Wickerham assimilation broth and incorporates an indicator, bromcresol green, that has a low pH range (3.8–5.4). *C. glabrata* utilizes the trehalose and produces acid more quickly than do other yeast isolates. (Image Appendix Figure 39.)

Preparation of Reagents

Yeast nitrogen base

A. Stock solution

1. Add 6.7 g of yeast nitrogen base to 100 ml of distilled water.
2. Dissolve by gently heating.
3. Filter sterilize.

B. Working solution

Dilute by combining 20 ml of the stock yeast nitrogen base solution with 80 ml of sterile distilled water.

40% Trehalose

1. Add 4 g of trehalose to 10 ml of distilled water.
2. Dissolve by gently heating at 56°C.
3. Filter sterilize.

Bromcresol green

1. Add 0.1 g of bromcresol green to 7.1 ml of 0.01 N NaOH. (Prepare 0.01 N NaOH by adding 0.4 g of NaOH to 1,000 ml [1 liter] of distilled water. Mix to dissolve.)
2. Dilute by adding 117.9 ml of distilled water.
3. Filter sterilize.

Cycloheximide

1. Add 0.1 g of cycloheximide to 10 ml of distilled water.
2. Gently heat to dissolve.
3. Filter sterilize.
4. Aliquot in 0.5-ml amounts. Store at –30°C (stable for 6 months).

Preparation of Rat Broth

Yeast nitrogen base (working solution)	80 ml
40% trehalose	10 ml
Bromcresol green	10 ml
Cycloheximide	0.4 ml

1. Combine ingredients and mix well.
2. Adjust pH to 5.4–5.5.
3. Dispense into sterile screw-cap tubes.

Test Procedure

1. Dispense 3 drops of RAT broth into as many microtiter wells as are needed for tests and controls.
2. Using a microtiter grid form, label each space as to culture number or control.
3. Emulsify a **<u>HEAVY</u>** inoculum of the yeast into the broth in the appropriate well.
4. Incubate plate for 1 h at 37°C in ambient air; do not cover with tape.

(When the test is finished, the used wells can be covered with tape and held until the remainder of the wells have been used.)

Interpretation

Positive: Broth changes from a blue to yellow; *C. glabrata*.
Negative: Broth remains blue or green; isolate is NOT *C. glabrata* (further testing is required for complete identification).

Quality Control

Positive control: *C. glabrata*
Negative control: *C. albicans*

> *Notes:*

- This method is approved by the Clinical and Laboratory Standards Institute (CLSI, M35-A2, 2008).
- Do not incubate longer than 1 h at 37°C. Depending on the source medium, false positives can occur if overincubated; CHROMagar Candida is a better source medium than Sabouraud dextrose agar (see Murray et al., 2005).
- Some reports indicate that incubation at 42°C for 3 h may increase the specificity of the test; this is not necessary if the yeasts to be tested are properly selected as described above. Only those meeting the criteria should be tested by this method.
- Beware: bacteria and *Prototheca* spp. can give positive results.

A commercially available RAT test is available (Remel, Lenexa, KS). It is performed in small tubes and incubated at 42°C for 3 h.

Sabouraud Brain Heart Infusion Agar (SABHI Agar)

SABHI agar combines two commonly used media. It has the glucose content of Sabouraud dextrose agar and the calf brain and beef heart infusions (albeit half as much) found in brain heart infusion agar. Antibiotic and/or sheep blood can be added to the formulation. It is favored as a medium for primary isolation of fungi in a number of clinical mycology laboratories.

Glucose	21.00 g
Neopeptone	5.00 g
Proteose peptone	5.00 g
Calf brains, infusion	100.00 g
Beef heart, infusion	125.00 g
Sodium chloride	2.50 g
Disodium phosphate	1.25 g
Agar	15.00 g
Distilled water	1,000 ml
(Optional: Chloramphenicol	50 mg
Sheep blood	100 ml)

1. Mix reagents (without antibiotic or blood) and bring to boil.
2. Autoclave at 15 lb/in² for 15 min.
3. If antibiotic and/or blood is to be added, cool medium to 50–52°C.
4. Add chloramphenicol (in 10 ml of sterile distilled water).

5. Add the sheep blood.

6. Dispense into plates, or tubes for slants, and cool.

Sabouraud Dextrose Agar (SDA)

SDA is much used in mycology laboratories but has limitations as a medium for primary isolation of fungi directly from specimens (see Scognamiglio et al., 2010).

Emmons modification

The Emmons modification differs from the original formula in that it has an approximately neutral pH and contains only 2% dextrose.

Most mycologists no longer consider it necessary or desirable to use 4% sugar, as in the original formula, and a pH near neutrality has been found to be better for some fungi. The very acid original formula once recommended for suppression of bacterial contaminants can now be replaced by media containing antibiotics.

Dextrose	20 g
Peptone	10 g
Agar	17 g
Distilled water	1,000 ml

Final pH, 6.9.

Original formula

Some workers still prefer the original formula.

Dextrose	40 g
Peptone	10 g
Agar	15 g
Distilled water	1,000 ml

Final pH, 5.6.

1. To prepare either of the formulas, dissolve the ingredients by boiling, and dispense in tubes if slants are to be made. Leave in bulk if plates are to be poured.

2. Autoclave at 15 lb/in^2 for 10 min.

3. Allow tubes to cool in slanted position or pour plates.

4. Store in refrigerator.

Both formulations of SDA are commercially available in prepared or dehydrated form.

Note: Can also be formulated with chloramphenicol and gentamicin to inhibit bacterial growth for non-sterile specimens.

Sabouraud Dextrose Agar with 15% NaCl

Testing for tolerance to 15% sodium chloride (NaCl) can be valuable for identifying some dematiaceous (black) fungi.

SDA ....500 ml
NaCl..75 g

1. Heat to dissolve.
2. Dispense in tubes; autoclave at 15 lb/in^2 for 10 min.
3. Allow to solidify as butts to be melted and slanted as needed.

Test Procedure

1. Place a pinpoint inoculum of the organism to be tested on a slant of the agar.
2. Incubate at room temperature.

The organism is considered to be strongly inhibited if its colony diameter is <2 mm at 21 days. If the colony surpasses 2 mm, the organism is considered tolerant of 15% NaCl. For application to "black yeasts" see Table 2.16 (p. 246).

Sabouraud Dextrose Broth

Dextrose... 20 g
Peptone.. 10 g
Distilled water .... 1,000 ml

Final pH, 5.7.

1. Dissolve ingredients; dispense into tubes.
2. Autoclave (15 lb/in^2) for 10 min.

Noting the manner in which yeasts grow in this broth can assist in their identification (see Table 2.2 [p. 124] and Table 2.3 [p. 126]). Sabouraud dextrose broth is also used for the detection of fungal contaminants in various products.

Starch Hydrolysis Agar

For aerobic actinomycetes.

Nutrient agar....................................... 23 g
Potato starch....................................... 10 g
Demineralized water................................. 1,000 ml

1. Dissolve agar in 500 ml of water by boiling.
2. Dissolve starch in 250 ml of water by boiling.
3. Combine and add 250 ml of water.
4. Dispense into screw-cap tubes.
5. Autoclave (15 lb/in^2) for 30 min.
6. Allow to cool as butts; melt down and pour into petri plates as needed.

Test Procedure

1. Inoculate a 10-mm-diameter round area of agar heavily with a pure culture of the organism to be tested.
2. Incubate at optimal growth temperature until good growth occurs.
3. Flood the area around the growth with Gram iodine.

Starch hydrolysis is demonstrated by a colorless (complete hydrolysis) or red (partial hydrolysis) area around the growth.

Unhydrolyzed starch in the medium will produce a deep blue to purple color in the presence of iodine (see Table 2.1 [p. 110]).

Trichophyton Agars

The set of seven media tests the growth factor requirements of the species of *Trichophyton*. They are often helpful in differentiating the species. It is seldom necessary to utilize the entire battery; ordinarily, no. 1 and no. 4 are the most commonly required.

Trichophyton agars are available commercially, either prepared or in dehydrated form. Their compositions are as follows.

No. 1, casein agar base (vitamin free)
No. 2, casein agar base plus inositol
No. 3, casein agar base plus inositol and thiamine
No. 4, casein agar base plus thiamine
No. 5, casein agar base plus nicotinic acid
No. 6, ammonium nitrate agar base
No. 7, ammonium nitrate agar base plus histidine

Inoculation of Media

The center of a slant of each medium must be inoculated with a small and equal-size amount of pure culture grown on routine medium with or without antibiotics. It is important that the culture be free of bacteria, for many bacteria synthesize vitamins that may invalidate the test. Care must also be taken not to transfer any of the source medium with the organism, as this may supply carryover nutrients and cause false reactions.

The following method of inoculation dilutes possible carryover nutrients and ensures that each slant receives an equal inoculum.

1. Make a homogeneous suspension of fuzzy or granular colonies in sterile saline or water.
2. Place 2 drops of the suspension on each slant of medium.

Test Procedure

1. Incubate tubes at 25–30°C for 2 weeks, preferably in a reclining position for the first few days so that the inoculum remains evenly dispensed over the surface of the agar.
2. Examine periodically for growth.
3. The tube that shows maximum growth is recorded as 4+. Other tubes are graded by comparison.

For interpretation of results, see Table 2.19 (p. 302) and Table 2.20 (p. 310).

Tyrosine Agar

For characterization of the "black yeasts."

Nutrient agar	23 g
Tyrosine	5 g
Distilled water	1,000 ml

1. Dissolve the agar in the distilled water by boiling (swirl frequently).
2. Add tyrosine, taking care to distribute the crystals evenly throughout the agar.
3. Adjust to pH 7.0; autoclave at 15 lb/in² for 15 min.

If the agar is too hot when poured, the time required for solidification will be long enough to permit settling out of the tyrosine granules. To avoid this, the medium should be allowed to cool to 45–48°C before being poured and the flask should be mixed well while the plates are poured to ensure an even distribution of the crystals. If the medium is to be stored for a long period, pour well-mixed medium, with evenly distributed crystals, into tubes. Allow to solidify as butts and refrigerate.

Test Procedure

1. When needed, place tubes of agar in boiling water bath to melt, cool to 45–48°C, mix well to resuspend crystals, pour into petri plates, and allow to solidify.
2. Heavily inoculate an area of agar 10 mm in diameter with a pure culture.
3. Incubate at the temperature at which the isolate grows best, i.e., at 25–30°C or at 35–37°C, for 2–3 weeks.
4. Examine every 3 or 4 days for clearing of the medium, around or directly beneath the colony, which indicates hydrolysis.

For interpretation of results, see Table 2.16 (p. 246).

Urea Agar

This medium is used for the differentiation of the yeastlike fungi and also in the identification of yeasts and *Trichophyton* species. It is the same as used in bacteriology and is commercially available in prepared or dehydrated form.

A. Urea agar base (Christensen) .... 29 g
    Distilled water .... 100 ml

Dissolve the powder in the water and sterilize by filtration.

B. Agar .... 15 g
    Distilled water .... 900 ml

1. Dissolve the agar in the water, and sterilize by autoclaving at 15 lb/in^2 for 15 min.
2. Cool the agar to ~50°C.
3. Add the 100 ml of sterile urea agar base.
4. Mix well; dispense aseptically into sterile tubes.
5. Allow to cool in slanted position to form butt about 1 in. (2.5 cm) deep and slant ~1.5 in. (3.8 cm) long.

    Urease-positive organisms produce an alkaline reaction indicated by a pink-red color.

Water Agar

To induce sporulation of some mucormycetes that do not sporulate on solid media.
    Nutritionally deficient media are known to enhance production of spores and conidia. Water agar is used for that purpose.

    Agar .... 20 g
    Distilled water .... 1,000 ml

1. Mix reagents; bring to boil to dissolve agar.
2. Dispense into tubes.
3. Autoclave at 15 lb/in^2 for 15 min.
4. Cool in slanted position or store as butts to be melted down and used as slants or plates when needed.

Image Appendix

The photographs on the following pages are presented to help in gaining a better visual image and understanding of descriptions that appear in the text of this book. The first 37 images pertain to direct microscopic examination of specimens. The remaining 5 pertain to media and tests that contribute to identification.

Stain abbreviations: GMS, Gomori methenamine silver; H&E, hematoxylin and eosin; PAS, periodic acid-Schiff.

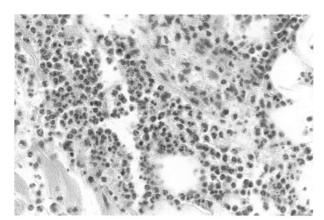

1. Suppurative inflammation/microabscess. Low magnification. H&E (see pp. 21, 24, and 26).

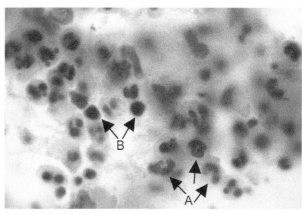

2. Suppurative inflammation: (A) polymorphonuclear leukocytes (neutrophils); (B) few lymphocytes. High magnification. H&E (see pp. 23 and 24).

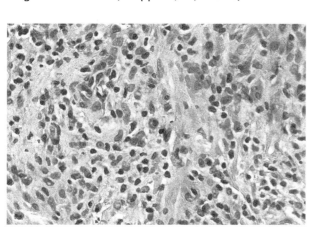

3. Chronic inflammation. Low magnification. H&E (see p. 26).

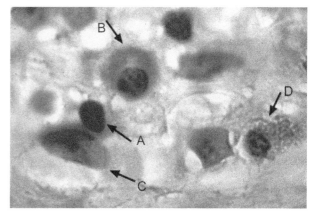

4. Chronic inflammation showing (A) lymphocyte, (B) plasma cell, (C) histiocyte, (D) eosinophil. High magnification. H&E (see pp. 22–24 and 26).

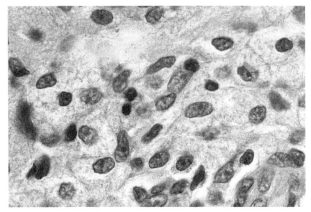

5. Epithelioid histiocytes and few lymphocytes. H&E (see p. 22).

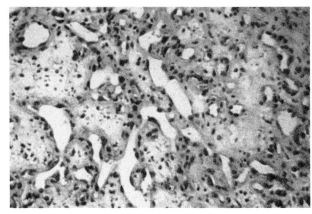

6. Granulation tissue. H&E (see p. 23).

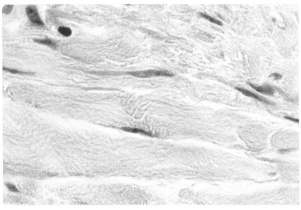

7. Collagen and fibroblasts. High magnification. H&E (see pp. 21 and 22).

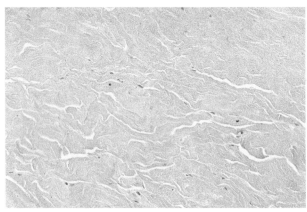

8. Fibrosis. Low magnification. H&E (see p. 22).

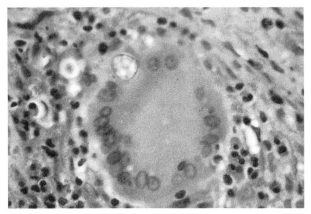

9. Langhans giant cell with engulfed immature spherule of *Coccidioides*. H&E (see pp. 22 and 26). (Courtesy of Joan Barenfanger.)

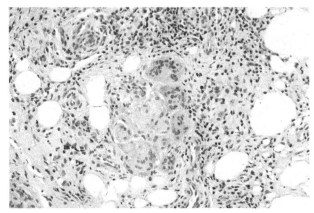

10. Granuloma composed of giant cells. H&E (see pp. 22, 23, and 27).

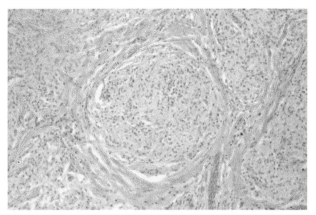

11. Granuloma with epithelioid histiocytes. H&E (see pp. 23 and 27).

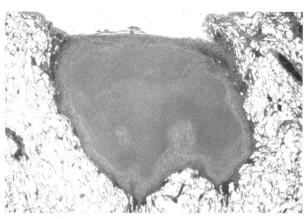

12. Granuloma with caseous necrosis in center. H&E. Low magnification (see pp. 21, 23, 24, and 27). (Courtesy of Douglas Flieder.)

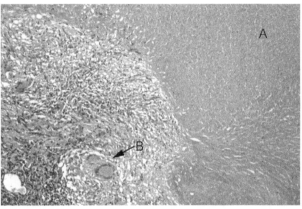

13. Granuloma with caseous necrosis (A); higher magnification of Image Appendix Figure 12. Giant cell (B, at arrow) in rim. H&E (see pp. 21–24 and 27). (Courtesy of Douglas Flieder.)

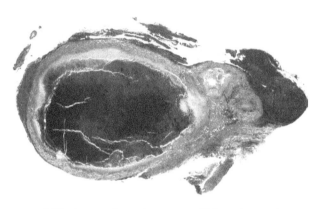

14. Calcified granuloma in a case of histoplasmosis. Low magnification. H&E (see pp. 21 and 55). (Courtesy of Douglas Flieder.)

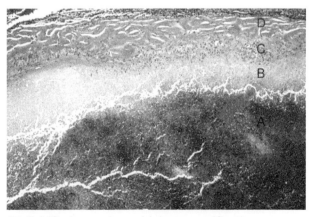

15. Calcified granuloma; higher magnification of Image Appendix Figure 14. (A) Calcification; (B) necrosis; (C) histiocytes; (D) fibrosis. H&E (see pp. 21, 22, 24, and 55). (Courtesy of Douglas Flieder.)

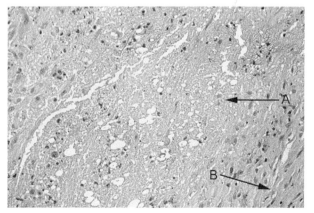

16. (A) Necrotic tissue. (B) Nonnecrotic tissue. H&E (see pp. 24 and 27).

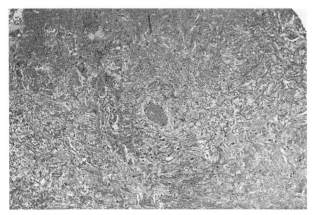

17. Angioinvasion and necrosis. Low magnification. H&E (see pp. 24 and 28).

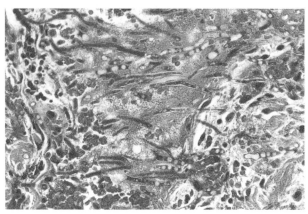

18. Angioinvasion and infarction. High magnification of Image Appendix Figure 17. H&E (see p. 28).

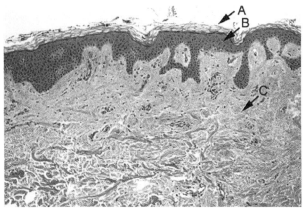

19. Skin: (A) stratum corneum; (B) epidermis; (C) dermis. H&E (see pp. 22 and 24).

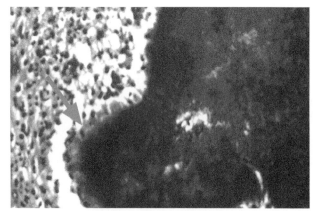

20. Splendore-Hoeppli phenomenon (at arrow) surrounding an actinomycotic granule (see pp. 24 and 28). (Courtesy of Joan Barenfanger.)

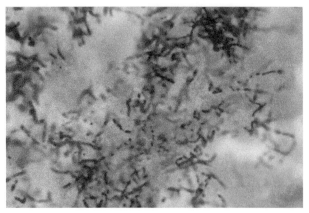

21. *Actinomyces* in liver aspirate. Gram stain (see p. 40). (Courtesy of Joan Barenfanger.)

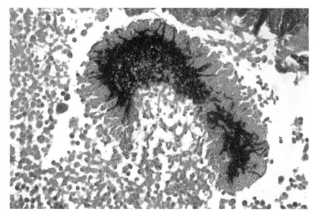

22. Eumycotic mycetoma granule. GMS (see p. 41). (Courtesy of Evelyn Koestenblatt.)

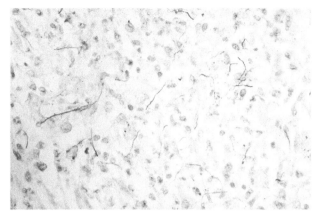

23. *Nocardia* in lung. Coates-Fite acid-fast stain (see p. 43). (Courtesy of Ron C. Neafie.)

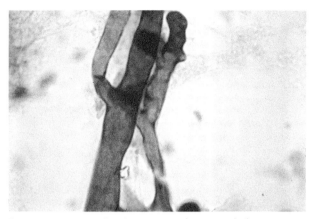

24. Mucormycete in tissue. GMS (see p. 44). (Courtesy of Joan Barenfanger.)

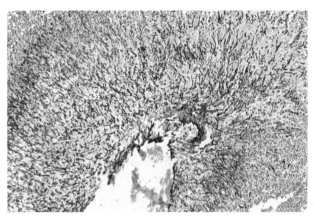

25. *Aspergillus* in lung. Low magnification. GMS (see p. 45).

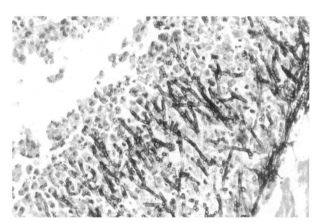

26. *Aspergillus* in lung. High magnification. GMS (see p. 45).

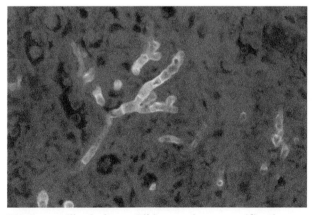

27. *Aspergillus* in lung. Oil immersion magnification. Calcofluor white stain (see p. 45).

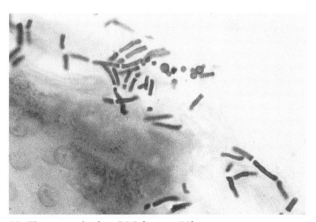

28. Tinea versicolor. PAS (see p. 50).

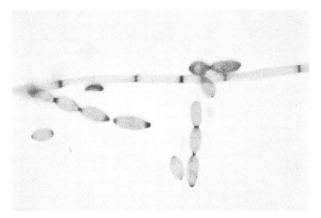

29. Fontana-Masson stain. *Cladosporium* in sputum smear (see p. 52).

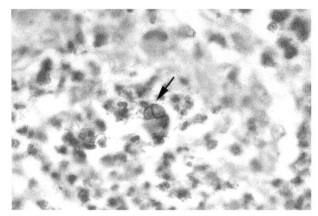

30. Chromoblastomycosis; brown sclerotic body in center. H&E (see p. 53). (Courtesy of Ron C. Neafie.)

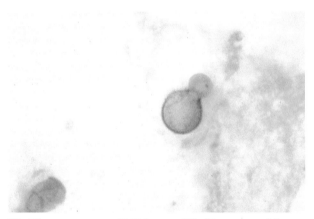

31. *Blastomyces* sp. GMS (see p. 59). (Courtesy of Joan Barenfanger.)

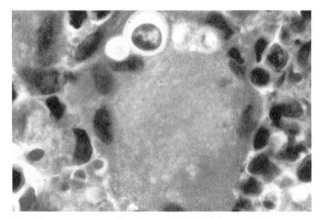

32. *Blastomyces* sp. in giant cell. H&E (see p. 59). (Courtesy of Joan Barenfanger.)

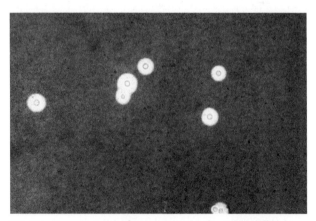

33. *Cryptococcus neoformans* in cerebrospinal fluid. India ink preparation (see p. 65).

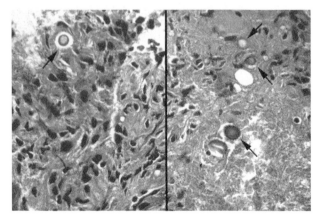

34. *Cryptococcus neoformans* (at arrows) in tissue. H&E (left). Mucicarmine (right) (see p. 65). (Courtesy of Douglas Flieder.)

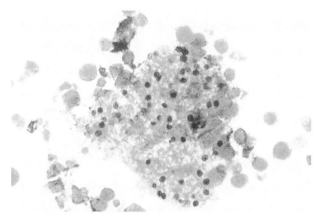

35. *Pneumocystis jirovecii* (formerly *Pneumocystis carinii*) in lung. GMS (see p. 67).

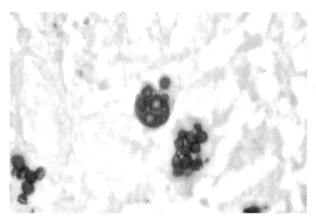

36. *Coccidioides* sp. in lung. GMS (see p. 69).

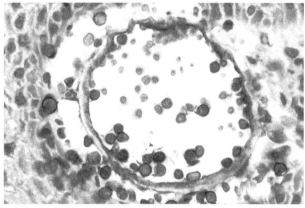

37. *Rhinosporidium seeberi* in nasal tissue. Mucicarmine (see p. 70). (Courtesy of Douglas Flieder.)

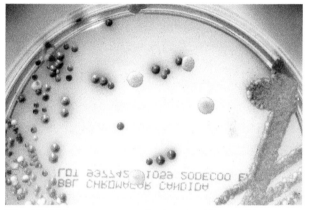

38. CHROMagar: green colonies, *C. albicans*; blue colonies, *C. tropicalis*; pink, dry colonies, *C. krusei* (see p. 123).

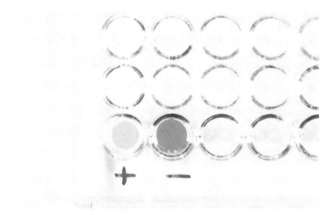

39. Rapid assimilation of trehalose (RAT) test, Mayo Clinic method: *C. glabrata* (positive) and *C. tropicalis* (negative); 37°C, 1 h (see p. 460).

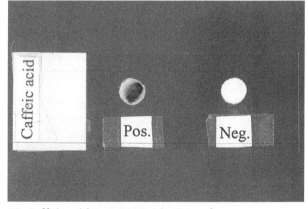

40. Caffeic acid test, 30°C, 4 h. *C. neoformans* or *C. gattii* (positive) and other *Cryptococcus* sp. (negative); (see p. 426).

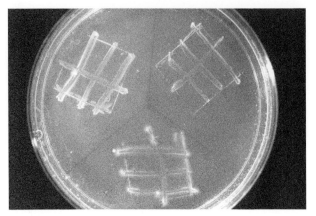

41. Dalmau plate. Three yeastlike fungi inoculated onto cornmeal-Tween 80 agar (see p. 454).

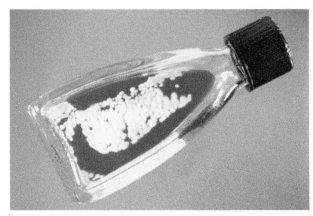

42. Dermatophyte test medium. Dermatophytes turn medium red (see p. 455).

Glossary

Abscess   Localized collection of pus in cavity formed by dissolution of tissue.

Aerial hyphae   Hyphae above the agar surface.

Aerobic   Able to grow in the presence of atmospheric oxygen.

Aleurioconidium (pl. *aleurioconidia*)   A conidium produced by the extrusion from the lateral aspect of a conidiophore or hyphal structure that is released by rupture of the attachment base.

Anaerobic   Able to grow in the absence of free or atmospheric oxygen.

Anamorph   An asexual form of a fungus.

Annellide   A cell that produces and extrudes conidia; the tip tapers, lengthens, and acquires a ring of cell wall material as each conidium is released; oil immersion magnification may be required to see the rings.

Anthropophilic   Pertaining to dermatophytes that preferentially colonize and infect humans.

Apex (pl. *apices*)   The tip or the top (often referring to the upper part of a conidia-bearing structure).

Apophysis   The swelling of a sporangiophore immediately below the columella.

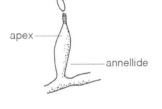

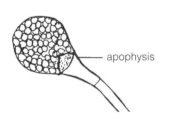

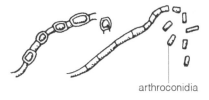

arthroconidia

Arthroconidium   An asexual spore formed by the breaking up of a hypha at the point of septation. The resulting cell may be rectangular or barrel shaped and thick or thin walled, depending on the genus.

Ascospore   A sexual spore produced in a saclike structure known as an *ascus*.

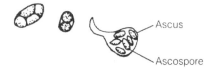

Ascus

Ascospore

Ascus (pl. *asci*)   A round or elongate saclike structure usually containing two to eight ascospores. The asci are often formed within a fruiting body, such as a cleistothecium or perithecium.

Asexual   Reproduction of an organism by division or redistribution of nuclei, but without nuclear fusion, i.e., not by the union of two compatible haploid nuclei. Also known as the *imperfect state*. This form of the fungus is called an *anamorph*.

Assimilation   The ability of a fungus to use a specific carbon or nitrogen source for growth; assimilation is read by the presence or the absence of growth.

Ballistospore   A spore that is forcibly discharged from a fungal cell.

Basidiospore   A sexual spore formed on a structure known as a *basidium*. Characteristic of the class Basidiomycetes.

Beak   A terminal extension of a conidium.

Biseriate   With reference to the genus *Aspergillus*, the phialide is supported by a metula as opposed to a uniseriate phialide, wherein the phialide forms directly on the vesicle. (See "Uniseriate.")

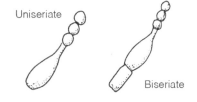

Uniseriate

Biseriate

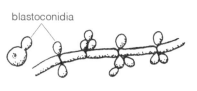

blastoconidia

Blastoconidium   A conidium formed by budding along a hypha, pseudohypha, or single cell, as in the yeasts.

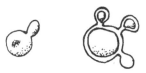

Budding   A process of asexual reproduction in which the new cell develops as a smaller outgrowth from the older parent cell. Characteristic of yeasts or yeastlike fungi.

Capsule   A colorless, transparent mucopolysaccharide sheath on the wall of a cell. Characteristic of *Cryptococcus*.

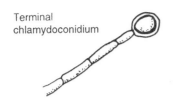

Terminal
chlamydoconidium

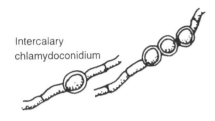

Intercalary
chlamydoconidium

Chlamydoconidium   An enlarged, rounded conidium that is thick walled and contains stored food, enabling it to function as a survival propagule. It may be located at the end of the hypha (terminal) or inserted along the hypha (intercalary), singly or in chains. Characteristically, it is greater in diameter than the hypha on which it is borne. Unlike other conidia, it does not readily separate from the hypha.

Chlamydospore   The misnomer applied to the thick-walled vesicle formed by *Candida albicans* and *Candida dubliniensis*. The more accepted term is *chlamydoconidium*.

Chloramphenicol   An antibiotic produced by *Streptomyces venezuelae* but usually prepared synthetically. It is a useful additive to mycology media, as it inhibits the growth of many bacteria that might contaminate the cultures.

Chromoblastomycosis   A cutaneous or subcutaneous disease caused by various black (dematiaceous) fungi that develop in tissue as dark sclerotic bodies (Medlar bodies).

Clade   A group of organisms having similar features inherited from a common ancestor.

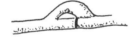

Clamp connection   A specialized bridge over a hyphal septum in the Basidiomycetes. During the formation of a new cell, it allows postmitosis nuclear migration.

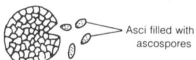

Asci filled with
ascospores

Cleistothecium   A large, fairly round, closed, many-celled structure in which asci and ascospores are formed and held until the structure bursts.

Coenocytic   Describing mucormycetes with pauciseptate hyphae containing multiple nuclei within the cytoplasm.

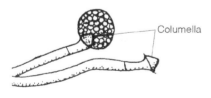

Columella

Columella   The enlarged, dome-shaped tip of a sporangiophore that extends into the sporangium. Often the sporangium bursts, leaving the columella bare and readily visible upon microscopic examination.

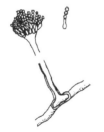

Columnar   Forming a column-like arrangement; the term is most commonly used to describe the phialides that form fairly parallel to the axis of the conidiophore in some species of *Aspergillus*, rather than radiating in many directions.

Conidiogenous cell   The cell that produces the conidia.

Conidiophore   A specialized hyphal structure that serves as a stalk on which conidia are formed. The shape and arrangement of the conidiophores and the conidia are generally characteristic of a genus. The suffix *phore* means "carrying" and is added to the word that denotes what is being carried; e.g., conidiophores bear conidia and sporangiophores bear sporangia.

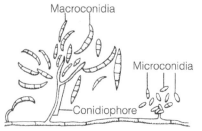

Macroconidia

Microconidia

Conidiophore

Conidium (pl. *conidia*)   An asexual propagule that forms on the side or the end of the hypha or conidiophore. It may consist of one or more cells, and the size, shape, and arrangement in groups are generally characteristic of the organism. It is always borne externally, i.e., not enclosed within a saclike structure such as a sporangium. If a fungus produces two types of conidia, those that are small and usually single celled are referred to as *microconidia*, whereas the larger *macroconidia* are usually segmented into two or more cells.

Contaminant   An environmental organism that is growing on a patient's culture, but is not thought to be actively involved in the infection. Its source could be the laboratory, but it is far more likely to have been on the patient, at or near the infection site, when the specimen was collected.

Cryptic species   An organism that is morphologically identical to another species but can be distinguished by molecular methods.

Cutaneous   Pertaining to the skin.

Cycloheximide   An antibiotic (proprietary name, Actidione) used in selective mycology media to inhibit the growth of saprophytic fungi. Because it is also known to inhibit some pathogenic fungi, it must be used in conjunction with a medium without antibiotics.

Dematiaceous   Having structures that are brown to black; this is due to a melanotic pigment in the cell walls.

Denticle   Short, narrow projection bearing a conidium.

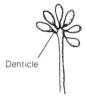

Denticle

Dermatophyte   A fungus belonging to the genus *Arthroderma*, *Epidermophyton*, *Lophophyton*, *Microsporum*, *Nannizzia*, *Paraphyton*, or *Trichophyton* with the ability to obtain nutrients from keratin and infect skin, hair, or nails of humans or animals.

Dichotomous   Branching (of hyphae) into two equal branches that are each equal in diameter to the hypha from which they originated.

Dikaryotic   A cell characterized by having two nuclei in each cell.

Dimorphic   Having two distinct morphological forms. In this guide, it refers to temperature-dependent changes in the organism on artificial culture media, i.e., fungi having a mould phase when cultured at 25–30°C and a yeast phase when cultured at 35–37°C and/or viewed directly in the host's specimen. Other sorts of dimorphism are not dependent on temperature, but exhibit different forms (i) in tissue versus artificial medium, regardless of temperature; (ii) or on routine media versus when grown under a coverslip (reducing the oxygen available).

Ectothrix Dermatophyte invasion of hair characterized by destruction of the cuticle, hyphae within the hair shaft, and a sheath of arthroconidia on the outer surface.

Endothrix Dermatophyte invasion of hair characterized by arthroconidia inside the hair shaft; the outer cuticle remains intact.

Favic chandeliers Terminal hyphal branches that are irregular, broad, and antlerlike in appearance. Especially characteristic of *Trichophyton schoenleinii*.

Fermentation The ability of a fungus to utilize a specific carbohydrate in the presence of other organic compounds, resulting in the production of gas. Therefore, the production of gas is the only indicator of a positive fermentation reaction; acid production (color change in indicator) may simply indicate that the carbohydrate has been assimilated. All carbohydrates fermented by a fungus are also assimilated, but many compounds that are assimilated are not necessarily fermented.

Filamentous Long, cylindrical, and threadlike; hyphae forming.

Floccose Cottony; like raw, fuzzy cotton.

Foot cell The base of the conidiophore, where it merges with the hyphae, giving the impression of a foot; typically seen in *Aspergillus* spp.

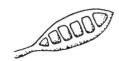

Fragmentation Breaking of the hyphae into pieces, each of which is capable of forming a new organism. Arthroconidia are formed in this manner.

Fungus (pl. *fungi*) An organism that is either filamentous or unicellular and lacks chlorophyll. It has a true nucleus enclosed in a membrane and chitin in the cell wall.

Fusiform Spindle shaped, i.e., being wider in the middle and narrowing toward the ends.

Geniculate Bent like a knee.

Genotype The genetic makeup, as distinguished from the physical appearance, of an organism or a group of organisms; deciphered by molecular testing.

Geophilic Pertaining to dermatophytes that grow in soil.

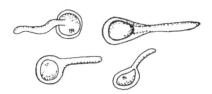

Germ tube A tubelike outgrowth from a conidium or spore; the beginning of a true hypha. A germ tube is not constricted at its point of origin from the parent cell (in contrast to a pseudohypha, which is constricted at its point of origin).

Glabrous Smooth; without or almost without aerial hyphae.

Globose Having a spherical shape.

Grain or granule An organized mass of hyphae or actinomycetous bacterial filaments in a mycetoma.

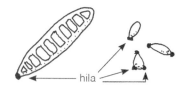

Hilum (pl. *hila*) Scar of attachment; it appears at the point(s) where the conidium was formerly attached to the conidiophore and/or another conidium.

Host The animal or plant that supports a parasite.

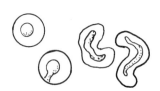

Hülle cells Thickened, large, sterile cells with a small lumen; they are associated with cleistothecia produced by the sexual stage of some *Aspergillus* spp. Droplets of exudate on the surface of a colony may indicate the site of Hülle cells.

Hyaline Clear, transparent, colorless.

Hypha (pl. *hyphae*) A filamentous structure of a fungus. Many together compose the mycelium.

Hyphomycete An asexual fungus that produces mycelium that may be colorless (hyaline) or darkly pigmented (dematiaceous).

Inflammation A local protective response of the body; characterized by redness, pain, heat, and swelling.

Intercalary Situated along the hypha, not at its end.

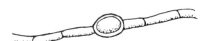

Intracellular Within cells.

Keratin A scleroprotein containing large amounts of sulfur, such as cystine; the primary component of skin, hair, and nails.

Keratitis Inflammation of the cornea of the eye.

Macroconidium (pl. *macroconidia*) The larger of two types of conidia in a fungus that produces both large and small conidia; may be single celled but usually is multicelled. (See "Conidium.")

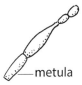

—metula

Metula (pl. *metulae*)   The separate structural portion of the conidiophore that supports the phialide (much like a pedestal) in genera such as *Aspergillus*, *Penicillium*, and *Paecilomyces*.

Microconidium (pl. *microconidia*)   The smaller of two types of conidia in a fungus that produces both large and small conidia; usually single celled and round, ovoid, pear shaped, or club shaped. (See "Conidium.")

Monokaryotic   A cell characterized by having one nucleus in each cell.

Monomorphic   In this guide, refers to fungi having the same type of morphology in culture at both 25–30°C and 35–37°C (i.e., if growth occurs at both temperature ranges; some saprophytes are inhibited at 35–37°C).

Monophyletic   Describing a group of organisms that share a close common ancestor.

Mould   A filamentous fungus composed of filaments that generally form a colony that may be fuzzy, powdery, woolly, velvety, or relatively smooth.

Muriform   Having transverse and longitudinal septations.

Mycelium (pl. *mycelia*)   A mat of intertwined hyphae that constitutes the colony surface of a mould.

Mycetoma   A localized, chronic, cutaneous or subcutaneous infection classically characterized by swollen tumorlike lesions that yield granular pus through draining sinuses.

Mycology   The study of fungi and their biology.

Mycosis (pl. *mycoses*)   A disease caused by a fungus.

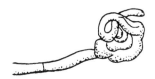

Nodular body   A round, knotlike structure formed by intertwined hyphae; seen especially in some dermatophytes.

Onychomycosis   Fungal infection of the nail caused by any fungus (a dermatophyte or other fungus). Tinea unguium differs by referring only to nail infection caused by dermatophytes.

Ostiole   An opening.

Pathogen   Any disease-producing microorganism.

Pectinate   Resembling a comb.

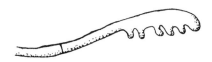

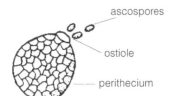

Pedicel   A slender stalk.

Pellicle   A firm or buttonlike mass formed on liquid medium by some fungi.

Perithecium (pl. *perithecia*)   A large, round or pear-shaped structure usually having a small, rounded opening (which differentiates it from a cleistothecium; the opening is called an *ostiole*) and containing asci and ascospores.

Phaeo-   A prefix meaning dark (brownish or blackish).

Phaeohyphomycosis   A subcutaneous or systemic disease caused by a variety of black fungi that develop in tissue as dark hyphae and/or yeastlike cells.

Phenotype   The observable physical or biochemical characteristics of an organism.

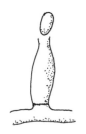

Phialide   A cell that produces and extrudes conidia without tapering or increasing in length with each new conidium produced. It is usually shaped like a flask, vase, or tenpin.

Phyletic   Relating to the evolutionary development or relationship of a group of species.

Phylogenic   Based on the lines of descent or evolutionary development of the organism.

Pleomorphism   The occurrence of two or more forms in the life cycle of an organism. Also refers to the occurrence of a form of dermatophyte that ceases to produce conidia (becomes sterile).

Polyphyletic   Describing a group of organisms that do not share a close common ancestor.

Propagule   A unit that can give rise to another organism.

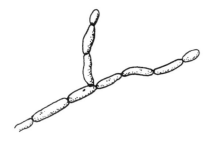

Pseudohypha   Chain of cells formed by budding that, when elongated, resembles a true hypha; differs from true hyphae by being constricted at the septa, forming branches that begin with a septation, and having terminal cells smaller than the other cells.

Pycnidium (pl. *pycnidia*)   A large, round or flask-shaped fruiting body containing conidia. Pycnidia usually have an opening (an ostiole).

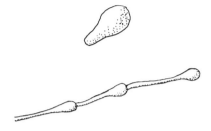

Pyriform   Pear shaped.

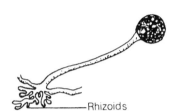

Racquet hypha   A hypha with club-shaped cells, the larger end of one cell being attached to the smaller end of an adjacent cell.

Radiate   Spreading out in all directions from a common center.

Rhizoid   Rootlike, branched hypha extending into the medium.

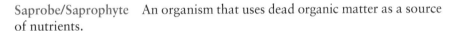

Rhizoids

Ringworm   Superficial skin disease caused by dermatophytes. Term derived from the ringlike, circular form of the lesions and from the belief that these infections were caused by wormlike organisms. The current accepted term is *tinea*.

Saprobe/Saprophyte   An organism that uses dead organic matter as a source of nutrients.

Septate   Having cross walls.

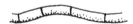

Sexual state   The portion of the life cycle in which the organism reproduces by the union of two compatible haploid nuclei. Also known as the *perfect state*. This form is called the *teleomorph*.

Sino-orbital   Pertaining to the paranasal sinuses and adjacent socket of the eye (often used in describing mucormycosis, aspergillosis, or other mould infection involving these structures).

Species complex   Composed of phylogenetically related species that are essentially indistinguishable by their morphology, but can be distinguished by molecular methods.

Spherule   Large (20–100 μm), round, thick-walled structure containing spores; characteristic of *Coccidioides* spp. in infected host material under direct microscopic examination. Spherules do not grow on routine artificial mycology media.

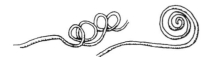

Spiral hypha   Hypha forming coiled or corkscrewlike turns.

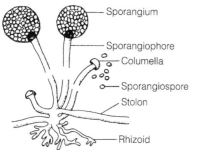

Sporangiophore   A specialized hyphal branch or stalk bearing a sporangium.

Sporangiospore   An asexual spore produced in a sporangium.

Sporangium (pl. *sporangia*)   A closed, saclike structure in which asexual spores (sporangiospores) are formed by cleavage.

Spore   Propagule that develops by sexual reproduction (ascospore, basidiospore, or zygospore) or by asexual means within a sporangium (sporangiospore). Those most commonly seen in the clinical laboratory are usually enclosed in a saclike structure (as opposed to conidia, which are free, not enclosed).

Sporodochium (pl. *sporodochia*)   A cushion-shaped mat of hyphae covered with conidiophores.

Sterigmata   Term formerly used to denote phialides of *Aspergillus* and other genera. More accurately refers to denticles produced by Basidiomycetes.

Stolon   A horizontal hypha, or runner, that grows along the surface of the medium, often bearing rhizoids that penetrate the medium and sporangiophores that ascend into the air (see drawing at Sporangiophore).

Subcutaneous   Situated or occurring directly under the skin.

Subhyaline   Neither clear nor strongly pigmented.

Suppurative   Producing pus.

Sympodial growth   Conidiogenous structure that continues to increase in length by forming a new growing point just below each new terminal conidium, often resulting in a geniculate (bent) appearance.

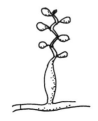

Synanamorph   One of two or more anamorphs of the same fungus; e.g., the zoophilic (formerly *Microsporum gallinae*) and geophilic (formerly *Microsporum vanbreuseghemii*) forms of *Lophophyton gallinae*.

Synnema (pl. *synnemata*)   A bundle of erect conidiophores that are cemented together producing conidia at the apex and/or along the sides.

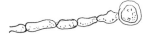

Teleomorph   The sexual form of a fungus; demonstrates sexual structures, such as ascospores or large fruiting bodies, e.g., cleistothecia.

Terminal   At the end.

Thallus   The vegetative body of a fungus; the colony surface.

Tinea barbae   Infection of the bearded areas of the face and neck by a dermatophyte.

Tinea capitis   Infection of the scalp and hair shaft by a dermatophyte.

Tinea corporis   Infection of the glabrous skin on body parts not otherwise specified (usually the trunk of the body) by a dermatophyte.

Tinea cruris   Infection of the groin, perineum, and perianal region by a dermatophyte.

Tinea manuum   Infection of the hand by a dermatophyte.

Tinea pedis   Infection of the feet by a dermatophyte.

Tinea unguium   Infection of the nails by a dermatophyte (onychomycosis is infection of the nail caused by any fungus, not necessarily caused by a dermatophyte).

Truncate   Cut off sharply; ending abruptly with a flattened edge.

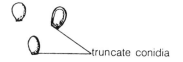

truncate conidia

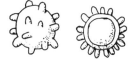

Tuberculate   Having knoblike projections.

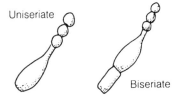

Uniseriate

Biseriate

Uniseriate   With reference to the genus *Aspergillus*, the phialide forms directly on the vesicle; a biseriate phialide is supported by a metula. (See "Biseriate.")

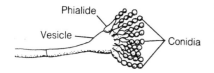

Vesicle Enlarged structure at the end of a conidiophore or sporangiophore. In *Aspergillus* spp. it bears the phialides (uniseriate) or metulae (biseriate), which in turn bear the conidia.

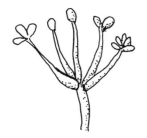

Whorl A group of cells radiating from a common point.

Yeastlike colony A soft, pasty, smooth colony; usually no filamentous (fuzzy) growth can be observed macroscopically.

Zoophilic Pertaining to dermatophytes that preferentially colonize and infect animals.

Zygospore Sexual spore that is characteristic of members of the Mucorales. They are usually large, dark, and rough walled.

References Cited

Abdolrasouli A, Bercusson AC, Rhodes JL, Hagen F, Buil JB, Tang AYY, de Boer LL, Shah A, Milburn AJ, Elborn JS, Jones AL, Meis JF, Fisher MC, Schelenz S, Simmonds NJ, Armstrong-James D. 2018. Airway persistence by the emerging multi-azole-resistant *Rasamsonia argillacea* complex in cystic fibrosis. *Mycoses* 61: 665–673. http://dx.doi.org/10.1111/myc.12789.

Abdolrasouli A, Howell S. 2023a. 8.2 Specimen Selection, Collection, and Transport. *In* Leber AL, Burnham CAB (ed), *Clinical Microbiology Procedures Handbook*, 5th Edition. ASM Press, Washington, DC.

Abdolrasouli A, Howell S. 2023b. 8.4 Processing Specimens for Fungal Culture. *In* Leber AL, Burnham CAB (ed), *Clinical Microbiology Procedures Handbook*, 5th Edition. ASM Press, Washington, DC.

Adams ED Jr, Cooper BH. 1974. Evaluation of a modified Wickerham medium for identifying medically important yeasts. *Am J Med Technol* 40:377–388.

Ajantha GS, Kulkarni RD. 2011. *Cladophialophora bantiana*, the neurotropic fungus—a mini review. *J Clin Diagn Res* 5:1301–1306.

Al Mosaid A, Sullivan D, Salkin IF, Shanley D, Coleman DC. 2001. Differentiation of *Candida dubliniensis* from *Candida albicans* on Staib agar and caffeic acid-ferric citrate agar. *J Clin Microbiol* 39:323–327. http://dx.doi.org/10.1128/JCM.39.1.323-327.2001.

Al-Obaid K, Ahmad S, Joseph L, Khan Z. 2018. *Lodderomyces elongisporus*: a bloodstream pathogen of greater clinical significance. *New Microbes New Infect* 26:20–24. http://dx.doi.org/10.1016/j.nmni.2018.07.004.

Alshehri B, Palanisamy M. 2020. Evaluation of molecular identification of *Aspergillus* species causing fungal keratitis. *Saudi J Biol Sci* 27:751–756. http://dx.doi.org/10.1016/j.sjbs.2019.12.030.

Al-Tawfiq JA, Alhumaid S, Alshukairi AN, Temsah MH, Barry M, Al Mutair A, Rabaan AA, Al-Omari A, Tirupathi R, AlQahtani M, AlBahrani S, Dhama K. 2021. COVID-19 and mucormycosis superinfection: the perfect storm. *Infection* 49:833–853. http://dx.doi.org/10.1007/s15010-021-01670-1.

Aly R. 1994. Culture media for growing dermatophytes. *J Am Acad Dermatol* 31:S107–S108. http://dx.doi.org/10.1016/S0190-9622(08)81279-0.

Amaike S, Keller NP. 2011. *Aspergillus flavus*. *Annu Rev Phytopathol* 49:107–133. http://dx.doi.org/10.1146/annurev-phyto-072910-095221.

Anaissie EJ, McGinnis MR, Pfaller MA (ed). 2009. *Clinical Mycology*, 2nd ed. Churchill Livingstone, Elsevier, New York, NY.

Angoulvant A, Guitard J, Hennequin C. 2016. Old and new pathogenic *Nakaseomyces* species: epidemiology, biology, identification, pathogenicity and antifungal resistance. *FEMS Yeast Res* 16:fov114.

Arastehfar A, Carvalho A, Houbraken J, Lombardi L, Garcia-Rubio R, Jenks JD, Rivero-Menendez O, Aljohani R, Jacobsen ID, Berman J, Osherov N, Hedayati MT, Ilkit M, Armstrong-James D, Gabaldón T, Meletiadis J, Kostrzewa M, Pan W, Lass-Flörl C, Perlin DS, Hoenigl M. 2021. *Aspergillus fumigatus* and aspergillosis: from basics to clinics. *Stud Mycol* 100:100115. http://dx.doi.org/10.1016/j.simyco.2021.100115.

Ariyawansa HA, Hyde KD, Jayasiri SC, Buyck B, Chethana KT, Dai DQ, Dai YC, Daranagama DA, Jayawardena RS, Lücking R, Ghobad-Nejhad M. 2015. Fungal diversity notes 111–252—taxonomic and phylogenetic contributions to fungal taxa. *Fungal diversity* 75:27–274.

Arzanlou M, Groenewald JZ, Gams W, Braun U, Shin HD, Crous PW. 2007. Phylogenetic and morphotaxonomic revision of *Ramichloridium* and allied genera. *Stud Mycol* 58:57–93. http://dx.doi.org/10.3114/sim.2007.58.03.

Ashraf N, Kubat RC, Poplin V, Adenis AA, Denning DW, Wright L, McCotter O, Schwartz IS, Jackson BR, Chiller T, Bahr NC. 2020. Re-drawing the maps for endemic mycoses. *Mycopathologia* 185:843–865. http://dx.doi.org/10.1007/s11046-020-00431-2.

Asner SA, Giulieri S, Diezi M, Marchetti O, Sanglard D. 2015. Acquired multidrug antifungal resistance in *Candida lusitaniae* during therapy. *Antimicrob Agents Chemother* 59:7715–7722. http://dx.doi.org/10.1128/AAC.02204-15.

Association for Molecular Pathology. 2014. Molecular diagnostic assay validation. Association for Molecular Pathology, Rockville, MD. https://www.amp.org/AMP/assets/File/resources/201503032014AssayValidationWhitePaper.pdf?pass=80

Badali H, Najafzadeh MJ, van Esbroeck M, van den Enden E, Tarazooie B, Meis JF, de Hoog GS. 2010. The clinical spectrum of *Exophiala jeanselmei*, with a case report and in vitro antifungal susceptibility of the species. *Med Mycol* 48:318–327. http://dx.doi.org/10.3109/13693780903148353.

Baddley JW, Benjamin DK Jr, Patel M, Miró J, Athan E, Barsic B, Bouza E, Clara L, Elliott T, Kanafani Z, Klein J, Lerakis S, Levine D, Spelman D, Rubinstein E, Tornos P, Morris AJ, Pappas P, Fowler VG Jr, Chu VH, Cabell C, International Collaboration on Endocarditis-Prospective Cohort Study Group (ICE-PCS). 2008. *Candida* infective endocarditis. *Eur J Clin Microbiol Infect Dis* 27:519–529. http://dx.doi.org/10.1007/s10096-008-0466-x.

Bader O, Weig M, Taverne-Ghadwal L, Lugert R, Gross U, Kuhns M. 2011. Improved clinical laboratory identification of human pathogenic yeasts by matrix-assisted laser desorption ionization time-of-flight mass spectrometry. *Clin Microbiol Infect* 17:1359–1365. http://dx.doi.org/10.1111/j.1469-0691.2010.03398.x.

Barker AP, Horan JL, Slechta ES, Alexander BD, Hanson KE. 2014. Complexities associated with the molecular and proteomic identification of *Paecilomyces* species in the clinical mycology laboratory. *Med Mycol* 52:537–545. http://dx.doi.org/10.1093/mmy/myu001.

Barnes RA, Vale L. 2005. 'Spiking' as a rapid method for differentiation of *Candida albicans* from other yeast species. *J Hosp Infect* 60:78–80. http://dx.doi.org/10.1016/j.jhin.2004.09.040.

Barros MB, de Almeida Paes R, Schubach AO. 2011. *Sporothrix schenckii* and Sporotrichosis. *Clin Microbiol Rev* 24:633–654. http://dx.doi.org/10.1128/CMR.00007-11.

Bays DJ, Thompson GR III. 2021. Coccidioidomycosis. *Infect Dis Clin North Am* 35:453–469. http://dx.doi.org/10.1016/j.idc.2021.03.010.

Bennett A, Ponder MM, Garcia-Diaz J. 2018. Phoma infections: classification, potential food sources, and its clinical impact. *Microorganisms* 6:58. http://dx.doi.org/10.3390/microorganisms6030058.

Bensch K, Braun U, Groenewald JZ, Crous PW. 2012. The genus *Cladosporium*. *Stud Mycol* 72:1–401. http://dx.doi.org/10.3114/sim0003.

Berkow EL, Sexton DJ. 2023. Specimen collection, transport, and processing: mycology. *In* Carroll KC, Pfaller MA, Karlowsky JA, Landry ML, McAdam AJ, Patel R, Pritt BS (ed), *Manual of Clinical Microbiology*, 13th Edition. ASM Press, Washington, DC.

Bizzini A, Greub G. 2010. Matrix-assisted laser desorption ionization time-of-flight mass spectrometry, a revolution in clinical microbial identification. *Clin Microbiol Infect* 16:1614–1619. http://dx.doi.org/10.1111/j.1469-0691.2010.03311.x.

Borman AM, Johnson EM. 2021. Name changes for fungi of medical importance, 2018-2019. *J Clin Microbiol* 59:e01811–e01820. http://dx.doi.org/10.1128/JCM.01811-20.

Borman AM, Johnson EM. 2023. *Candida, Cryptococcus,* and other yeasts of medical importance. *In* Carroll KC, Pfaller MA, Karlowsky JA, Landry ML, McAdam AJ, Patel R, Pritt BS (ed), *Manual of Clinical Microbiology*, 13th Edition. ASM Press, Washington, DC.

Borman AM, Muller J, Walsh-Quantick J, Szekely A, Patterson Z, Palmer MD, Fraser M, Johnson EM. 2020. MIC distributions for amphotericin B, fluconazole, itraconazole, voriconazole, flucytosine and anidulafungin and 35 uncommon pathogenic yeast species from the UK determined using the CLSI broth microdilution method. *J Antimicrob Chemother* 75:1194–1205. http://dx.doi.org/10.1093/jac/dkz568.

Borman AM, Summerbell RC. 2023. The dermatophytes and their relatives (*Trichophyton, Microsporum, Epidermophyton, Arthroderma, Nannizzia, Paraphyton,* and *Lophophyton*) and other agents of superficial mycoses. *In* Carroll KC, Pfaller MA, Karlowsky JA, Landry ML, McAdam AJ, Patel R, Pritt BS (ed), *Manual of Clinical Microbiology*, 13th Edition. ASM Press, Washington, DC.

Bourbeau P, McGough DA, Fraser H, Shah N, Rinaldi MG. 1992. Fatal disseminated infection caused by *Myceliophthora thermophila*, a new agent of mycosis: case history and laboratory characteristics. *J Clin Microbiol* 30:3019–3023. http://dx.doi.org/10.1128/jcm.30.11.3019-3023.1992.

Brandt ME, Lockhart SR. 2012. Recent taxonomic developments with *Candida* and other opportunistic yeasts. *Curr Fungal Infect Rep* 6:170–177. http://dx.doi.org/10.1007/s12281-012-0094-x.

Brown-Elliott BA, Brown JM, Conville PS, Wallace RJ Jr. 2006. Clinical and laboratory features of the *Nocardia* spp. based on current molecular taxonomy. *Clin Microbiol Rev* 19:259–282. http://dx.doi.org/10.1128/CMR.19.2.259-282.2006.

Brown-Elliott BA, Zelazny AM, Conville PS. 2023. *Nocardia, Rhodococcus, Gordonia, Actinomadura, Streptomyces,* and other aerobic actinomycetes. *In* Carroll KC, Pfaller MA, Karlowsky JA, Landry ML, McAdam AJ, Patel R, Pritt BS (ed), *Manual of Clinical Microbiology*, 13th Edition. ASM Press, Washington, DC.

Brunner-Mendoza C, Guerrero-Guerra C, Villagómez-Figueroa O, Navarro-Barranco H, Pérez-Mejía A, Toriello C. 2022. A review of described cases of mycotic keratitis and sclerokeratitis related to entomopathogenic fungi from 1984 to 2021. *J Mycol Med* 32:101249. http://dx.doi.org/10.1016/j.mycmed.2022.101249.

Bryant S, Almahmoud I, Pierre I, Bardet J, Touati S, Maubon D, Cornet M, Richarme C, Maurin M, Pavese P, Caspar Y. 2020. Evaluation of microbiological performance and the potential clinical impact of the ePlex® blood culture identification panels for the rapid diagnosis of bacteremia and fungemia. *Front Cell Infect Microbiol* 10:594951.

Buchan BW, Ledeboer NA. 2013. Advances in identification of clinical yeast isolates by use of matrix-assisted laser desorption ionization-time of flight mass spectrometry. *J Clin Microbiol* 51:1359–1366. http://dx.doi.org/10.1128/JCM.03105-12.

Cabañes FJ. 2014. *Malassezia* yeasts: how many species infect humans and animals? *PLoS Pathog* 10:e1003892. http://dx.doi.org/10.1371/journal.ppat.1003892.

Cárdenas Del Castillo B, Bejarano JIC, DeLaGarza-Pineda O, Ruiz JAA, Villanueva Lozano H, Treviño-Rangel RJ, González M G, García Martínez JM. 2021. Case report: cerebral phaeohyphomycosis due to *Chaetomium strumarium* in a child with visceral heterotaxy syndrome. *Am J Trop Med Hyg* 106:574–577. http://dx.doi.org/10.4269/ajtmh.21-0277.

Castillo CG, Kauffman CA, Miceli MH. 2016. Blastomycosis. *Infect Dis Clin North Am* 30:247–264. http://dx.doi.org/10.1016/j.idc.2015.10.002.

Cavanna C, Pagella F, Esposto MC, Tamarozzi F, Clemente L, Marone P, Matti E, Lallitto F. 2019. Human infections due to *Schizophyllum commune*: case report and review of the literature. *J Mycol Med* 29:365–371. http://dx.doi.org/10.1016/j.mycmed.2019.100897.

Cendejas-Bueno E, Kolecka A, Alastruey-Izquierdo A, Theelen B, Groenewald M, Kostrzewa M, Cuenca-Estrella M, Gómez-López A, Boekhout T. 2012. Reclassification of the *Candida haemulonii* complex as *Candida haemulonii* (*C. haemulonii* group I), *C. duobushaemulonii* sp. nov. (*C. haemulonii* group II), and *C. haemulonii* var. *vulnera* var. nov.: three multiresistant human pathogenic yeasts. *J Clin Microbiol* 50:3641–3651. http://dx.doi.org/10.1128/JCM.02248-12.

Chakrabarti A, Bonifaz A, Gutierrez-Galhardo MC, Mochizuki T, Li S. 2015. Global epidemiology of sporotrichosis. *Med Mycol* 53:3–14. http://dx.doi.org/10.1093/mmy/myu062.

Chandler FW, Watts JC. 1987. *Pathologic Diagnosis of Fungal Infections*. American Society of Clinical Pathology Press, Chicago, IL.

Chen AJ, Frisvad JC, Sun BD, Varga J, Kocsubé S, Dijksterhuis J, Kim DH, Hong SB, Houbraken J, Samson RA. 2016. *Aspergillus* section *Nidulantes* (formerly *Emericella*): polyphasic taxonomy, chemistry and biology. *Stud Mycol* 84:1–118. http://dx.doi.org/10.1016/j.simyco.2016.10.001.

Chen SC-A, Halliday CL, Hoenigl M, Cornely OA, Meyer W. 2021a. *Scedosporium* and *Lomentospora* infections: contemporary microbiological tools for the diagnosis of invasive disease. *J Fungi (Basel)* 7:23. http://dx.doi.org/10.3390/jof7010023.

Chen SC-A, Meyer W, Sorrell TC, Halliday CL. 2023. *Aspergillus*, *Talaromyces*, and *Penicillium*. *In* Carroll KC, Pfaller MA, Karlowsky JA, Landry ML, McAdam AJ, Patel R, Pritt BS (ed), *Manual of Clinical Microbiology*, 13th Edition. ASM Press, Washington, DC.

Chen SC-A, Meyer W, Sorrell TC. 2014. *Cryptococcus gattii infections. Clin Microbiol Rev* 27:980–1024. http://dx.doi.org/10.1128/CMR.00126-13.

Chen SC-A, Perfect J, Colombo AL, Cornely OA, Groll AH, Seidel D, Albus K, de Almedia JN Jr, Garcia-Effron G, Gilroy N, Lass-Flörl C, Ostrosky-Zeichner L, Pagano L, Papp T, Rautemaa-Richardson R, Salmanton-García J, Spec A, Steinmann J, Arikan-Akdagli S, Arenz DE, Sprute R, Duran-Graeff L, Freiberger T, Girmenia C, Harris M, Kanj SS, Roudbary M, Lortholary O, Meletiadis J, Segal E, Tuon FF, Wiederhold N, Bicanic T, Chander J, Chen YC, Hsueh PR, Ip M, Munoz P, Spriet I, Temfack E, Thompson L, Tortorano AM, Velegraki A, Govender NP. 2021b. Global guideline for the diagnosis and management of rare yeast infections: an initiative of the ECMM in cooperation with ISHAM and ASM. *Lancet Infect Dis* 21:e375–e386. http://dx.doi.org/10.1016/S1473-3099(21)00203-6.

Choi H, Kim YI, Na CH, Kim MS, Shin BS. 2019. Primary cutaneous *Pseudallescheria angusta* infection successfully treated with voriconazole in an immunocompetent patient. *J Dermatol* 46:e420–e421. http://dx.doi.org/10.1111/1346-8138.15018.

Chowdhary A, Kathuria S, Agarwal K, Meis JF. 2014a. Recognizing filamentous basidiomycetes as agents of human disease: A review. *Med Mycol* 52:782–797. http://dx.doi.org/10.1093/mmy/myu047.

Chowdhary A, Perfect J, de Hoog GS. 2014b. Black molds and melanized yeasts pathogenic to humans. *Cold Spring Harb Perspect Med* 5:a019570. http://dx.doi.org/10.1101/cshperspect.a019570.

Clinical and Laboratory Standards Institute. 2008. Abbreviated identification of bacteria and yeast, 2nd edition. CLSI document M35-A2. Clinical and Laboratory Standards Institute, Wayne, PA.

Clinical and Laboratory Standards Institute. 2014. Nucleic acid sequencing methods in diagnostic laboratory medicine, 2nd edition. CLSI guideline MM09. Clinical and Laboratory Standards Institute, Wayne, PA.

Clinical and Laboratory Standards Institute. 2021. Principles and procedures for detection and culture of fungi in clinical specimens, 2nd edition. CLSI guideline M54. Clinical and Laboratory Standards Institute, Wayne, PA.

Clinical and Laboratory Standards Institute. 2022. Performance standards for antifungal susceptibility testing of filamentous fungi, 3rd edition. CLSI supplement M38M51S, Clinical and Laboratory Standards Institute, Malvern, PA.

Clinical and Laboratory Standards Institute. 2022. Epidemiological cutoff values for antifungal susceptibility testing, 4th edition. CLSI document M57S. Clinical and Laboratory Standards Institute, Malvern, PA.

Colombo AL, Guimarães T, Silva LR, de Almeida Monfardini LP, Cunha AK, Rady P, Alves T, Rosas RC. 2007. Prospective observational study of candidemia in São Paulo, Brazil: incidence rate, epidemiology, and predictors of mortality. *Infect Control Hosp Epidemiol* 28:570–576. http://dx.doi.org/10.1086/513615.

Colombo AL, Júnior JNA, Guinea J. 2017. Emerging multidrug-resistant *Candida* species. *Curr Opin Infect Dis* **30**:528–538. http://dx.doi.org/10.1097/QCO.0000000000000411.

Colombo AL, Padovan AC, Chaves GM. 2011. Current knowledge of *Trichosporon* spp. and trichosporonosis. *Clin Microbiol Rev* **24**:682–700. http://dx.doi.org/10.1128/CMR.00003-11.

Conen A, Weisser M, Hohler D, Frei R, Stern M. 2011. *Hormographiella aspergillata*: an emerging mould in acute leukaemia patients? *Clin Microbiol Infect* **17**:273–277. http://dx.doi.org/10.1111/j.1469-0691.2010.03266.x.

Connor DH, Chandler FW, Schwartz DA, Manz H, Lack EE. 1997. *Pathology of Infectious Diseases*. Appleton & Lange, Stamford, CT.

Conville PS, Brown-Elliott BA, Smith T, Zelazny AM. 2017. The complexities of *Nocardia* taxonomy and identification. *J Clin Microbiol* **56**:e01419–e17.

Cooper CR Jr, Haycocks NG. 2000. *Penicillium marneffei*: an insurgent species among the penicillia. *J Eukaryot Microbiol* **47**:24–28. http://dx.doi.org/10.1111/j.1550-7408.2000.tb00006.x.

Cornely OA Alastruey-Izquierdo A, Arenz D, Chen SCA, Dannaoui E, Hochhegger B, Hoenigl M, Jensen HE, Lagrou K, Lewis RE, Mellinghoff SC, Mer M, Pana ZD, Seidel D, Sheppard DC, Wahba R, Akova M, Alanio A, Al-Hatmi AMS, Arikan-Akdagli S, Badali H, Ben-Ami R, Bonifaz A, Bretagne S, Castagnola E, Chayakulkeeree M, Colombo AL, Corzo-León DE, Drgona L, Groll AH, Guinea J, Heussel CP, Ibrahim AS, Kanj SS, Klimko N, Lackner M, Lamoth F, Lanternier F, Lass-Floerl C, Lee DG, Lehrnbecher T, Lmimouni BE, Mares M, Maschmeyer G, Meis JF, Meletiadis J, Morrissey CO, Nucci M, Oladele R, Pagano L, Pasqualotto A, Patel A, Racil Z, Richardson M, Roilides E, Ruhnke M, Seyedmousavi S, Sidharthan N, Singh N, Sinko J, Skiada A, Slavin M, Soman R, Spellberg B, Steinbach W, Tan BH, Ullmann AJ, Vehreschild JJ, Vehreschild MJGT, Walsh TJ, White PL, Wiederhold NP, Zaoutis T, Chakrabarti A; Mucormycosis ECMM MSG Global Guideline Writing Group.2019. Global guideline for the diagnosis and management of mucormycosis: an initiative of the European Confederation of Medical Mycology in cooperation with the Mycoses Study Group Education and Research Consortium. *Lancet Infect Dis* **19**:e405–e421. http://dx.doi.org/10.1016/S1473-3099(19)30312-3.

Cortez KJ, Roilides E, Quiroz-Telles F, Meletiadis J, Antachopoulos C, Knudsen T, Buchanan W, Milanovich J, Sutton DA, Fothergill A, Rinaldi MG, Shea YR, Zaoutis T, Kottilil S, Walsh TJ. 2008. Infections caused by *Scedosporium* spp. *Clin Microbiol Rev* **21**:157–197. http://dx.doi.org/10.1128/CMR.00039-07.

da Cunha KC, Sutton DA, Fothergill AW, Cano J, Gené J, Madrid H, De Hoog S, Crous PW, Guarro J. 2012. Diversity of *Bipolaris* species in clinical samples in the United States and their antifungal susceptibility profiles. *J Clin Microbiol* **50**:4061–4066.

da Cunha KC, Sutton DA, Gené J, Cano J, Capilla J, Madrid H, Decock C, Wiederhold NP, Guarro J. 2014. *Pithomyces* species (Montagnulaceae) from clinical specimens: identification and antifungal susceptibility profiles. *Med Mycol* **52**:748–757. http://dx.doi.org/10.1093/mmy/myu044.

D'Antonio D, Romano F, Pontieri E, Fioritoni G, Caracciolo C, Bianchini S, Olioso P, Staniscia T, Sferra R, Boccia S, Vetuschi A, Federico G, Gaudio E, Carruba G. 2002. Catheter-related candidemia caused by *Candida lipolytica* in a patient receiving allogeneic bone marrow transplantation. *J Clin Microbiol* **40**:1381–1386. http://dx.doi.org/10.1128/JCM.40.4.1381-1386.2002.

de Almeida Junior JN, Hennequin C. 2016. Invasive *Trichosporon* infection: a systematic review on a re-emerging fungal pathogen. *Front Microbiol* **7**:1629.

de Azevedo CM, Gomes RR, Vicente VA, Santos DW, Marques SG, do Nascimento MM, Andrade CE, Silva RR, Queiroz-Telles F, de Hoog GS. 2015. *Fonsecaea pugnacius*, a novel agent of disseminated chromoblastomycosis. *J Clin Microbiol* **53**:2674–2685. http://dx.doi.org/10.1128/JCM.00637-15.

Degreef H. 2008. Clinical forms of dermatophytosis (ringworm infection). *Mycopathologia* **166**:257–265. http://dx.doi.org/10.1007/s11046-008-9101-8.

de Hoog GS, Chaturvedi V, Denning DW, Dyer PS, Frisvad JC, Geiser D, Gräser Y, Guarro J, Haase G, Kwon-Chung KJ, Meis JF, Meyer W, Pitt JI, Samson RA, Taylor JW, Tintelnot K, Vitale RG, Walsh TJ, Lackner M, ISHAM Working Group on Nomenclature of Medical Fungi. 2015. Name changes in medically important fungi and their implications for clinical practice. *J Clin Microbiol* **53**:1056–1062. http://dx.doi.org/10.1128/JCM.02016-14.

de Hoog GS, Dukik K, Monod M, Packeu A, Stubbe D, Hendrickx M, Kupsch C, Stielow JB, Freeke J, Göker M, Rezaei-Matehkolaei A, Mirhendi H, Gräser Y. 2017. Toward a novel multilocus phylogenetic taxonomy for the dermatophytes. *Mycopathologia* **182**:5–31.

de Hoog GS, Guarro J, Gené J, Ahmed SA, Al-Hatmi AMS, Figueras MJ, Vitale RG. 2020. *Atlas of Clinical Fungi: The Ultimate Benchtool for Diagnostics*, 4th ed. Foundation Atlas of Clinical Fungi, Hilversum, The Netherlands.

de Hoog GS, Haase G, Chaturvedi V, Walsh TJ, Meyer W, Lackner M. 2013. Taxonomy of medically important fungi in the molecular era. *Lancet Infect Dis* **13**:385–386. http://dx.doi.org/10.1016/S1473-3099(13)70058-6.

de Hoog GS, Horré R. 2002. Molecular taxonomy of the *Alternaria* and *Ulocladium* species from humans and their identification in the routine laboratory. *Mycoses* **45**: 259–276.

de Hoog GS, Smith MT. 2004. Ribosomal gene phylogeny and species delimitation in *Geotrichum* and its teleomorphs. *Stud Mycol* **50**:489–515.

de Jong AW, Dieleman C, Carbia M, Mohd Tap R, Hagen F. 2021. Performance of two novel chromogenic media for the identification of multidrug-resistant *Candida auris* compared with other commercially available formulations. *J Clin Microbiol* **59**:e03220–e20. http://dx.doi.org/10.1128/JCM.03220-20.

DeLucca A, Walsh TJ. 2015. Mycotoxins of *Fusarium* spp.: biochemistry and toxicology, p 323–354. *In* Russell R, Paterson M, Lima N (ed), *Molecular Biology of Food and Water Borne Mycotoxigenic and Mycotic Fungi*. CRC Press, Boca Raton, FL.

De Ravin SS, Challipalli M, Anderson V, Shea YR, Marciano B, Hilligoss D, Marquesen M, Decastro R, Liu Y-C, Sutton DA, Wickes BL, Kammeyer PL, Sigler L, Sullivan K, Kang EM, Malech HL, Holland SM, Zelazny AM. 2011. *Geosmithia argillacea*: an emerging cause of invasive mycosis in human chronic granulomatous disease. *Clin Infect Dis* 52:e136–e143. http://dx.doi.org/10.1093/cid/ciq250.

Destino L, Sutton DA, Helon AL, Havens PL, Thometz JG, Willoughby RE Jr, Chusid MJ. 2006. Severe osteomyelitis caused by *Myceliophthora thermophila* after a pitchfork injury. *Ann Clin Microbiol Antimicrob* 5:21. http://dx.doi.org/10.1186/1476-0711-5-21.

Develoux M, Amona FM, Hennequin C. 2021. Histoplasmosis caused by *Histoplasma capsulatum* var. *duboisii*: a comprehensive review of cases from 1993 to 2019. *Clin Infect Dis* 73: e543–e549. http://dx.doi.org/10.1093/cid/ciaa1304.

Diekema DJ, Petroelje B, Messer SA, Hollis RJ, Pfaller MA. 2005. Activities of available and investigational antifungal agents against *Rhodotorula* species. *J Clin Microbiol* 43:476–478. http://dx.doi.org/10.1128/JCM.43.1.476-478.2005.

Du M, Hu W, Tamura T, Alshahni MM, Satoh K, Yamanishi C, Naito T, Makimura K. 2021. Investigation of the physiological, biochemical and antifungal susceptibility properties of *Candida auris*. *Mycopathologia* 186:189–198. http://dx.doi.org/10.1007/s11046-020-00526-w.

Dukik K, Muñoz JF, Jiang Y, Feng P, Sigler L, Stielow JB, Freeke J, Jamalian A, Gerrits van den Ende B, McEwen JG, Clay OK, Schwartz IS, Govender NP, Maphanga TG, Cuomo CA, Moreno LF, Kenyon C, Borman AM, de Hoog S. 2017. Novel taxa of thermally dimorphic systemic pathogens in the Ajellomycetaceae (Onygenales). *Mycoses* 60:296–309. http://dx.doi.org/10.1111/myc.12601.

El-Herte RI, Schouweiler KE, Farah RS, Arbulu R, Diekema D, Wanat KA, Ford BA. 2014. *Phaeoacremonium parasiticum* phaeohyphomycosis in a patient with systemic lupus erythematosus treated successfully with surgical debridement and voriconazole: a case report and review of the literature. *IDCases* 1:84–88. http://dx.doi.org/10.1016/j.idcr.2014.10.004.

Enache-Angoulvant A, Hennequin C. 2005. Invasive *Saccharomyces* infection: a comprehensive review. *Clin Infect Dis* 41:1559–1568. http://dx.doi.org/10.1086/497832.

Espinel-Ingroff A, Montero D, Martin-Mazuelos E. 2004. Long-term preservation of fungal isolates in commercially prepared cryogenic microbank vials. *J Clin Microbiol* 42:1257–1259. http://dx.doi.org/10.1128/JCM.42.3.1257-1259.2004.

Farina C, Russello G, Andreoni S, Bonetti C, Conte M, Fazi P, Lombardi G, Luzzaro F, Manso E, Marone P, Passera M, Rocchetti A, Sanna S, Viganò EF, Medical Mycology Committee (CoSM), Italian Society of Clinical Microbiology (AMCLI). 2012. Microarray technology for yeast identification directly from positive blood cultures. A multicenter Italian experience. *Med Mycol* 50:549–555. http://dx.doi.org/10.3109/13693786.2011.648216.

Fera MT, La Camera E, De Sarro A. 2009. New triazoles and echinocandins: mode of action, *in vitro* activity and mechanisms of resistance. *Expert Rev Anti Infect Ther* 7:981–998. http://dx.doi.org/10.1586/eri.09.67.

Frías-De-León MG, Hernández-Castro R, Conde-Cuevas E, García-Coronel IH, Vázquez-Aceituno VA, Soriano-Ursúa MA, Farfán-García ED, Ocharán-Hernández E, Rodríguez-Cerdeira C, Arenas R, Robledo-Cayetano M, Ramírez-Lozada T, Meza-Meneses P, Pinto-Almazán R, Martínez-Herrera E. 2021. *Candida glabrata* antifungal resistance and virulence factors, a perfect pathogenic combination. *Pharmaceutics* 13:1529. http://dx.doi.org/10.3390/pharmaceutics13101529.

Gaitanis G, Magiatis P, Hantschke M, Bassukas ID, Velegraki A. 2012. The *Malassezia* genus in skin and systemic diseases. *Clin Microbiol Rev* 25:106–141. http://dx.doi.org/10.1128/CMR.00021-11.

Garcia-Hermoso D, Alanio A, Lanternier F, Lortholary O. 2023. Agents of systemic and subcutaneous mucormycosis and entomophthoromycosis. *In* Carroll KC, Pfaller MA, Karlowsky JA, Landry ML, McAdam AJ, Patel R, Pritt BS (ed), *Manual of Clinical Microbiology*, 13th Edition. ASM Press, Washington, DC.

Géry A, Séguin V, Eldin de Pécoulas P, Bonhomme J, Garon D. 2022. *Aspergilli* series *Versicolores*: importance of species identification in the clinical setting. *Crit Rev Microbiol* 26:1–14. http://dx.doi.org/10.1080/1040841X.2022.2082267.

Gianni C, Caretta G, Romano C. 2003. Skin infection due to *Geomyces pannorum* var. *pannorum*. *Mycoses* 46:430–432. http://dx.doi.org/10.1046/j.1439-0507.2003.00897.x.

Gilgado F, Cano J, Gené J, Sutton DA, Guarro J. 2008. Molecular and phenotypic data supporting distinct species statuses for *Scedosporium apiospermum* and *Pseudallescheria boydii* and the proposed new species *Scedosporium dehoogii*. *J Clin Microbiol* 46:766–771. http://dx.doi.org/10.1128/JCM.01122-07.

Giraldo A, Sutton DA, Samerpitak K, de Hoog GS, Wiederhold NP, Guarro J, Gené J. 2014. Occurrence of *Ochroconis* and *Verruconis* species in clinical specimens from the United States. *J Clin Microbiol* 52:4189–4201. http://dx.doi.org/10.1128/JCM.02027-14.

Girard V, Mailler S, Polsinelli S, Jacob D, Saccomani MC, Celliere B, Monnin V, van Belkum A, Hagen F, Meis JF, Durand G. 2017. Routine identification of *Nocardia* species by MALDI-TOF mass spectrometry. *Diagn Microbiol Infect Dis* 87:7–10. http://dx.doi.org/10.1016/j.diagmicrobio.2016.09.024.

Girmenia C, Pizzarelli G, Cristini F, Barchiesi F, Spreghini E, Scalise G, Martino P. 2006. *Candida guilliermondii* fungemia in patients with hematologic malignancies. *J Clin Microbiol* 44:2458–2464.

Glampedakis E, Cassaing S, Fekkar A, Dannaoui E, Bougnoux ME, Bretagne S, Neofytos D, Schreiber PW, Hennequin C, Morio F, Shadrivova O, Bongomin F, Fernández-Ruiz M, Bellanger AP, Arikan-Akdagli S, Erard V, Aigner M, Paolucci M, Khanna N, Charpentier E, Bonnal C, Brun S, Gabriel F, Riat A, Zbinden R, Le Pape P, Klimko N, Lewis RE, Richardson M, İnkaya AC, Coste AT, Bochud PY, Lamoth F. 2021. Invasive aspergillosis due to *Aspergillus* section *Usti*: a multicenter retrospective study. *Clin Infect Dis* **72**:1379–1385. http://dx.doi.org/10.1093/cid/ciaa230.

Glampedakis E, Erard V, Lamoth F. 2020. Clinical relevance and characteristics of *Aspergillus calidoustus* and other *Aspergillus* species of section *Usti*. *J Fungi (Basel)* **6**:84. http://dx.doi.org/10.3390/jof6020084.

Glass NL, Donaldson GC. 1995. Development of primer sets designed for use with the PCR to amplify conserved genes from filamentous ascomycetes. *Appl Environ Microbiol* **61**:1323–1330. http://dx.doi.org/10.1128/aem.61.4.1323-1330.1995.

Gonçalves FG, Rosa PS, Belone AFF, Carneiro LB, de Barros VLQ, Bispo RF, Sbardelott YADS, Neves SAVM, Vittor AY, Woods WJ, Laporta GZ. 2022. Lobomycosis epidemiology and management: the quest for a cure for the most neglected of neglected tropical diseases. *J Fungi (Basel)* **8**:494.

González-Durán E, Contreras-Pérez CU, Caceres DH, Ríos-Rosas C, Piñón-Ortega JJ, Téllez-Saucedo MD, Marín-Suro ES, Wong-Arámbula CE, Moreno-Escobar EA, Ramírez-González JE, Ramírez-Barrios JG, Montes-Colima NA, Lockhart SR, Martínez-Montiel N, Martínez-Contreras RD, García-Ruíz P, Salazar-Sánchez MI, Hernández-Rivas L, López-Martínez I. 2022. The use of readily available laboratory tests for the identification of the emerging yeast *Candida auris* in Mexico. *Arch Microbiol* **204**:592. http://dx.doi.org/10.1007/s00203-022-03159-3.

Gonzales Zamora JA, Varadarajalu Y. 2019. Fatal *Curvularia* brain abscess in a heart and kidney transplant recipient. *IDCases* **17**:e00576. http://dx.doi.org/10.1016/j.idcr.2019.e00576.

Goodwin S, McPherson JD, McCombie WR. 2016. Coming of age: ten years of next-generation sequencing technologies. *Nat Rev Genet* **17**:333–351. http://dx.doi.org/10.1038/nrg.2016.49.

Gräser Y, Kuijpers AF, Presber W, de Hoog GS. 2000. Molecular taxonomy of the *Trichophyton* rubrum complex. *J Clin Microbiol* **38**:3329–3336. http://dx.doi.org/10.1128/JCM.38.9.3329-3336.2000.

Grava S, Lopes FA, Cavallazzi RS, Grassi MF, Svidzinski TI. 2016. A rare case of hemorrhagic pneumonia due to *Cladosporium cladosporioides*. *J Bras Pneumol* **42**:392–394. http://dx.doi.org/10.1590/S1806-37562016000000079.

Gregory TR. 2008. Understanding evolutionary trees. *Evo Edu Outreach* **1**:121–137. http://dx.doi.org/10.1007/s12052-008-0035-x.

Guarner J, Brandt ME. 2011. Histopathologic diagnosis of fungal infections in the 21st century. *Clin Microbiol Rev* **24**:247–280. http://dx.doi.org/10.1128/CMR.00053-10.

Guarro J, Madrid H, de Hoog S. 2023. *Curvularia, Exophiala, Scedosporium, Sporothrix*, and other melanized fungi. *In* Carroll KC, Pfaller MA, Karlowsky JA, Landry ML, McAdam AJ, Patel R, Pritt BS (ed), *Manual of Clinical Microbiology*, 13th Edition. ASM Press, Washington, DC.

Gupta AK, Venkataraman M, Hall DC, Cooper EA, Summerbell RC. 2022. The emergence of *Trichophyton indotineae*: implications

for clinical practice. *Int J Dermatol*ijd.16362. http://dx.doi.org/10.1111/ijd.16362.

Gushiken AC, Saharia KK, Baddley JW. 2021. Cryptococcosis. *Infect Dis Clin North Am* **35**:493–514. http://dx.doi.org/10.1016/j.idc.2021.03.012.

Hagen F, Khayhan K, Theelen B, Kolecka A, Polacheck I, Sionov E, Falk R, Parnmen S, Lumbsch HT, Boekhout T. 2015. Recognition of seven species in the *Cryptococcus gattii/Cryptococcus neoformans* species complex. *Fungal Genet Biol* **78**:16–48. http://dx.doi.org/10.1016/j.fgb.2015.02.009.

Hall BG. 2007. *Phylogenetic Trees Made Easy: A How-To Manual*, 3rd ed. Sinauer Associates, Sunderland, MA.

Harrington BJ, Hageage GJ Jr. 2003. Calcofluor white: a review of its uses and applications in clinical mycology and parasitology. *Lab Med* **34**:361–367. http://dx.doi.org/10.1309/EPH2TDT8335GH0R3.

Harrington TL, Eldredge D, Benson EK. 2018. Immigration brings new pathology with no standardized treatment protocol. *J Am Podiatr Med Assoc* **108**:517–522. http://dx.doi.org/10.7547/17-058.

Harris JL. 2000. Safe, low-distortion tape touch method for fungal slide mounts. *J Clin Microbiol* **38**:4683–4684. http://dx.doi.org/10.1128/JCM.38.12.4683-4684.2000.

Hassan Y, Chew SY, Than LTL. 2021. *Candida glabrata*: pathogenicity and resistance mechanisms for adaptation and survival. *J Fungi (Basel)* **7**:667. http://dx.doi.org/10.3390/jof7080667.

Havlickova B, Czaika VA, Friedrich M. 2008. Epidemiological trends in skin mycoses worldwide. *Mycoses* **51**(Suppl 4):2–15. http://dx.doi.org/10.1111/j.1439-0507.2008.01606.x.

Hawksworth DL. 2011. A new dawn for the naming of fungi: impacts of decisions made in Melbourne in July 2011 on the future publication and regulation of fungal names. *IMA Fungus* **2**:155–162. http://dx.doi.org/10.5598/imafungus.2011.02.02.06.

Heelan JS, Siliezar D, Coon K. 1996. Comparison of rapid testing methods for enzyme production with the germ tube method for presumptive identification of *Candida albicans*. *J Clin Microbiol* **34**:2847–2849. http://dx.doi.org/10.1128/jcm.34.11.2847-2849.1996.

Henriet SS, Verweij PE, Warris A. 2012. *Aspergillus nidulans* and chronic granulomatous disease: a unique host-pathogen interaction. *J Infect Dis* **206**:1128–1137. http://dx.doi.org/10.1093/infdis/jis473.

Hernandez-Ramirez G, Barber D, Tome-Amat J, Garrido-Arandia M, Diaz-Perales A. 2021. *Alternaria* as an inducer of allergic sensitization. *J Fungi (Basel)* **7**:838. http://dx.doi.org/10.3390/jof7100838.

Hettick JM, Green BJ, Buskirk AD, Kashon ML, Slaven JE, Janotka E, Blachere FM, Schmechel D, Beezhold DH. 2008. Discrimination of *Aspergillus* isolates at the species and strain level by matrix-assisted laser desorption/ionization time-of-flight mass spectrometry fingerprinting. *Anal Biochem* **380**:276–281. http://dx.doi.org/10.1016/j.ab.2008.05.051.

Hibbett D, Abarenkov K, Kõljalg U, Öpik M, Chai B, Cole J, Wang Q, Crous P, Robert V, Helgason T, Herr JR, Kirk P, Lueschow S, O'Donnell K, Nilsson RH, Oono R, Schoch C, Smyth C, Walker DM, Porras-Alfaro A, Taylor JW, Geiser DM. 2016. Sequence-based classification and identification of Fungi. *Mycologia* **108**:1049–1068.

Hickey PW, Sutton DA, Fothergill AW, Rinaldi MG, Wickes BL, Schmidt HJ, Walsh TJ. 2009. *Trichosporon mycotoxinivorans*, a novel respiratory pathogen in patients with cystic fibrosis. *J Clin Microbiol* **47**:3091–3097. http://dx.doi.org/10.1128/JCM.00460-09.

Hoenigl M, Egger M, Price J, Krause R, Prattes J, White PL. 2023. Metagenomic next-generation sequencing of plasma for diagnosis of COVID-19-associated pulmonary aspergillosis. *J Clin Microbiol* **21**:e0185922.

Hospenthal DR, Beckius ML, Floyd KL, Horvath LL, Murray CK. 2006. Presumptive identification of *Candida* species other than *C. albicans, C. krusei,* and *C. tropicalis* with the chromogenic medium CHROMagar Candida. *Ann Clin Microbiol Antimicrob* **5**:1–5. http://dx.doi.org/10.1186/1476-0711-5-1.

Houbraken J, Giraud S, Meijer M, Bertout S, Frisvad JC, Meis JF, Bouchara JP, Samson RA. 2013. Taxonomy and antifungal susceptibility of clinically important *Rasamsonia* species. *J Clin Microbiol* **51**:22–30. http://dx.doi.org/10.1128/JCM.02147-12.

Houbraken J, Kocsubé S, Visagie CM, Yilmaz N, Wang XC, Meijer M, Kraak B, Hubka V, Bensch K, Samson RA, Frisvad JC. 2020. Classification of *Aspergillus, Penicillium, Talaromyces* and related genera (*Eurotiales*): an overview of families, genera, subgenera, sections, series and species. *Stud Mycol* **95**:5–169. http://dx.doi.org/10.1016/j.simyco.2020.05.002.

Houbraken J, Spierenburg H, Frisvad JC. 2012. *Rasamsonia*, a new genus comprising thermotolerant and thermophilic *Talaromyces* and *Geosmithia* species. *Antonie van Leeuwenhoek* **101**:403–421. http://dx.doi.org/10.1007/s10482-011-9647-1.

Hsieh TT, Tseng HK, Sun PL, Wu YH, Chen GS. 2013. Disseminated zygomycosis caused by *Cunninghamella bertholletiae* in patient with hematological malignancy and review of published case reports. *Mycopathologia* **175**:99–106. http://dx.doi.org/10.1007/s11046-012-9595-y.

Huber WM, Caplin SM. 1947. Simple plastic mount for permanent preservation of fungi and small arthropods. *Arch Derm Syphilol* **56**:763–765. http://dx.doi.org/10.1001/archderm.1947.01520120051003.

Hubka V, Mencl K, Skorepova M, Lyskova P, Zalabska E. 2011. Phaeohyphomycosis and onychomycosis due to *Chaetomium* spp., including the first report of *Chaetomium brasiliense* infection. *Med Mycol* **49**:724–733.

Ioannou P, Vamvoukaki R, Samonis G. 2019. *Rhodotorula* species infections in humans: a systematic review. *Mycoses* **62**:90–100. http://dx.doi.org/10.1111/myc.12856.

Jang MS, Park JB, Yang MH, Jang JY, Kim JH, Kim SH, Kim YK, Suh KS. 2018. Superficial mycosis of the foot caused by *Cladophialophora boppii. J Dermatol* **45**:e144–e145. http://dx.doi.org/10.1111/1346-8138.14195.

Jeffery-Smith A, Taori SK, Schelenz S, Jeffery K, Johnson EM, Borman A, Manuel R, Brown CS, Candida auris Incident Management Team. 2017. *Candida auris:* a review of the literature. *Clin Microbiol Rev* **31**:e00029–e17.

Jeong W, Keighley C, Wolfe R, Lee WL, Slavin MA, Kong DCM, Chen SC-A. 2019. The epidemiology and clinical manifestations of mucormycosis: a systematic review and meta-analysis of case reports. *Clin Microbiol Infect* **25**:26–34. http://dx.doi.org/10.1016/j.cmi.2018.07.011.

Jiang Y, Dukik K, Muñoz JF, Sigler L, Schwartz IS, Govender NP, Kenyon C, Feng P, van den Ende BG, Stielow JB, Stchigel AM, Lu H, de Hoog S. 2018. Phylogeny, ecology and taxonomy of systemic pathogens and their relatives in Ajellomycetaceae (Onygenales): *Blastomyces, Emergomyces, Emmonsia, Emmonsiellopsis. Fungal Divers* **90**:245–291. http://dx.doi.org/10.1007/s13225-018-0403-y.

Jo SY, Lee S, Kim KH, Yi J. 2021. A case of brain abscess caused by the dematiaceous mold *Neoscytalidium dimidiatum* in a Korean man. *Ann Lab Med* **41**:247–249. http://dx.doi.org/10.3343/alm.2021.41.2.247.

Kane J, Summerbell R, Sigler L, Krajden S, Land G. 1997. *Laboratory Handbook of Dermatophytes.* Star Publishing Co, Belmont, CA.

Kaneko T, Makimura K, Abe M, Shiota R, Nakamura Y, Kano R, Hasegawa A, Sugita T, Shibuya S, Watanabe S, Yamaguchi H, Abe S, Okamura N. 2007. Revised culture-based system for identification of *Malassezia* species. *J Clin Microbiol* **45**:3737–3742. http://dx.doi.org/10.1128/JCM.01243-07.

Kannan A, Asner SA, Trachsel E, Kelly S, Parker J, Sanglard D. 2019. Comparative genomics for the elucidation of multidrug resistance in *Candida lusitaniae. MBio* **10**:e02512–e02519. http://dx.doi.org/10.1128/mBio.02512-19.

Kano R. 2020. Emergence of fungal-like organisms: *Prototheca. Mycopathologia* **185**:747–754.

Kano R, Kimura U, Kakurai M, Hiruma J, Kamata H, Suga Y, Harada K. 2020. *Trichophyton indotineae* sp. nov.: a new highly terbinafine-resistant anthropophilic dermatophyte species. *Mycopathologia* **185**:947–958. http://dx.doi.org/10.1007/s11046-020-00455-8.

Kantarcioglu AS, de Hoog GS, Guarro J. 2012. Clinical characteristics and epidemiology of pulmonary pseudallescheriasis. *Rev Iberoam Micol* **29**:1–13. http://dx.doi.org/10.1016/j.riam.2011.04.002.

Kantarcioğlu AS, Yücel A, de Hoog GS. 2002. Case report. Isolation of *Cladosporium cladosporioides* from cerebrospinal fluid. *Mycoses* **45**:500–503.

Kapadia M, Rolston KVI, Han XY. 2007. Invasive *Streptomyces* infections: six cases and literature review. *Am J Clin Pathol* **127**:619–624. http://dx.doi.org/10.1309/QJEBXP0BCGR54L15.

Kathuria S, Singh PK, Sharma C, Prakash A, Masih A, Kumar A, Meis JF, Chowdhary A. 2015. Multidrug-resistant *Candida auris* misidentified as *Candida haemulonii*: characterization by matrix-assisted laser desorption ionization-time of flight mass spectrometry and DNA sequencing and its antifungal susceptibility profile variability by Vitek 2, CLSI broth microdilution, and Etest method. *J Clin Microbiol* 53:1823–1830. http://dx.doi.org/10.1128/JCM.00367-15.

Katragkou A, Pana ZD, Perlin DS, Kontoyiannis DP, Walsh TJ, Roilides E. 2014. *Exserohilum* infections: review of 48 cases before the 2012 United States outbreak. *Med Mycol* 52:376–386. http://dx.doi.org/10.1093/mmy/myt030.

Kauffman CA. 2007. Histoplasmosis: a clinical and laboratory update. *Clin Microbiol Rev* 20:115–132. http://dx.doi.org/10.1128/CMR.00027-06.

Kaur R, Wadhwa A, Gulati A, Agrawal A. 2010. An unusual phaeoid fungi: *Ulocladium*, as a cause of chronic allergic fungal sinusitis. *Iran J Microbiol* 2:95–97.

Kemna ME, Neri RC, Ali R, Salkin IF. 1994. *Cokeromyces recurvatus*, a mucoraceous zygomycete rarely isolated in clinical laboratories. *J Clin Microbiol* 32:843–845. http://dx.doi.org/10.1128/jcm.32.3.843-845.1994.

Kent D, Wong T, Osgood R, Kosinski K, Coste G, Bor D. 1998. Fungemia due to *Hormonema dematioides* following intense avian exposure. *Clin Infect Dis* 26:759–760. http://dx.doi.org/10.1086/517116.

Kenyon C, Bonorchis K, Corcoran C, Meintjes G, Locketz M, Lehloenya R, Vismer HF, Naicker P, Prozesky H, van Wyk M, Bamford C, du Plooy M, Imrie G, Dlamini S, Borman AM, Colebunders R, Yansouni CP, Mendelson M, Govender NP. 2013. A dimorphic fungus causing disseminated infection in South Africa. *N Engl J Med* 369:1416–1424. http://dx.doi.org/10.1056/NEJMoa1215460.

Khan Z, Gené J, Ahmad S, Cano J, Al-Sweih N, Joseph L, Chandy R, Guarro J. 2013. Coniochaeta polymorpha, a new species from endotracheal aspirate of a preterm neonate, and transfer of *Lecythophora* species to *Coniochaeta*. *Antonie van Leeuwenhoek* 104:243–252. http://dx.doi.org/10.1007/s10482-013-9943-z.

Khunnamwong P, Lertwattanasakul N, Jindamorakot S, Limtong S, Lachance MA. 2015. Description of *Diutina* gen. nov., *Diutina siamensis*, f.a. sp. nov., and reassignment of *Candida catenulata*, *Candida mesorugosa*, *Candida neorugosa*, *Candida pseudorugosa*, *Candida ranongensis*, *Candida rugosa* and *Candida scorzettiae* to the genus *Diutina*. *Int J Syst Evol Microbiol* 65:4701–4709. http://dx.doi.org/10.1099/ijsem.0.000634.

Kidd SE, Abdolrasouli A, Hagen F. 2023a. Fungal nomenclature: managing change is the name of the game. *Open Forum Infect Dis* 10:ofac559.

Kidd S, Halliday C, Ellis D. 2023b. *Descriptions of Medical Fungi*, 4th ed. CABI, Oxfordshire, UK.

Kimura M, McGinnis MR. 1998. Fontana-Masson--stained tissue from culture-proven mycoses. *Arch Pathol Lab Med* 122:1107–1111.

Kimura M, Smith MB, McGinnis MR. 1999. Zygomycosis due to *Apophysomyces elegans*: report of 2 cases and review of the literature. *Arch Pathol Lab Med* 123:386–390. http://dx.doi.org/10.5858/1999-123-0386-ZDTAE.

Kirchhoff L, Olsowski M, Rath PM, Steinmann J. 2019. *Exophiala dermatitidis*: key issues of an opportunistic fungal pathogen. *Virulence* 10:984–998. http://dx.doi.org/10.1080/21505594.2019.1596504.

Klein KR, Hall L, Deml SM, Rysavy JM, Wohlfiel SL, Wengenack NL. 2009. Identification of *Cryptococcus gattii* by use of L-canavanine glycine bromothymol blue medium and DNA sequencing. *J Clin Microbiol* 47:3669–3672. http://dx.doi.org/10.1128/JCM.01072-09.

Kousha M, Tadi R, Soubani AO. 2011. Pulmonary aspergillosis: a clinical review. *Eur Respir Rev* 20:156–174. http://dx.doi.org/10.1183/09059180.00001011.

Kravitz JN, Steed LL, Judson MA. 2011. Intracavitary voriconazole for the treatment of hemoptysis complicating *Pseudallescheria angusta* pulmonary mycetomas in fibrocystic sarcoidosis. *Med Mycol* 49:198–201. http://dx.doi.org/10.3109/13693786.2010.512619.

Kuhn DM, Ghannoum MA. 2003. Indoor mold, toxigenic fungi, and *Stachybotrys chartarum*: infectious disease perspective. *Clin Microbiol Rev* 16:144–172. http://dx.doi.org/10.1128/CMR.16.1.144-172.2003.

Kurtzmann CP, Fell JW, Boekhout T (ed). 2011. *The Yeasts, A Taxonomic Study*, 5th ed. Elsevier, Amersterdam, The Netherlands.

Kurtzman CP, Robnett CJ. 1991. Phylogenetic relationships among species of *Saccharomyces*, *Schizosaccharomyces*, *Debaryomyces* and *Schwanniomyces* determined from partial ribosomal RNA sequences. *Yeast* 7:61–72. http://dx.doi.org/10.1002/yea.320070107.

Kurtzman CP, Suzuki M. 2010. Phylogenetic analysis of ascomycete yeasts that form coenzyme Q-9 and the proposal of the new genera *Babjeviella*, *Meyerozyma*, *Millerozyma*, *Priceomyces*, and *Scheffersomyces*. *Mycoscience* 51:2–14. http://dx.doi.org/10.1007/S10267-009-0011-5.

Kwon-Chung KJ, Bennett JE, Wickes BL, Meyer W, Cuomo CA, Wollenburg KR, Bicanic TA, Castañeda E, Chang YC, Chen J, Cogliati M, Dromer F, Ellis D, Filler SG, Fisher MC, Harrison TS, Holland SM, Kohno S, Kronstad JW, Lazera M, Levitz SM, Lionakis MS, May RC, Ngamskulrongroj P, Pappas PG, Perfect JR, Rickerts V, Sorrell TC, Walsh TJ, Williamson PR, Xu J, Zelazny AM, Casadevall A. 2017. The case for adopting the "species complex" nomenclature for the etiologic agents of cryptococcosis. *MSphere* 2:e00357–e16. http://dx.doi.org/10.1128/mSphere.00357-16.

Kwon-Chung KJ, Polacheck I, Bennett JE. 1982. Improved diagnostic medium for separation of *Cryptococcus neoformans* var. *neoformans* (serotypes A and D) and *Cryptococcus neoformans* var. *gattii* (serotypes B and C). *J Clin Microbiol* 15:535–537. http://dx.doi.org/10.1128/jcm.15.3.535-537.1982.

Lackner M, de Hoog GS, Verweij PE, Najafzadeh MJ, Curfs-Breuker I, Klaassen CH, Meis JF. 2012. Species-specific antifungal susceptibility patterns of *Scedosporium* and *Pseudallescheria* species. *Antimicrob Agents Chemother* 56:2635–2642. http://dx.doi.org/10.1128/AAC.05910-11.

Lackner M de Hoog GS, Yang L, Ferreira Moreno L, Ahmed SA, Andreas F, Kaltseis J, Nagl M, Lass-Flörl C, Risslegger B, Rambach G. 2014. Proposed nomenclature for *Pseudallescheria*, *Scedosporium* and related genera. *Fungal Divers* 67:1–10. http://dx.doi.org/10.1007/s13225-014-0295-4.

Larone DH. 1989. The identification of dematiaceous fungi. *Clin Microbiol Newsl* 11:145–150.

Larone DH, Walsh TJ. 2013. *Exserohilum rostratum*: anatomy of a national outbreak of fungal meningitis. *Clin Microbiol Newsl* 35:185–193. http://dx.doi.org/10.1016/j.clinmicnews.2013.11.001.

Lass-Flörl C, Dietl AM, Kontoyiannis DP, Brock M. 2021. *Aspergillus terreus* species complex. *Clin Microbiol Rev* 34:e0031120. http://dx.doi.org/10.1128/CMR.00311-20.

Lass-Flörl C, Mayr A. 2007. Human protothecosis. *Clin Microbiol Rev* 20:230–242. http://dx.doi.org/10.1128/CMR.00032-06.

Latgé JP, Chamilos G. 2019. *Aspergillus fumigatus* and aspergillosis in 2019. *Clin Microbiol Rev* 33:e00140–e18. http://dx.doi.org/10.1128/CMR.00140-18.

Lawrence DP, Gannibal PB, Peever TL, Pryor BM. 2013. The sections of *Alternaria*: formalizing species-group concepts. *Mycologia* 105:530–546. http://dx.doi.org/10.3852/12-249.

Leber AL, Everhart K, Balada-Llasat JM, Cullison J, Daly J, Holt S, Lephart P, Salimnia H, Schreckenberger PC, DesJarlais S, Reed SL, Chapin KC, LeBlanc L, Johnson JK, Soliven NL, Carroll KC, Miller JA, Dien Bard J, Mestas J, Bankowski M, Enomoto T, Hemmert AC, Bourzac KM. 2016. Multicenter evaluation of BioFire FilmArray Meningitis/Encephalitis Panel for detection of bacteria, viruses, and yeast in cerebrospinal fluid specimens. *J Clin Microbiol* 54:2251–2261. http://dx.doi.org/10.1128/JCM.00730-16.

Leek R, Aldag E, Nadeem I, Gunabushanam V, Sahajpal A, Kramer DJ, Walsh TJ. 2016. Scedosporiosis in a combined kidney and liver transplant recipient: a case report of possible transmission from a near-drowning donor. *Case Rep Transplant* 2016:1879529. http://dx.doi.org/10.1155/2016/1879529.

Leeming JP, Notman FH. 1987. Improved methods for isolation and enumeration of *Malassezia furfur* from human skin. *J Clin Microbiol* 25:2017–2019. http://dx.doi.org/10.1128/jcm.25.10.2017-2019.1987.

Levenson D, Pfaller MA, Smith MA, Hollis R, Gerarden T, Tucci CB, Isenberg HD. 1991. *Candida zeylanoides*: another opportunistic yeast. *J Clin Microbiol* 29:1689–1692. http://dx.doi.org/10.1128/jcm.29.8.1689-1692.1991.

Levenstadt JS, Poutanen SM, Mohan S, Zhang S, Silverman M. 2012. *Pleurostomophora richardsiae* - an insidious fungus presenting in a man 44 years after initial inoculation: a case report and review of the literature. *Can J Infect Dis Med Microbiol* 23:110–113. http://dx.doi.org/10.1155/2012/406982.

Liesman RM, Strasburg AP, Heitman AK, Theel ES, Patel R, Binnicker MJ. 2018. Evaluation of a commercial multiplex molecular panel for diagnosis of infectious meningitis and encephalitis. *J Clin Microbiol* 56:e01927–17.

Lipner SR, Scher RK. 2019. Onychomycosis: clinical overview and diagnosis. *J Am Acad Dermatol* 80:835–851. http://dx.doi.org/10.1016/j.jaad.2018.03.062.

Litvintseva AP, Brandt ME, Mody RK, Lockhart SR. 2015. Investigating fungal outbreaks in the 21st century. *PLoS Pathog* 11:e1004804. http://dx.doi.org/10.1371/journal.ppat.1004804.

Liu K, Howell DN, Perfect JR, Schell WA. 1998. Morphologic criteria for the preliminary identification of *Fusarium, Paecilomyces*, and *Acremonium* species by histopathology. *Am J Clin Pathol* 109:45–54. http://dx.doi.org/10.1093/ajcp/109.1.45.

Liu WC, Chan MC, Lin TY, Hsu CH, Chiu SK. 2013. *Candida lipolytica* candidemia as a rare infectious complication of acute pancreatitis: a case report and literature review. *J Microbiol Immunol Infect* 46:393–396. http://dx.doi.org/10.1016/j.jmii.2013.04.007.

Liu X-Z, Wang Q-M, Göker M, Groenewald M, Kachalkin AV, Lumbsch HT, Millanes AM, Wedin M, Yurkov AM, Boekhout T, Bai F-Y. 2015. Towards an integrated phylogenetic classification of the Tremellomycetes. *Stud Mycol* 81:85–147. http://dx.doi.org/10.1016/j.simyco.2015.12.001.

Lockhart SR, Ghannoum MA, Alexander BD. 2017. Establishment and use of epidemiological cutoff values for molds and yeasts by use of the Clinical and Laboratory Standards Institute M57 Standard. *J Clin Microbiol* 55:1262–1268. http://dx.doi.org/10.1128/JCM.02416-16.

Lockhart SR, Toda M, Benedict K, Caceres DH, Litvintseva AP. 2021. Endemic and other dimorphic mycoses in the Americas. *J Fungi (Basel)* 7:151. http://dx.doi.org/10.3390/jof7020151.

Lücking R, Aime MC, Robbertse B, Miller AN, Aoki T, Ariyawansa HA, Cardinali G, Crous PW, Druzhinina IS, Geiser DM, Hawksworth DL, Hyde KD, Irinyi L, Jeewon R, Johnston PR, Kirk PM, Malosso E, May TW, Meyer W, Nilsson HR, Öpik M, Robert V, Stadler M, Thines M, Vu D, Yurkov AM, Zhang N, Schoch CL. 2021. Fungal taxonomy and sequence-based nomenclature. *Nat Microbiol* 6:540–548. http://dx.doi.org/10.1038/s41564-021-00888-x.

Lyman M, Forsberg K, Reuben J, Dang T, Free R, Seagle EE, Sexton DJ, Soda E, Jones H, Hawkins D, Anderson A, Bassett J, Lockhart SR, Merengwa E, Iyengar P, Jackson BR, Chiller T. 2021. Notes from the field: transmission of pan-resistant and echinocandin-resistant *Candida auris* in health care facilities – Texas and the District of Columbia, January-April 2021. *MMWR Morb Mortal Wkly Rep* 70:1022–1023. http://dx.doi.org/10.15585/mmwr.mm7029a2.

Lyon GM, Smilack JD, Komatsu KK, Pasha TM, Leighton JA, Guarner J, Colby TV, Lindsley MD, Phelan M, Warnock DW, Hajjeh RA. 2001. Gastrointestinal basidiobolomycosis in Arizona: clinical and epidemiological characteristics and review of the literature. *Clin Infect Dis* 32:1448–1455. http://dx.doi.org/10.1086/320161.

Lyons JL, Gireesh ED, Trivedi JB, Bell WR, Cettomai D, Smith BR, Karram S, Chang T, Tochen L, Zhang SX, McCall CM, Pearce DT, Carroll KC, Chen L, Ratchford JN, Harrison DM, Ostrow LW, Stevens RD. 2012. Fatal exserohilum meningitis and central nervous system vasculitis after cervical epidural methylprednisolone injection. *Ann Intern Med* 157:835–836. http://dx.doi.org/10.7326/0003-4819-158-1-201212040-00557.

Mahan CT, Sale GE. 1978. Rapid methenamine silver stain for *Pneumocystis* and fungi. *Arch Pathol Lab Med* 102:351–352.

Manamgoda DS, Cai L, McKenzie EHC, Crous PW, Madrid H, Chukeatirote E, Shivas G, Tan YP, Hyde KD. 2012. A phylogenetic and taxonomic reevaluation of the *Bipolaris - Cochliobolus - Curvularia* complex. *Fungal Divers* 56:131–144. http://dx.doi.org/10.1007/s13225-012-0189-2.

Marimon R, Cano J, Gené J, Sutton DA, Kawasaki M, Guarro J. 2007. *Sporothrix brasiliensis*, *S. globosa*, and *S. mexicana*, three new Sporothrix species of clinical interest. *J Clin Microbiol* 45:3198–3206. http://dx.doi.org/10.1128/JCM.00808-07.

Marin-Felix Y, Stchigel AM, Miller AN, Guarro J, Cano-Lira JF. 2015. A re-evaluation of the genus *Myceliophthora* (Sordariales, Ascomycota): its segregation into four genera and description of *Corynascus fumimontanus* sp. nov. *Mycologia* 107:619–632. http://dx.doi.org/10.3852/14-228.

Marques SA. 2012. Paracoccidioidomycosis. *Clin Dermatol* 30:610–615. http://dx.doi.org/10.1016/j.clindermatol.2012.01.006.

Mazzocato S, Marchionni E, Fothergill AW, Sutton DA, Staffolani S, Gesuita R, Skrami E, Fiorentini A, Manso E, Barchiesi F. 2015. Epidemiology and outcome of systemic infections due to *Saprochaete capitata*: case report and review of the literature. *Infection* 43:211–215. http://dx.doi.org/10.1007/s15010-014-0668-3.

McCarthy M, Rosengart A, Schuetz AN, Kontoyiannis DP, Walsh TJ. 2014. Mold infections of the central nervous system. *N Engl J Med* 371:150–160. http://dx.doi.org/10.1056/NEJMra1216008.

McCarthy MW, Walsh TJ. 2017. Containment strategies to address the expanding threat of multidrug-resistant *Candida auris*. *Expert Rev Anti Infect Ther* 15:1095–1099.

McCarty TP, White CM, Pappas PG. 2021. Candidemia and invasive candidiasis. *Infect Dis Clin North Am* 35:389–413. http://dx.doi.org/10.1016/j.idc.2021.03.007.

McGinnis MR. 1980. *Laboratory Handbook of Medical Mycology*. Academic Press, New York, NY.

McGough DA, Fothergill AW, Rinaldi MG. 1990. *Cokeromyces recurvatus* Poitras, a distinctive zygomycete and potential pathogen: criteria for identification. *Clin Microbiol Newsl* 12:113–117. http://dx.doi.org/10.1016/0196-4399(90)90053-E.

McNeil MM, Brown JM. 1994. The medically important aerobic actinomycetes: epidemiology and microbiology. *Clin Microbiol Rev* 7:357–417. http://dx.doi.org/10.1128/CMR.7.3.357.

Meechan PJ, Potts J (ed). 2020. *Biosafety in Microbiological and Biomedical Laboratories*, 6th ed. U.S. Department of Health and Human Services, Washington, DC. https://www.cdc.gov/labs/pdf/SF__19_308133-A_BMBL6_00-BOOK-WEB-final-3.pdf.

Mehta V, Nayyar C, Gulati N, Singla N, Rai S, Chandar J. 2021. A comprehensive review of *Trichosporon* spp.: an invasive and emerging fungus. *Cureus* 13:e17345. http://dx.doi.org/10.7759/cureus.17345.

Mhmoud NA, Ahmed SA, Fahal AH, de Hoog GS, Gerrits van den Ende AH, van de Sande WW. 2012. *Pleurostomophora ochracea*, a novel agent of human eumycetoma with yellow grains. *J Clin Microbiol* 50:2987–2994. http://dx.doi.org/10.1128/JCM.01470-12.

Miller JM, Astles R, Baszler T, Chapin K, Carey R, Garcia L, Gray L, Larone D, Pentella M, Pollock A, Shapiro DS, Weirich E, Wiedbrauk D, Biosafety Blue Ribbon Panel, Centers for Disease Control and Prevention (CDC). 2012. Guidelines for safe work practices in human and animal medical diagnostic laboratories. Recommendations of a CDC-convened, Biosafety Blue Ribbon Panel. *MMWR Suppl* 61(MMWR Suppl):1–102.

Miller JM, Binnicker MJ, Campbell S, Carroll KC, Chapin KC, Gilligan PH, Gonzalez MD, Jerris RC, Kehl SC, Patel R, Pritt BS, Richter SS, Robinson-Dunn B, Schwartzman JD, Snyder JW, Telford S III, Theel ES, Thomson RB Jr, Weinstein MP, Yao JD. 2018. A guide to utilization of the microbiology laboratory for diagnosis of infectious diseases: 2018 update by the Infectious Diseases Society of America and the American Society for Microbiology. *Clin Infect Dis* 67:e1–e94. http://dx.doi.org/10.1093/cid/ciy381.

Miller MB, Tang YW. 2009. Basic concepts of microarrays and potential applications in clinical microbiology. *Clin Microbiol Rev* 22:611–633. http://dx.doi.org/10.1128/CMR.00019-09.

Mills R, Rautemaa-Richardson R, Wilkinson S, Patel L, Maitra A, Horsley A. 2021. Impact of airway *Exophiala* spp. on children with cystic fibrosis. *J Cyst Fibros* 20:702–707. http://dx.doi.org/10.1016/j.jcf.2021.03.012.

Mir F, Shakoor S, Khan MJ, Minhas K, Zafar A, Zaidi AK. 2013. *Madurella mycetomatis* as an agent of brain abscess: case report and review of literature. *Mycopathologia* 176:429–434. http://dx.doi.org/10.1007/s11046-013-9707-3.

Mittal J, Szymczak WA, Pirofski LA, Galen BT. 2018. Fungemia caused by *Aureobasidium pullulans* in a patient with advanced AIDS: a case report and review of the medical literature. *JMM Case Rep* 5:e005144. http://dx.doi.org/10.1099/jmmcr.0.005144.

Mochon AB, Sussland D, Saubolle MA. 2016. Aerobic actinomycetes of clinical significance. *Microbiol Spectr* 4:DMIH2-0021-2015.

Mongkolsamrit S, Khonsanit A, Thanakitpipattana D, Tasanathai K, Noisripoom W, Lamlertthon S, Himaman W, Houbraken J, Samson RA, Luangsa-Ard J. 2020. Revisiting *Metarhizium* and the description of new species from Thailand. *Stud Mycol* 95:171–251. http://dx.doi.org/10.1016/j.simyco.2020.04.001.

Moniot M, Lavergne RA, Morel T, Guieze R, Morio F, Poirier P, Nourrisson C. 2020. *Hormographiella aspergillata*: an emerging basidiomycete in the clinical setting? A case report and literature review. *BMC Infect Dis* 20:945. http://dx.doi.org/10.1186/s12879-020-05679-z.

Morales-López SE, Garcia-Effron G. 2021. Infections due to rare *Cryptococcus* species. A literature review. *J Fungi (Basel)* 7:279. http://dx.doi.org/10.3390/jof7040279.

Morhaime JL, Scognamiglio T, Chung SM, Larone DH. 2004. Growth characteristics of moulds on BBL CHROMagar Candida Medium. BD, Franklin Lakes, NJ. https://legacy.bd.com/ds/technicalCenter/whitepapers/LR810.pdf

Morris DO, O'Shea K, Shofer FS, Rankin S. 2005. *Malassezia pachydermatis* carriage in dog owners. *Emerg Infect Dis* 11: 83–88. http://dx.doi.org/10.3201/eid1101.040882.

Mulet Bayona JV, Salvador García C, Tormo Palop N, Valentín Martín A, González Padrón C, Colomina Rodríguez J, Pemán J, Gimeno Cardona C. 2022. Novel chromogenic medium CHROMagar Candida Plus for detection of *Candida auris* and other *Candida* species from surveillance and environmental samples: a multicenter study. *J Fungi (Basel)* 8:281. http://dx.doi.org/10.3390/jof8030281.

Murray MP, Zinchuk R, Larone DH. 2005. CHROMagar Candida as the sole primary medium for isolation of yeasts and as a source medium for the rapid-assimilation-of-trehalose test. *J Clin Microbiol* 43:1210–1212. http://dx.doi.org/10.1128/JCM.43.3.1210-1212.2005.

Mylonakis E, Clancy CJ, Ostrosky-Zeichner L, Garey KW, Alangaden GJ, Vazquez JA, Groeger JS, Judson MA, Vinagre YM, Heard SO, Zervou FN, Zacharioudakis IM, Kontoyiannis DP, Pappas PG. 2015. T2 magnetic resonance assay for the rapid diagnosis of candidemia in whole blood: a clinical trial. *Clin Infect Dis* 60:892–899. http://dx.doi.org/10.1093/cid/ciu959.

Narayanasamy S, Dat VQ, Thanh NT, Ly VT, Chan JF, Yuen KY, Ning C, Liang H, Li L, Chowdhary A, Youngchim S, Supparatpinyo K, Aung NM, Hanson J, Andrianopoulos A, Dougherty J, Govender NP, Denning DW, Chiller T, Thwaites G, van Doorn HR, Perfect J, Le T. 2021. A global call for talaromycosis to be recognised as a neglected tropical disease. *Lancet Glob Health* 9:e1618–e1622.

Nargesi S, Jafarzadeh J, Najafzadeh MJ, Nouripour-Sisakht S, Haghani I, Abastabar M, Ilkit M, Hedayati MT. 2022. Molecular identification and antifungal susceptibility of clinically relevant and cryptic species of *Aspergillus* sections *Flavi* and *Nigri*. *J Med Microbiol* 71: http://dx.doi.org/10.1099/jmm.0.001480.

Normand AC, Packeu A, Cassagne C, Hendrickx M, Ranque S, Piarroux R. 2018. Nucleotide sequence database comparison for routine dermatophyte identification by internal transcribed spacer 2 genetic region DNA barcoding. *J Clin Microbiol* 56:e00046–e18. http://dx.doi.org/10.1128/JCM.00046-18.

Nourrisson C, Garcia-Hermoso D, Morio F, Kauffmann-Lacroix C, Berrette N, Bonhomme J, Poirier P, Lortholary O, Cazenave Roblot F, Hoinard D, Launay E, Lavergne RA, Le Naourès Méar C, Penn P, Rammaert B, Sitbon K, Vidal-Roux M, French Mycosis Study Group. 2017. *Thermothelomyces thermophila* human infections. *Clin Microbiol Infect* 23:338–341. http://dx.doi.org/10.1016/j.cmi.2016.10.025.

Nucci M, Anaissie E. 2007. *Fusarium* infections in immunocompromised patients. *Clin Microbiol Rev* 20:695–704. http://dx.doi.org/10.1128/CMR.00014-07.

Obana Y, Sano M, Jike T, Homma T, Nemoto N. 2010. Differential diagnosis of trichosporonosis using conventional histopathological stains and electron microscopy. *Histopathology* 56:372–383. http://dx.doi.org/10.1111/j.1365-2559.2010.03477.x.

Odds FC, Bernaerts R. 1994. CHROMagar Candida, a new differential isolation medium for presumptive identification of clinically important *Candida* species. *J Clin Microbiol* 32:1923–1929. http://dx.doi.org/10.1128/jcm.32.8.1923-1929.1994.

O'Donnell K, Sarver BA, Brandt M, Chang DC, Noble-Wang J, Park BJ, Sutton DA, Benjamin L, Lindsley M, Padhye A, Geiser DM, Ward TJ. 2007. Phylogenetic diversity and microsphere array-based genotyping of human pathogenic Fusaria, including isolates from the multistate contact lens-associated U.S. keratitis outbreaks of 2005 and 2006. *J Clin Microbiol* 45:2235–2248. http://dx.doi.org/10.1128/JCM.00533-07.

Padhye AA, Ajello L. 1988. Simple method of inducing sporulation by *Apophysomyces elegans* and *Saksenaea vasiformis*. *J Clin Microbiol* 26:1861–1863. http://dx.doi.org/10.1128/jcm.26.9.1861-1863.1988.

Padovan AC, Melo AS, Colombo AL. 2013. Systematic review and new insights into the molecular characterization of the *Candida rugosa* species complex. *Fungal Genet Biol* 61:33–41. http://dx.doi.org/10.1016/j.fgb.2013.10.007.

Pammi M, Holland L, Butler G, Gacser A, Bliss JM. 2013. *Candida parapsilosis* is a significant neonatal pathogen: a systematic review and meta-analysis. *Pediatr Infect Dis J* 32:e206–e216. http://dx.doi.org/10.1097/INF.0b013e3182863a1c.

Pancholi P, Carroll KC, Buchan BW, Chan RC, Dhiman N, Ford B, Granato PA, Harrington AT, Hernandez DR, Humphries RM, Jindra MR, Ledeboer NA, Miller SA, Mochon AB, Morgan MA, Patel R, Schreckenberger PC, Stamper PD, Simner PJ, Tucci NE, Zimmerman C, Wolk DM. 2018. Multicenter evaluation of the Accelerate PhenoTest BC kit for rapid identification and phenotypic antimicrobial susceptibility testing using morphokinetic cellular analysis. *J Clin Microbiol* 56:e01329-17.

Pappas PG, Kauffman CA, Andes DR, Clancy CJ, Marr KA, Ostrosky-Zeichner L, Reboli AC, Schuster MG, Vazquez JA, Walsh TJ, Zaoutis TE, Sobel JD. 2016. Clinical practice guideline for the management of candidiasis: 2016 update by the Infectious Diseases Society of America. *Clin Infect Dis* 62:e1–e50. http://dx.doi.org/10.1093/cid/civ933.

Pappas PG, Lionakis MS, Arendrup MC, Ostrosky-Zeichner L, Kullberg BJ. 2018. Invasive candidiasis. *Nat Rev Dis Primers* 4:18026. http://dx.doi.org/10.1038/nrdp.2018.26.

Pastor FJ, Guarro J. 2006. Clinical manifestations, treatment and outcome of *Paecilomyces lilacinus* infections. *Clin Microbiol Infect* 12:948–960. http://dx.doi.org/10.1111/j.1469-0691.2006.01481.x.

Pastor FJ, Guarro J. 2008. *Alternaria* infections: laboratory diagnosis and relevant clinical features. *Clin Microbiol Infect* 14:734–746.

Patel R. 2019. A moldy application of MALDI: MALDI-TOF mass spectrometry for fungal identification. *J Fungi (Basel)* 5:4. http://dx.doi.org/10.3390/jof5010004.

Patterson TF, Thompson GR III, Denning DW, Fishman JA, Hadley S, Herbrecht R, Kontoyiannis DP, Marr KA, Morrison VA, Nguyen MH, Segal BH, Steinbach WJ, Stevens DA, Walsh TJ, Wingard JR, Young JA, Bennett JE. 2016. Practice guidelines for the diagnosis and management of aspergillosis: 2016 update by the Infectious Diseases Society of America. *Clin Infect Dis* 63:e1–e60. http://dx.doi.org/10.1093/cid/ciw326.

Pérez-Cantero A, Guarro J. 2020a. Current knowledge on the etiology and epidemiology of *Scopulariopsis* infections. *Med Mycol* 58:145–155.

Pérez-Cantero A, Guarro J. 2020b. *Sarocladium* and *Acremonium* infections: new faces of an old opportunistic fungus. *Mycoses* 63:1203–1214. http://dx.doi.org/10.1111/myc.13169.

Pérez-Hansen A, Lass-Flörl C, Lackner M, Aigner M, Alastruey-Izquierdo A, Arikan-Akdagli S, Bader O, Becker K, Boekhout T, Buzina W, Cornely OA, Hamal P, Kidd SE, Kurzai O, Lagrou K, Lopes Colombo A, Mares M, Masoud H, Meis JF, Oliveri S, Rodloff AC, Orth-Höller D, Guerrero-Lozano I, Sanguinetti M, Segal E, Taj-Aldeen SJ, Tortorano AM, Trovato L, Walther G, Willinger B, Rare Yeast Study Group. 2019. Antifungal susceptibility profiles of rare ascomycetous yeasts. *J Antimicrob Chemother* 74:2649–2656. http://dx.doi.org/10.1093/jac/dkz231.

Peri AM, Bauer MJ, Bergh H, Butkiewicz D, Paterson DL, Harris PN. 2022. Performance of the BioFire Blood Culture Identification 2 panel for the diagnosis of bloodstream infections. *Heliyon* 8:e09983.

Persing DH, Tenover FC, Hayden RT, Ieven M, Miller MB, Nolte FS, Tang YW, van Belkum A. 2016. *Molecular Microbiology: Diagnostic Principles and Practice*, 3rd ed. ASM Press, Washington, DC. http://dx.doi.org/10.1128/9781555819071

Petraitis V, Petraitiene R, Antachopoulos C, Hughes JE, Cotton MP, Kasai M, Harrington S, Gamaletsou MN, Bacher JD, Kontoyiannis DP, Roilides E, Walsh TJ. 2013. Increased virulence of *Cunninghamella bertholletiae* in experimental pulmonary mucormycosis: correlation with circulating molecular biomarkers, sporangiospore germination and hyphal metabolism. *Med Mycol* 51:72–82. http://dx.doi.org/10.3109/13693786.2012.690107.

Pfaller MA, Diekema DJ, Colombo AL, Kibbler C, Ng KP, Gibbs DL, Newell VA, Global Antifungal Surveillance Group. 2006. *Candida rugosa*, an emerging fungal pathogen with resistance to azoles: geographic and temporal trends from the ARTEMIS DISK antifungal surveillance program. *J Clin Microbiol* 44:3578–3582. http://dx.doi.org/10.1128/JCM.00863-06.

Pincus DH, Coleman DC, Pruitt WR, Padhye AA, Salkin IF, Geimer M, Bassel A, Sullivan DJ, Clarke M, Hearn V. 1999. Rapid identification of *Candida dubliniensis* with commercial yeast identification systems. *J Clin Microbiol* 37:3533–3539. http://dx.doi.org/10.1128/JCM.37.11.3533-3539.1999.

Pincus DH, Salkin IF, Hurd NJ, Levy IL, Kemna MA. 1988. Modification of potassium nitrate assimilation test for identification of clinically important yeasts. *J Clin Microbiol* 26:366–368. http://dx.doi.org/10.1128/jcm.26.2.366-368.1988.

Pinheiro BG, Hahn RC, Camargo ZP, Rodrigues AM. 2020. Molecular tools for detection and identification of *Paracoccidioides* species: current status and future perspectives. *J Fungi (Basel)* 6:293. http://dx.doi.org/10.3390/jof6040293.

Pitt JI, Hocking AD. 2009. *Fungi and Food Spoilage*, 3rd ed. Springer, New York, NY. http://dx.doi.org/10.1007/978-0-387-92207-2.

Polack FM, Siverio C, Bresky RH. 1976. Corneal chromomycosis: double infection by *Phialophora verrucosa* (Medlar) and *Cladosporium cladosporioides* (Frescenius). *Ann Ophthalmol* 8:139–144.

Pont-Kingdon G, Gedge F, Wooderchak-Donahue W, Schrijver I, Weck KE, Kant JA, Oglesbee D, Bayrak-Toydemir P, Lyon E, Biochemical and Molecular Genetic Resource Committee of the College of American Pathologists. 2012. Design and analytical validation of clinical DNA sequencing assays. *Arch Pathol Lab Med* 136:41–46. http://dx.doi.org/10.5858/arpa.2010-0623-OA.

Posch W, Blatzer M, Wilflingseder D, Lass-Flörl C. 2018. *Aspergillus terreus:* Novel lessons learned on amphotericin B resistance. *Med Mycol* 56(suppl_1):73–82.

Procop GW, Pritt B. 2014. *Pathology of Infectious Diseases*. Elsevier, New York, NY.

Proia LA, Hayden MK, Kammeyer PL, Ortiz J, Sutton DA, Clark T, Schroers HJ, Summerbell RC. 2004. *Phialemonium:* an emerging mold pathogen that caused 4 cases of hemodialysis-associated endovascular infection. *Clin Infect Dis* 39:373–379. http://dx.doi.org/10.1086/422320.

Queiroz-Telles F, de Hoog S, Santos DW, Salgado CG, Vicente VA, Bonifaz A, Roilides E, Xi L, Azevedo CM, da Silva MB, Pana ZD, Colombo AL, Walsh TJ. 2017. Chromoblastomycosis. *Clin Microbiol Rev* 30:233–276. http://dx.doi.org/10.1128/CMR.00032-16.

Radic M, Goic-Barisic I, Novak A, Rubic Z, Tonkic M. 2016. Evaluation of PNA FISH® Yeast Traffic Light in identification of *Candida* species from blood and non-blood culture specimens. *Med Mycol* 54:654–658. http://dx.doi.org/10.1093/mmy/myw012.

Ramani R, Newman R, Salkin IF, Li K, Slim M, Arlievsky N, Gedris C, Chaturvedi V. 2000. *Cokeromyces recurvatus* as a human pathogenic fungus: case report and critical review of the published literature. *Pediatr Infect Dis J* 19:155–158. http://dx.doi.org/10.1097/00006454-200002000-00014.

Ramirez-Garcia A, Pellon A, Rementeria A, Buldain I, Barreto-Bergter E, Rollin-Pinheiro R, de Meirelles JV, Xisto MIDS, Ranque S, Havlicek V, Vandeputte P, Govic YL, Bouchara J-P, Giraud S, Chen S, Rainer J, Alastruey-Izquierdo A, Martin-Gomez MT, López-Soria LM, Peman J, Schwarz C, Bernhardt A, Tintelnot K, Capilla J, Martin-Vicente A, Cano-Lira J, Nagl M, Lackner M, Irinyi L, Meyer W, de Hoog S, Hernando FL. 2018. *Scedosporium* and *Lomentospora:* an updated overview of underrated opportunists. *Med Mycol* 56(suppl_1):102–125. http://dx.doi.org/10.1093/mmy/myx113.

Rath P-M, Steinmann J. 2018. Overview of commercially available PCR assays for the detection of *Aspergillus* spp. DNA in patient samples. *Front Microbiol* 9:740. http://dx.doi.org/10.3389/fmicb.2018.00740.

Rebell G, Taplin D. 1970. *Dermatophytes, Their Recognition and Identifications*, 2nd ed. University of Miami Press, Coral Gables, FL.

Revankar SG, Sutton DA. 2010. Melanized fungi in human disease. *Clin Microbiol Rev* 23:884–928. http://dx.doi.org/10.1128/CMR.00019-10.

Rezusta A, Gilaberte Y, Betran A, Gene J, Querol I, Arias M, Revillo MJ. 2010. Tinea nigra: a rare imported infection. *J Eur Acad Dermatol Venereol* 24:89–91. http://dx.doi.org/10.1111/j.1468-3083.2009.03300.x.

Ribes JA, Vanover-Sams CL, Baker DJ. 2000. Zygomycetes in human disease. *Clin Microbiol Rev* 13:236–301. http://dx.doi.org/10.1128/CMR.13.2.236.

Rigby S, Procop GW, Haase G, Wilson D, Hall G, Kurtzman C, Oliveira K, Von Oy S, Hyldig-Nielsen JJ, Coull J, Stender H. 2002. Fluorescence in situ hybridization with peptide nucleic acid probes for rapid identification of *Candida albicans* directly from blood culture bottles. *J Clin Microbiol* 40:2182–2186. http://dx.doi.org/10.1128/JCM.40.6.2182-2186.2002.

Rihs JD, Padhye AA, Good CB. 1996. Brain abscess caused by *Schizophyllum commune*: an emerging basidiomycete pathogen. *J Clin Microbiol* 34:1628–1632. http://dx.doi.org/10.1128/jcm.34.7.1628-1632.1996.

Rippon JW. 1988. *Medical Mycology: the Pathogenic Fungi and the Pathogenic Actinomycetes*, 3rd ed. WB Saunders Co, Philadelphia, PA.

Roden MM, Zaoutis TE, Buchanan WL, Knudsen TA, Sarkisova TA, Schaufele RL, Sein M, Sein T, Chiou CC, Chu JH, Kontoyiannis DP, Walsh TJ. 2005. Epidemiology and outcome of zygomycosis: a review of 929 reported cases. *Clin Infect Dis* 41:634–653. http://dx.doi.org/10.1086/432579.

Rodrigues AM, de Hoog GS, de Camargo ZP. 2015. Molecular diagnosis of pathogenic *Sporothrix* species. *PLoS Negl Trop Dis* 9:e0004190. http://dx.doi.org/10.1371/journal.pntd.0004190.

Rodrigues de Miranda L. 1979. *Clavispora*, a new yeast genus of the Saccharomycetales. *Antonie van Leeuwenhoek* 45:479–483. http://dx.doi.org/10.1007/BF00443285.

Rodríguez-Gutiérrez G, Carrillo-Casas EM, Arenas R, García-Méndez JO, Toussaint S, Moreno-Morales ME, Schcolnik-Cabrera AA, Xicohtencatl-Cortes J, Hernández-Castro R. 2015. Mucormycosis in a non-Hodgkin lymphoma patient caused by *Syncephalastrum racemosum*: case report and review of literature. *Mycopathologia* 180:89–93. http://dx.doi.org/10.1007/s11046-015-9878-1.

Saito T, Hayashi M, Yaguchi Y, Okamura K, Araki Y, Yamaguchi S, Sano A, Ohe R, Suzuki T. 2020. Case of phaeohyphomycosis caused by *Cladophialophora boppii* successfully treated with local hyperthermia and systemic terbinafine. *J Dermatol* 47:e250–e251. http://dx.doi.org/10.1111/1346-8138.15357.

Sal E, Stemler J, Salmanton-García J, Falces-Romero I, Kredics L, Meyer E, Würstl B, Lass-Flörl C, Racil Z, Klimko N, Cesaro S, Kindo AJ, Wisplinghoff H, Koehler P, Cornely OA, Seidel D. 2022. Invasive *Trichoderma* spp. infections: clinical presentation and outcome of cases from the literature and the FungiScope® registry. *J Antimicrob Chemother* 77:2850–2858. http://dx.doi.org/10.1093/jac/dkac235.

Salfelder K. 1990. *Atlas of Fungal Pathology*. Kluwer Academic Publishers, Dordrecht, The Netherlands.

Salkin IF, Hollick GE, Hurd NJ, Kemna ME. 1985. Evaluation of human hair sources for the in vitro hair perforation test. *J Clin Microbiol* 22:1048–1049. http://dx.doi.org/10.1128/jcm.22.6.1048-1049.1985.

Samson RA, Yilmaz N, Houbraken J, Spierenburg H, Seifert KA, Peterson SW, Varga J, Frisvad JC. 2011. Phylogeny and nomenclature of the genus *Talaromyces* and taxa accommodated in *Penicillium* subgenus *Biverticillium*. *Stud Mycol* 70:159–183. http://dx.doi.org/10.3114/sim.2011.70.04.

Sandoval-Denis M, Sutton DA, Cano-Lira JF, Gené J, Fothergill AW, Wiederhold NP, Guarro J. 2014. Phylogeny of the clinically relevant species of the emerging fungus *Trichoderma* and their antifungal susceptibilities. *J Clin Microbiol* 52:2112–2125. http://dx.doi.org/10.1128/JCM.00429-14.

Sandoval-Denis M, Sutton DA, Martin-Vicente A, Cano-Lira JF, Wiederhold N, Guarro J, Gené J. 2015. *Cladosporium* species recovered from clinical samples in the United States. *J Clin Microbiol* 53:2990–3000. http://dx.doi.org/10.1128/JCM.01482-15.

Sangoi AR, Rogers WM, Longacre TA, Montoya JG, Baron EJ, Banaei N. 2009. Challenges and pitfalls of morphologic identification of fungal infections in histologic and cytologic specimens: a ten-year retrospective review at a single institution. *Am J Clin Pathol* 131:364–375. http://dx.doi.org/10.1309/AJCP99OOOZSNISCZ.

Sanguinetti M, Posteraro B. 2017. Identification of molds by matrix-assisted laser desorption ionization–time of flight mass spectrometry. *J Clin Microbiol* 55:369–379. http://dx.doi.org/10.1128/JCM.01640-16.

Satoh K, Makimura K, Hasumi Y, Nishiyama Y, Uchida K, Yamaguchi H. 2009. *Candida auris* sp. nov., a novel ascomycetous yeast isolated from the external ear canal of an inpatient in a Japanese hospital. *Microbiol Immunol* 53:41–44. http://dx.doi.org/10.1111/j.1348-0421.2008.00083.x.

Savini V, Catavitello C, Onofrillo D, Masciarelli G, Astolfi D, Balbinot A, Febbo F, D'Amario C, D'Antonio D. 2011. What do we know about *Candida guilliermondii*? A voyage throughout past and current literature about this emerging yeast. *Mycoses* 54:434–441. http://dx.doi.org/10.1111/j.1439-0507.2010.01960.x.

Schlaberg R, Fisher MA, Hanson KE. 2014. Susceptibility profiles of *Nocardia* isolates based on current taxonomy. *Antimicrob Agents Chemother* **58**:795–800. http://dx.doi.org/10.1128/AAC.01531-13.

Schnadig VJ, Woods GL. 2009. Histopathology of fungal infections, p 79–108. *In* Anaissie EJ, McGinnis MR, Pfaller MA (ed), *Clinical Mycology*, 2nd ed. Elsevier, New York, NY. http://dx.doi.org/10.1016/B978-1-4160-5680-5.00005-0.

Schoch CL, Seifert KA, Huhndorf S, Robert V, Spouge JL, Levesque CA, Chen W; Fungal Barcoding Consortium; Fungal Barcoding Consortium Author List. 2012. Nuclear ribosomal internal transcribed spacer (ITS) region as a universal DNA barcode marker for Fungi. *Proc Natl Acad Sci USA* **109**:6241–6246. http://dx.doi.org/10.1073/pnas.1117018109.

Scholer HJ, Muller E, Schipper MA. 1983. Mucorales, p 9–59. *In* Howard DH (ed), *Fungi Pathogenic for Humans and Animals*, part A. Marcel Dekker, New York, NY.

Schuetz AN, Pisapia D, Yan J, Hoda RS. 2012. An atypical morphologic presentation of *Coccidioides* spp. in fine-needle aspiration of lung. *Diagn Cytopathol* **40**:163–167. http://dx.doi.org/10.1002/dc.21613.

Schuetz AN, Walsh TJ. 2015. Importance of fungal histopathology in immunocompromised pediatric patients: it's not just "*Aspergillus*" anymore. *Am J Clin Pathol* **144**:185–187.

Schwartz IS, Govender NP, Sigler L, Jiang Y, Maphanga TG, Toplis B, Botha A, Dukik K, Hoving JC, Muñoz JF, de Hoog S, Cuomo CA, Colebunders R, Kenyon C. 2019a. *Emergomyces*: the global rise of new dimorphic fungal pathogens. *PLoS Pathog* **15**:e1007977. http://dx.doi.org/10.1371/journal.ppat.1007977.

Schwartz IS, Kenyon C, Feng P, Govender NP, Dukik K, Sigler L, Jiang Y, Stielow JB, Muñoz JF, Cuomo CA, Botha A, Stchigel AM, de Hoog GS. 2015. 50 years of *Emmonsia* disease in humans: the dramatic emergence of a cluster of novel fungal pathogens. *PLoS Pathog* **11**:e1005198. http://dx.doi.org/10.1371/journal.ppat.1005198.

Schwartz IS, Sanche S, Wiederhold NP, Patterson TF, Sigler L. 2018. *Emergomyces canadensis*, a dimorphic fungus causing fatal systemic human disease in North America. *Emerg Infect Dis* **24**:758–761. http://dx.doi.org/10.3201/eid2404.171765.

Schwartz IS, Wiederhold NP, Hanson KE, Patterson TF, Sigler L. 2019b. *Blastomyces helicus*, a new dimorphic fungus causing fatal pulmonary and systemic disease in humans and animals in Western Canada and the United States. *Clin Infect Dis* **68**:188–195. http://dx.doi.org/10.1093/cid/ciy483.

Schwartz RA. 2004. Superficial fungal infections. *Lancet* **364**:1173–1182. http://dx.doi.org/10.1016/S0140-6736(04)17107-9.

Schwartze VU, Jacobsen ID. 2014. *Mucormycoses* caused by *Lichtheimia* species. *Mycoses* **57**(Suppl 3):73–78. http://dx.doi.org/10.1111/myc.12239.

Scognamiglio T, Zinchuk R, Gumpeni P, Larone DH. 2010. Comparison of inhibitory mold agar to Sabouraud dextrose agar as a primary medium for isolation of fungi. *J Clin Microbiol* **48**:1924–1925. http://dx.doi.org/10.1128/JCM.01814-09.

Segal BH. 2009. Aspergillosis. *N Engl J Med* **360**:1870–1884. http://dx.doi.org/10.1056/NEJMra0808853.

Segal E, Elad D. 2021. Human and zoonotic dermatophytosis: epidemiological aspects. *Front Microbiol* **12**:713532. http://dx.doi.org/10.3389/fmicb.2021.713532.

Shaikh N, Hussain KA, Petraitiene R, Schuetz AN, Walsh TJ. 2016. Entomophthoramycosis: a neglected tropical mycosis. *Clin Microbiol Infect* **22**:688–694. http://dx.doi.org/10.1016/j.cmi.2016.04.005.

Shimono LH, Hartman B. 1986. A simple and reliable rapid methenamine silver stain for *Pneumocystis carinii* and fungi. *Arch Pathol Lab Med* **110**:855–856.

Shin JH, Lee SK, Suh SP, Ryang DW, Kim NH, Rinaldi MG, Sutton DA. 1998. Fatal *Hormonema dematioides* peritonitis in a patient on continuous ambulatory peritoneal dialysis: criteria for organism identification and review of other known fungal etiologic agents. *J Clin Microbiol* **36**:2157–2163. http://dx.doi.org/10.1128/JCM.36.7.2157-2163.1998.

Sigler L, Bartley JR, Parr DH, Morris AJ. 1999. Maxillary sinusitis caused by medusoid form of *Schizophyllum commune*. *J Clin Microbiol* **37**:3395–3398. http://dx.doi.org/10.1128/JCM.37.10.3395-3398.1999.

Sigler L, de la Maza LM, Tan G, Egger KN, Sherburne RK. 1995. Diagnostic difficulties caused by a nonclamped *Schizophyllum commune* isolate in a case of fungus ball of the lung. *J Clin Microbiol* **33**:1979–1983. http://dx.doi.org/10.1128/jcm.33.8.1979-1983.1995.

Singh AK, Chandra A, Islahi S, Das A, Malhotra K, Rao N. 2021. *Phialemonium obovatum* infection of the renal allograft: case report and review of the literature. *Exp Clin Transplant* **19**:871–876. http://dx.doi.org/10.6002/ect.2020.0313.

Siqueira JP, Sutton DA, García D, Gené J, Thomson P, Wiederhold N, Guarro J. 2016. Species diversity of *Aspergillus* section *Versicolores* in clinical samples and antifungal susceptibility. *Fungal Biol* **120**:1458–1467. http://dx.doi.org/10.1016/j.funbio.2016.02.006.

Skovrlj B, Haghighi M, Smethurst ME, Caridi J, Bederson JB. 2014. Curvularia abscess of the brainstem. *World Neurosurg* **82**:241. e9–241.e13. http://dx.doi.org/10.1016/j.wneu.2013.07.014.

Slatko BE, Gardner AF, Ausubel FM. 2018. Overview of next-generation sequencing technologies. *Curr Protoc Mol Biol* **122**:e59. http://dx.doi.org/10.1002/cpmb.59.

Sleator RD. 2011. Phylogenetics. *Arch Microbiol* **193**:235–239. http://dx.doi.org/10.1007/s00203-011-0677-x.

Southwick K, Adams EH, Greenko J, Ostrowsky B, Fernandez R, Patel R, Quinn M, Vallabhaneni S, Denis RJ, Erazo R, Chaturvedi S, Haley VB, Leach L, Zhu YC, Giardina R, Lutterloh EC, Blog

DS. 2018. New York State 2016–2018: progression from *Candida auris* colonization to bloodstream infection. *Open Forum Infect Dis* 5(suppl_1):S594–S595. http://dx.doi.org/10.1093/ofid/ofy210.1695.

Sprute R, Salmanton-García J, Sal E, Malaj X, Falces-Romero I, Hatvani L, Heinemann M, Klimko N, López-Soria L, Meletiadis J, Shruti M, Steinmann J, Seidel D, Cornely OA, Stemler J. 2021a. Characterization and outcome of invasive infections due to *Paecilomyces variotii*: analysis of patients from the FungiScope® registry and literature reports. *J Antimicrob Chemother* 76:765–774. http://dx.doi.org/10.1093/jac/dkaa481.

Sprute R, Salmanton-García J, Sal E, Malaj X, Ráčil Z, Ruiz de Alegría Puig C, Falces-Romero I, Barać A, Desoubeaux G, Kindo AJ, Morris AJ, Pelletier R, Steinmann J, Thompson GR III, Cornely OA, Seidel D, Stemler J, FungiScope® ECMM/ISHAM Working Group. 2021b. Invasive infections with *Purpureocillium lilacinum*: clinical characteristics and outcome of 101 cases from FungiScope® and the literature. *J Antimicrob Chemother* 76:1593–1603. http://dx.doi.org/10.1093/jac/dkab039.

Steinbrink JM, Miceli MH. 2021. Mucormycosis. *Infect Dis Clin North Am* 35:435–452. http://dx.doi.org/10.1016/j.idc.2021.03.009.

Stemler J, Salmanton-García J, Seidel D, Alexander BD, Bertz H, Hoenigl M, Herbrecht R, Meintker L, Meißner A, Mellinghoff SC, Sal E, Zarrouk M, Koehler P, Cornely OA. 2020. Risk factors and mortality in invasive *Rasamsonia* spp. infection: analysis of cases in the FungiScope® registry and from the literature. *Mycoses* 63:265–274. http://dx.doi.org/10.1111/myc.13039.

Stevenson LG, Drake SK, Shea YR, Zelazny AM, Murray PR. 2010. Evaluation of matrix-assisted laser desorption ionization-time of flight mass spectrometry for identification of clinically important yeast species. *J Clin Microbiol* 48:3482–3486. http://dx.doi.org/10.1128/JCM.00687-09.

St-Germain G, Summerbell R. 2011. *Identifying Fungi: A Clinical Laboratory Handbook*, 2nd ed. Star Publishing Company, Inc, Belmont, CA.

Stockman L, Roberts G. 1985. Rapid screening method for the identification of *C. glabrata*, abstr F-80, p 377. Abstr 85th Annu Meet Am Soc Microbiol. American Society for Microbiology, Washington, DC.

Sugita T, Nakajima M, Ikeda R, Matsushima T, Shinoda T. 2002. Sequence analysis of the ribosomal DNA intergenic spacer 1 regions of *Trichosporon* species. *J Clin Microbiol* 40:1826–1830. http://dx.doi.org/10.1128/JCM.40.5.1826-1830.2002.

Sugui JA, Peterson SW, Clark LP, Nardone G, Folio L, Riedlinger G, Zerbe CS, Shea Y, Henderson CM, Zelazny AM, Holland SM, Kwon-Chung KJ. 2012. *Aspergillus tanneri* sp. nov., a new pathogen that causes invasive disease refractory to antifungal therapy. *J Clin Microbiol* 50:3309–3317. http://dx.doi.org/10.1128/JCM.01509-12.

Sullivan D, Coleman D. 1998. *Candida dubliniensis*: characteristics and identification. *J Clin Microbiol* 36:329–334. http://dx.doi.org/10.1128/JCM.36.2.329-334.1998.

Sullivan DJ, Moran GP, Coleman DC. 2005. *Candida dubliniensis*: ten years on. *FEMS Microbiol Lett* 253:9–17. http://dx.doi.org/10.1016/j.femsle.2005.09.015.

Summerbell RC, Gueidan C, Schroers HJ, de Hoog GS, Starink M, Rosete YA, Guarro J, Scott JA. 2011. *Acremonium* phylogenetic overview and revision of *Gliomastix*, *Sarocladium*, and *Trichothecium*. *Stud Mycol* 68:139–162. http://dx.doi.org/10.3114/sim.2011.68.06.

Taj-Aldeen SJ, Almaslamani M, Alkhalf A, Al Bozom I, Romanelli AM, Wickes BL, Fothergill AW, Sutton DA. 2010. Cerebral phaeohyphomycosis due to *Rhinocladiella mackenziei* (formerly *Ramichloridium mackenziei*): a taxonomic update and review of the literature. *Med Mycol* 48:546–556. http://dx.doi.org/10.3109/13693780903383914.

Taj-Aldeen SJ, Rammaert B, Gamaletsou M, Sipsas NV, Zeller V, Roilides E, Kontoyiannis DP, Miller AO, Petraitis V, Walsh TJ, Lortholary O, International Osteoarticular Mycoses Consortium. 2015. Osteoarticular infections caused by non-*Aspergillus* filamentous fungi in adult and pediatric patients: a systematic review. *Medicine (Baltimore)* 94:e2078. http://dx.doi.org/10.1097/MD.0000000000002078.

Tamsikara J, Naidu J, Singh SM. 2006. Phaeohyphomycotic sebaceous cyst due to *Cladosporium cladosporioides*: case report and review of literature. *J Mycol Med* 16:55–57. http://dx.doi.org/10.1016/j.mycmed.2005.12.002.

Tang C, Kong X, Ahmed SA, Thakur R, Chowdhary A, Nenoff P, Uhrlass S, Verma SB, Meis JF, Kandemir H, Kang Y, de Hoog GS. 2021. Taxonomy of the *Trichophyton mentagrophytes/T. interdigitale* species complex harboring the highly virulent, multiresistant genotype *T. indotineae*. *Mycopathologia* 186:315–326. http://dx.doi.org/10.1007/s11046-021-00544-2.

Tavanti A, Davidson AD, Gow NA, Maiden MC, Odds FC. 2005. *Candida orthopsilosis* and *Candida metapsilosis* spp. nov. to replace *Candida parapsilosis* groups II and III. *J Clin Microbiol* 43:284–292. http://dx.doi.org/10.1128/JCM.43.1.284-292.2005.

Thompson GR III, Gomez BL. 2023. *Histoplasma, Blastomyces, Coccidioides, Paracoccidioides* and other dimorphic fungi causing systemic mycoses. *In* Carroll KC, Pfaller MA, Karlowsky JA, Landry ML, McAdam AJ, Patel R, Pritt BS (ed), *Manual of Clinical Microbiology*, 13th ed. ASM Press, Washington, DC.

Thompson GR III, Young JH. 2021. Aspergillus Infections. *N Engl J Med* 385:1496–1509. http://dx.doi.org/10.1056/NEJMra2027424.

Thygesen JB, Glerup H, Tarp B. 2012. *Saccharomyces boulardii* fungemia caused by treatment with a probioticum. *BMJ Case Rep* 2012(mar26 1):bcr0620114412. http://dx.doi.org/10.1136/bcr.06.2011.4412.

Trilles L, Fernández-Torres B, Lazéra MS, Wanke B, Guarro J. 2004. in vitro antifungal susceptibility of *Cryptococcus gattii. J Clin Microbiol* 42:4815–4817. http://dx.doi.org/10.1128/JCM.42.10.4815-4817.2004.

Vachharajani TJ, Zaman F, Latif S, Penn R, Abreo KD. 2005. Curvularia geniculata fungal peritonitis: a case report with review of literature. *Int Urol Nephrol* 37:781–784. http://dx.doi.org/10.1007/s11255-004-0628-4.

Vallabhaneni S, Kallen A, Tsay S, Chow N, Welsh R, Kerins J, Kemble SK, Pacilli M, Black SR, Landon E, Ridgway J, Palmore TN, Zelzany A, Adams EH, Quinn M, Chaturvedi S, Greenko J, Fernandez R, Southwick K, Furuya EY, Calfee DP, Hamula C, Patel G, Barrett P, Lafaro P, Berkow EL, Moulton-Meissner H, Noble-Wang J, Fagan RP, Jackson BR, Lockhart SR, Litvintseva AP, Chiller TM, MSD. 2016. Investigation of the first seven reported cases of *Candida auris*, a globally emerging invasive, multidrug-resistant fungus—United States, May 2013–August 2016. *MMWR Morb Mortal Wkly Rep* 65:1234–1237. http://dx.doi.org/10.15585/mmwr.mm6544e1.

Vance PH, Weissfeld AS. 2007. The controversies surrounding sick building syndrome. *Clin Microbiol Newsl* 29:73–76. http://dx.doi.org/10.1016/j.clinmicnews.2007.04.007.

Varga J, Houbraken J, Van Der Lee HAL, Verweij PE, Samson RA. 2008. *Aspergillus calidoustus* sp. nov., causative agent of human infections previously assigned to *Aspergillus ustus. Eukaryot Cell* 7:630–638. http://dx.doi.org/10.1128/EC.00425-07.

Vaughan-Martini A, Kurtzman CP, Meyer SA, O'Neill EB. 2005. Two new species in the *Pichia guilliermondii* clade: *Pichia caribbica* sp. nov., the ascosporic state of *Candida fermentati*, and *Candida carpophila* comb. nov. *FEMS Yeast Res* 5:463–469. http://dx.doi.org/10.1016/j.femsyr.2004.10.008.

Velegraki A, Cafarchia C, Gaitanis G, Iatta R, Boekhout T. 2015. *Malassezia* infections in humans and animals: pathophysiology, detection, and treatment. *PLoS Pathog* 11:e1004523. http://dx.doi.org/10.1371/journal.ppat.1004523.

Verma P, Jha A. 2019. Mycetoma: reviewing a neglected disease. *Clin Exp Dermatol* 44:123–129. http://dx.doi.org/10.1111/ced.13642.

Verweij PE, Chowdhary A, Melchers WJ, Meis JF. 2016. Azole resistance in *Aspergillus fumigatus:* can we retain the clinical use of mold-active antifungal azoles? *Clin Infect Dis* 62:362–368. http://dx.doi.org/10.1093/cid/civ885.

Vieira MR, Milheiro A, Pacheco FA. 2001. Phaeohyphomycosis due to *Cladosporium cladosporioides. Med Mycol* 39:135–137. http://dx.doi.org/10.1080/mmy.39.1.135.137.

Vilela R, Mendoza L. 2018. Human pathogenic entomophthorales. *Clin Microbiol Rev* 31:e00014–e00018. http://dx.doi.org/10.1128/CMR.00014-18.

Walsh TJ, Hospenthal DR, Petraitis V, Kontoyiannis DP. 2019. Necrotizing mucormycosis of wounds following combat injuries, natural disasters, burns, and other trauma. *J Fungi (Basel)* 5:57.

Walsh TJ, Lee JW, Melcher GP, Navarro E, Bacher J, Callender D, Reed KD, Wu T, Lopez-Berestein G, Pizzo PA. 1992. Experimental *Trichosporon* infection in persistently granulocytopenic rabbits: implications for pathogenesis, diagnosis, and treatment of an emerging opportunistic mycosis. *J Infect Dis* 166:121–133. http://dx.doi.org/10.1093/infdis/166.1.121.

Walsh TJ, McCarthy MW. 2019. The expanding use of matrix-assisted laser desorption/ionization-time of flight mass spectroscopy in the diagnosis of patients with mycotic diseases. *Expert Rev Mol Diagn* 19:241–248.

Wang QM, Yurkov AM, Göker M, Lumbsch HT, Leavitt SD, Groenewald M, Theelen B, Liu XZ, Boekhout T, Bai FY. 2015. Phylogenetic classification of yeasts and related taxa within Pucciniomycotina. *Stud Mycol* 81:149–189. http://dx.doi.org/10.1016/j.simyco.2015.12.002.

Warnock DW. 2017. Name changes for fungi of medical importance, 2012 to 2015. *J Clin Microbiol* 55:53–59. http://dx.doi.org/10.1128/JCM.00829-16.

Warnock DW. 2019. Name changes for fungi of medical importance, 2016–2017. *J Clin Microbiol* 57:e01183–e18. http://dx.doi.org/10.1128/JCM.01183-18.

Weber RW. 2005. Helminthosporium. *Ann Allergy Asthma Immunol* 95:A6. http://dx.doi.org/10.1016/S1081-1206(10)61179-9.

White TC, Findley K, Dawson TL Jr, Scheynius A, Boekhout T, Cuomo CA, Xu J, Saunders CW. 2014. Fungi on the skin: dermatophytes and *Malassezia. Cold Spring Harb Perspect Med* 4:a019802. http://dx.doi.org/10.1101/cshperspect.a019802.

White TJ, Bruns T, Lee S, Taylor J. 1990. Amplification and direct sequencing of fungal ribosomal RNA genes for phylogenetics, p 315–322. *In* Innis MA, Gelfand DH, Sninsky JJ, White TJ (ed), *PCR Protocols: A Guide to Methods and Applications.* Academic Press, San Diego, CA.

Wiederhold NP, Verweij PE. 2020. *Aspergillus fumigatus* and pan-azole resistance: who should be concerned? *Curr Opin Infect Dis* 33:290–297. http://dx.doi.org/10.1097/QCO.0000000000000662.

Wilhelmus KR, Jones DB. 2001. Curvularia keratitis. *Trans Am Ophthalmol Soc* 99:111–130, discussion 130–132.

Wooley DP, Byers KB (ed). 2017. *Biological Safety: Principles and Practices*, 5th ed. ASM Press, Washington, DC. http://dx.doi.org/10.1128/9781555819637.

Yassin AF, Rainey FA, Burghardt J, Gierth D, Ungerechts J, Lux I, Seifert P, Bal C, Schaal KP. 1997. Description of *Nocardiopsis synnemataformans* sp. nov., elevation of *Nocardiopsis alba* subsp. prasine to *Nocardiopsis antarctica* and *Nocardiopsis alborubida* as later subjective synonyms of *Nocardiopsis dassonvillei. Int J Syst Bacteriol* 47:983–988. http://dx.doi.org/10.1099/00207713-47-4-983.

Yu HY, Qu TT, Yang Q, Hu JH, Sheng JF. 2021. A fatal case of *Exophiala dermatitidis* meningoencephalitis in an immunocompetent host: A case report and literature review. *J Infect Chemother* 27:1520–1524. http://dx.doi.org/10.1016/j.jiac.2021.06.014.

Zaid DM, Bakheet OE, Ahmed ES, Abdalati F, Mhmoud NA, Mohamed ESW, Bakhiet SM, Siddig EE, Fahal AH. 2021. Multiple extensive *Madurella mycetomatis* eumycetoma lesions: a case report and review of the literature. *Trans R Soc Trop Med Hyg* 115:411–414. http://dx.doi.org/10.1093/trstmh/traa164.

Zeng JS, Sutton DA, Fothergill AW, Rinaldi MG, Harrak MJ, de Hoog GS. 2007. Spectrum of clinically relevant *Exophiala* species in the United States. *J Clin Microbiol* 45:3713–3720. http://dx.doi.org/10.1128/JCM.02012-06.

Zhang SX, Babady NE, Hanson KE, Harrington AT, Larkin PMK, Leal SM Jr, Luethy PM, Martin IW, Pancholi P, Procop GW, Riedel S, Seyedmousavi S, Sullivan KV, Walsh TJ, Lockhart SR, Fungal Diagnostics Laboratories Consortium (FDLC). 2021. Recognition of diagnostic gaps for laboratory diagnosis of fungal diseases: expert opinion from the Fungal Diagnostics Laboratories Consortium (FDLC). *J Clin Microbiol* 59:e0178420. http://dx.doi.org/10.1128/JCM.01784-20.

Zuza-Alves DL, Silva-Rocha WP, Chaves GM. 2017. An update on *Candida tropicalis* based on basic and clinical approaches. *Front Microbiol* 8:1927. http://dx.doi.org/10.3389/fmicb.2017.01927.

Index

Page numbers in **bold** indicate descriptive details, numbers in *italics* indicate image appendix figures, and a t follows page numbers with a table.

507